# Practice of Intramedullary Locked Nails

Advanced Techniques and Special Applications

Recommended by AIOD

Springer

*Berlin*
*Heidelberg*
*New York*
*Barcelona*
*Hong Kong*
*London*
*Milan*
*Paris*
*Tokyo*

Chief Editors I. Kempf · K. S. Leung

Co-Editors A. Grosse · H. J. T. M. Haarman
H. Seidel · G. Taglang

# Practice of Intramedullary Locked Nails

## Advanced Techniques and Special Applications Recommended by "Association Internationale pour l'Ostéosynthèse Dynamique" (AIOD)

With 235 Figures
and 10 Tables

Springer

*Chief Editors*

Professor Dr. I. Kempf
AIOD, 16 Rue du Parc
67205 Straßbourg, France

Professor Dr. K.S. Leung
The Chinese University of Hong Kong
Department of Orthopaedics
and Traumatology
Shatin, Hong Kong SAR
China

*Co-Editors*

Dr. A. Grosse
Centre de Traumatologie et d'Orthopédie
10 Avenue A. Baumann
67400 Straßbourg, France

Professor Dr. H.J.T.M. Haarman
Academisch Ziekenhuis
Department of Surgery
De Boelelaan 1117, P.O. Box 7057
1007 MB Amsterdam, The Netherlands

Dr. H. Seidel
Allgemeines Krankenhaus Wandsbeck
Abteilung für Unfallchirurgie
Alphonsstraße 14
22043 Hamburg, Germany

Dr. G. Taglang
Centre de Traumatologie et d'Orthopédie
10 Avenue A. Baumann
67400 Straßbourg, France

ISBN 3-540-64080-0
Springer-Verlag Berlin Heidelberg New York

Library of Congress Cataloging-in-Publication Data
applied for

Die Deutsche Bibliothek – CIP-Einheitsaufnahme
Practice of intramedullary locked nails / [I. Kempf; K.S. Leung chief ed.]. – Berlin; Heidelberg; New York; Barcelona; Hong Kong; London; Milan; Paris; Tokyo: Springer
Advanced techniques and special applications. – 2002
ISBN 3-540-64080-0



Springer-Verlag Berlin Heidelberg New York
a member of BertelsmannSpringer Science+Business Media GmbH

http://www.springer.de



Production: PRO EDIT GmbH, Heidelberg, Germany
Cover design: Erich Kirchner, Heidelberg, Germany
Typesetting: K + V Fotosatz GmbH, Beerfelden, Germany

Printed on acid-free paper
SPIN 10497453 24/3130/Di 5 4 3 2 1 0

# Foreword

Medullary nailing is one of the oldest types of surgical fracture treatment. Splinting a fracture by insertion of plugs made of ebony dates back to the ancient Egyptian culture. As for many other types of fracture treatment, some outstanding but lone pioneers performed what was in their hands an art based on intuition. But most of them remained lonely pioneers since they could teach neither the basics nor the surgical art without a deeper understanding of the underlying science. It took the tenacity of Küntscher to establish medullary nailing as an accepted method of treatment world-wide. It is a method that is attractive because of its apparent simplicity and tolerance of the procedures. Küntscher's great achievements were certainly crowned by his success in convincing other pioneers, such as L. Böhler and M.E. Müller, to accept his procedure and to use it in addition to their own special approaches.

It is interesting to note that in respect to what we today understand to be the state of the art in locked medullary nailing. Küntscher had visionary ideas that led the way but did not come to fruition. This gave the next generation the opportunity to made an essential contribution. Küntscher's "detention nail" remained a Cinderella until Klemm and Schellman proved the clinical merits of locked nailing. This technology widened the spectrum of indications for nailing and improved its safety. As impressive as their achievements were, it took the vision and determination of Ivan Kempfs to grasp the idea and to push for its realization. To Arsène Grosse, an ingenious developer and surgeon, we owe a technology that would be accepted and soon find world-wide recognition.

Early on, I was impressed not only by the technology, its simplicity and its safety, but even more so by the school of thought of the Strasbourg team that devised a way of teaching the system to encourage general acceptance. An important factor that contributed to this acceptance was the fact that this school reported clinical experience in a way that did not allow the surgeon to be carried away by enthusiasm. They impressed by reporting merits and pitfalls alike in a very realistic and convincing manner.

When we consider the past, we automatically confront the question, "What is next?" Where are today's problems and what could the solutions be? The present book discusses the view that medullary nailing is able to compensate for the disturbance to blood circulation brought by the fracture, the surgical procedures, the instruments and the implants. On the one hand, it is apparent that there is potential for biological improvements, specifical in terms of avoiding or reducing traumata due to reaming. But this will invariably be achieved at the expense of stability or strength of the fixation. Similar to the possibilities for improving the afferent blood supply, the effects of nailing on a patient local circulation and general, disseminated, microvascular aggregation must be resolved, especially for patients with thoracic trauma. We are convinced that the spirit established by the group in Strasbourg and Hong Kong and maintained by their colleagues and pupils provides good reason to hope that the next step forward is not far beyond the horizon. The present book will not only help the clinically active surgeon and his team, but will serve as a guide to the researcher and developer in the insatiable urge to strive for improvements.

It is obvious that no single method can solve all the problems of fracture treatment. Progress and success depend on clean concepts and optimal employment of each single method. This is where the present book, made with care, deep insight and great experience concerning the important technology of medullary nailing by the authors and editors I. Kempf and K.S. Leung, contributes in an outstanding way.

Stephan Perren
Davos, 16 December 2000

# Preface

Following the steps of Gerhard Küntscher, the father of intramedullary fixation of fractures, Dr. Klemm and Dr. Schellmann from Frankfurt am Main, Germany, took up the idea of locking the nail to the bone in the early 1970s. Professor Ivan Kempf and Dr. Arsène Grosse from Strasbourg, France, further developed these concepts, putting intramedullary locked nails into clinical practice in a systemic and scientific manner for the first time. In fact, the introduction of the intramedullary locked nail system to musculoskeletal trauma was considered to be one of the major advancements of the 1970s. Throughout these years, hundreds of training courses were organised to promote the concept and practice of the closed treatment of long bone fractures with this technique. Numerous clinical results have proven the beneficial effect of the technique to patients. Intramedullary locked has nail become an indispensable instrument in fracture management as well as reconstructive surgery in orthopaedics. Fixing long bone fractures with intramedullary locked nails agrees with the modern concept of minimally invasive surgery.

Intramedullary fixation fulfils the biological requirement for fracture healing and minimises surgical trauma. Intramedullary locked nails provide a favourable biomechanical environment, from fracture stabilisation to post-operative rehabilitation. In accordance with the principles of closed biological treatment of fractures and minimally invasive techniques, most long bone fractures can be stabilised using this technique without embarking on more complicated and invasive methods. With many innovative modifications, this technique has been applied to managing difficult trauma conditions as well as a number of other orthopaedic conditions. Today, it is our strong belief that the use of intramedullary locked nails in the management of long bone fractures has become a well-established philosophy of patient management. The principles and applications are universal and far beyond the limit of any particular instrument or implant. Based on this faith, *Practice of Intramedullary Locked Nails* is written in the hope that this technique will evolve further for the betterment of patients.

This book describes the use and relevance of the closed technique of intramedullary locked nails in orthopaedic and trauma surgeries. *The Practice of Intramedullary Locked Nails* comprises of two volumes: Vol. 1 covers the scientific principles and standard surgical techniques of intramedullary locked nails; Vol. 2 covers the advanced surgical techniques in extended indications. This work would not have been possible without the contribution and collaboration of world-leading trauma centres. The contributions from surgeons with different areas of expertise throughout the world are essential in providing international and comprehensive views of these nailing techniques.

Ivan Kempf
Kwok-Sui Leung

# Acknowledgements

This book could not have been completed after such an exceptionally long period of preparation without the support and contribution of our friends and colleagues. Our special gratitude goes to:

- Our friends and colleagues who prepared the manuscripts based on the framework proposed by the editorial board. Without their patience and relentless support, this book could never have become a reality.
- Our co-editors and the members of the editorial board who share our vision in promoting the concept and practice of the closed treatment of fractures developed by Prof. Gerhard Küntscher with the intramedullary locked nails.
- Professor Stephan Perren, our dear friend and colleague, for his kind remarks in the Foreword.
- The council members of the AIOD who have supported the project throughout these years of preparation.
- The secretarial staff of the AIOD, especially Mrs. Margot Hamm, Mrs. Michèle Obringer and Ms. Audrey Muller for their patience, endurance and perseverance in making the project progress, for their excellent and professional secretarial support in preparing the manuscripts.
- Mrs. Christiane Schaeffer-Cinqualbre, who prepared the illustrations.
- Mr. Robert Cooley for improving the English of the manuscripts.
- The staff of Springer-Verlag in Heidelberg, especially Mrs. G. Schröder, who supported the project from the very beginning, and for their expertise in producing and publishing this book.

# Contents

# Contributors

Dr. F. C. Bakker
Academisch Ziekenhuis
Department of Surgery
De Boelelaan 1117, P.O. Box 7057
1007 MB Amsterdam, The Netherlands

Dr. S. Bandiera
Ospedale Maggiore
Azienda USL Citta di Bologna - Largo B.
Nigrisoli, 2, 40133 Bologna, Italy

Dr. S. Boriani
Ospedale Maggiore
Azienda USL Citta di Bologna - Largo B.
Nigrisoli, 2, 40133 Bologna, Italy

Dr. P. H. Breedveld
Academisch Ziekenhuis Maastricht
Chirurgie, P. Debylaan 25
6229 HX Maastricht, The Netherlands

Dr. D. Brinkert
Centre de Traumatologie et d'Orthopédie
10 Avenue A. Baumann
67400 Strasbourg, France

Prof. C. M. Court-Brown
Royal Infirmary of Edinburgh
Edinburgh Orthopaedic Trauma Unit
Lauriston Place
EH3 9YW Edinburgh, Scotland

Dr. D. Dagrenat
Cabinet de Chirurgie Orthopédique
16 Allée de la Robertsau
67000 Strasbourg, France

Dr. F. De Iure
Ospedale Maggiore
Azienda USL Citta di Bologna - Largo B.
Nigrisoli, 2, 40133 Bologna, Italy

Dr. G. J. Eggink
University Hospital Maastricht
Department of Surgery
Section Traumatology, P.O. Box 5800
6202 AZ Maastricht, The Netherlands

Dr. A. Gasbarrini
Ospedale Maggiore
Azienda USL Citta di Bologna - Largo B.
Nigrisoli, 2, 40133 Bologna, Italy

Dr. M. L. M. J. Goessens
University Hospital Maastricht
Department of Surgery
Section Traumatology, P.O. Box 5800
6202 AZ Maastricht, The Netherlands

Dr. A. Grosse
Centre de Traumatologie et d'Orthopédie
10 Avenue A. Baumann
67400 Strasbourg, France

Prof. H. J. T. M. Haarman
Academisch Ziekenhuis
Department of Surgery
De Boelelaan 1117, P.O. Box 7057
1007 MB Amsterdam, The Netherlands

Prof. I. Kempf
Association Internationale
pour l'Ostéosynthèse Dynamique
16 Rue du Parc
67205 Strasbourg, France

Prof. C. Lefèvre
Hôpital de la Cavale Blanche
Service d'Orthopédie
29200 Brest, France

Prof. D. Le Nen
Hôpital de la Cavale Blanche
Service d'Orthopédie,
29200 Brest, France

Prof. K.S. Leung
The Chinese University of Hong Kong
Department of Orthopaedics and Traumatology
Shatin, Hong Kong SAR, China

Prof. A.C. Masquelet
Hôpital Avicenne - Université Paris XIII
125 Rue de Stalingrad
93009 Bobigny Cedex, France

Dr. R. Pascarella
Ospedale Maggiore
Azienda USL Citta di Bologna - Largo B.
Nigrisoli, 2, 40133 Bologna, Italy

Dr. P. Patka
Academisch Ziekenhuis
Department of Surgery
De Boelelaan 1117, P.O. Box 7057
1007 MB Amsterdam, The Netherlands

Dr. B. Schenck
Centre de Traumatologie et d'Orthopédie
10 Avenue A. Baumann
67400 Strasbourg, France

Dr. M.J.M. Segers
Vrije Universiteit Medisch Centrum
Chirurgie, Postbus 7057
1007 MB Amsterdam, The Netherlands

Dr. H. Seidel
Allgemeines Krankenhaus Wandsbeck
Abteilung für Unfallchirurgie
Alphonsstraße 14
22043 Hamburg, Germany

Prof. J.W.J.L. Stapert
Academisch Ziekenhuis Maastricht
Heelkunde, P. Debylaan 25
6229 HX Maastricht, The Netherlands

Dr. G. Taglang
Centre de Traumatologie et d'Orthopédie
10 Avenue A. Baumann
67400 Strasbourg, France

Dr. J.P.A.M. Verbruggen
Academisch Ziekenhuis Maastricht
Traumatologie, P. Debylaan 25
6229 HX Maastricht, The Netherlands

CHAPTER 1

# Introduction

I. Kempf and H. Seidel

The first part of this volume is dedicated to specific problems related to acute fracture treatment: associated fractures of the femur, distal fractures of the femur, proximal and distal fractures of the tibia, complex proximal humerus fractures, and open fractures.

Closed, locked intramedullary nailing is not only an excellent method in the treatment of acute fractures, but it brings excellent solutions in reconstructive surgery, the subject of the second part of this volume.

Küntscher himself opened the way in the treatment of pseudarthrosis and malunions. He successfully treated a large number of midshaft pseudarthroses of the femur and tibia by rereaming and insertion of a larger nail, followed by immediate weight-bearing. Locked intramedullary nailing, mostly in a dynamic mode, allows the surgeon to extend the method to include the treatment of proximal and distal long-bone pseudarthrosis. These are very difficult to treat using other methods.

To fix a corrective osteotomy, solid fixation is needed. Locked intramedullary nailing addresses this need at all levels of the long bones. It was also Küntscher who imagined the fascinating technique of closed osteotomies with an intramedullary saw. To accomplish this he was able to perform reconstructive surgery for reaxation, derotation, lengthening, and shortening of long bones using closed techniques. Transarticular locked nailing also permits the arthrodesis of a joint.

Last but not least, locked intramedullary nailing is very helpful in modern reconstructive surgery after tumor excision, providing more solid fixation of massive grafts and allowing much earlier and more secure weight-bearing than plate fixation.

It is dangerous but exciting to predict the future development of a therapeutic method. Progress, improvements, and new developments are continuously brought to the forefront, and new perspectives will surely be imagined.

The success of this method requires illustration, and therefore an atlas of clinical cases will close this volume.

# CHAPTER 2

# Ipsilateral Hip and Diaphyseal Fractures

K. S. Leung

## Surgical Principles

Ipsilateral hip and femoral shaft fractures are not uncommon combination fractures in high-energy trauma. Most reports show that diaphyseal fractures are comminuted, as the energy of trauma dissipates through shaft fractures [1, 4, 9, 11, 12, 16], while hip fractures remain relatively undisplaced or minimally displaced. This is one of the reasons why hip fractures are quite frequently missed in polytrauma patients with femoral shaft fractures [13]. It becomes apparent that careful radiological examination of the hip should always be done in *all* patients with femoral shaft fractures [14].

### Fracture Characteristics

Hip fractures can be intracapsular and extracapsular fractures. Most of these fractures are either undisplaced or minimally displaced (Fig. 2.1). The result of closed treatment is good except in very proximal fractures with comminutions [7].

Most femoral shaft fractures are comminuted and unstable, Winquist Type II to IV, and stable fixation is indicated to maintain length and allow early mobilization [7].

Treatment of these complex combined fractures is difficult. Operative treatment is indicated in most cases [1, 3, 5, 6]. Treatment of these combined fractures can be considered in separate stages, but combined treatment is another viable option [17].

The closed-treatment technique with intramedullary locked nails is usually indicated in comminuted femoral shaft fractures to provide immediate stability. The hip fractures can be treated separately, e.g., with hip screws [2, 8], or in combination with the intramedullary locked nail system or the long gamma nail.

## Indications

All combine fractures should be treated with internal fixation.

Open fractures in the femur can be treated with intramedullary locked nails provided the principles of management for open fractures are observed.

## Preoperative Preparation

Preoperative preparation is similar to that for single femoral shaft fractures (see Chap. 9 "Femoral Fractures," other volume). Skeletal traction should always be applied to maintain length and control pain before the operation. Careful adjustment of the traction force is needed to prevent displacement in hip fractures.

Patients must be carefully assessed to exclude injuries in other systems. Life-threatening conditions must receive priority management. Skeletal fixation should be done as soon as the patient's condition is stabilized.

## Special Instruments and Implants

Combined fractures can be fixed with a single implant system [15], a long gamma nail (Fig. 2.2), or a combination of intramedullary locked nails and hip screws (Fig. 2.3). In general, we recommend the long gamma nail for ipsilateral trochanteric and shaft fractures and a combination of the intramedullary locked nail and hip screws for ipsilateral femoral neck and diaphyseal fractures [7].

The instruments required are standard instruments for intramedullary locked femoral nailing. When using the long gamma nail, the proximal targeting device for the gamma lag screw is needed (see Chap. 11 "Operative Technique for Peritrochanteric Fractures" in "Proximal Femoral Fractures," other volume). When using combina-

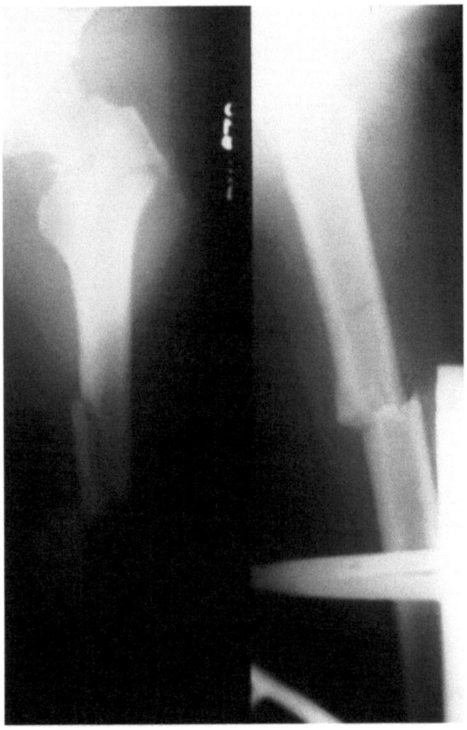

**Fig. 2.1.** X-ray showing ipsilateral hip and femoral shaft fracture. Note the relatively undisplaced hip fracture and the comminuted diaphyseal fracture

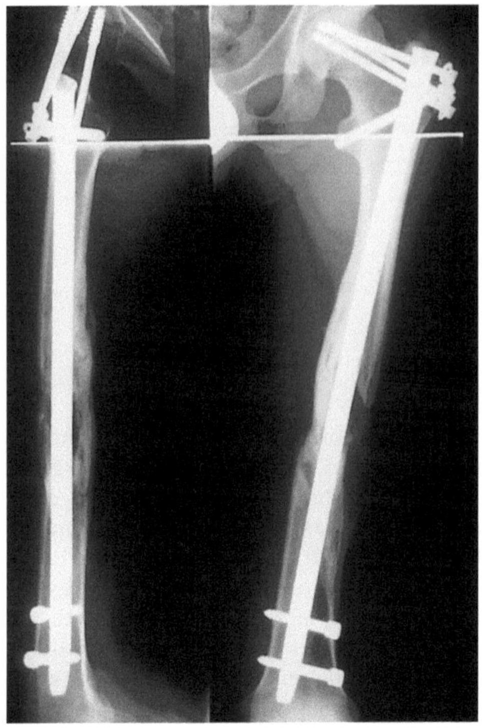

**Fig. 2.3.** Ipsilateral hip and femoral shaft fracture fixed with Grosse-Kempf locked nail and cannulated hip screws

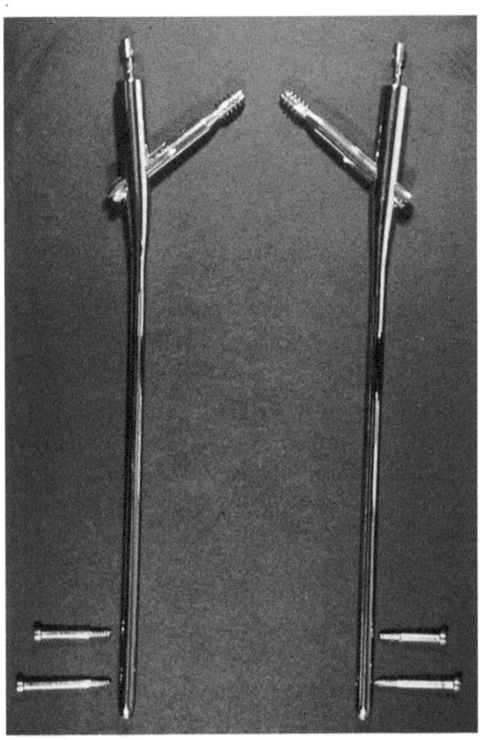

**Fig. 2.2.** The design of a long gamma nail. Lag screw to fix the hip fracture; long femoral component with left and right version and two distal locking screws

tion fixation with intramedullary locked nailing and hip screw fixation, an additional system of cannulated screws is preferred.

## Positioning

As for the intramedullary fixation of femur, the supine position on a traction table is preferred. Skeletal traction through the distal femur is set up to facilitate reduction of the femur. Adequate exposure of the hip region from the iliac crest is prepared (see Chap. 9 "Femoral Fractures," other volume).

The C-arm is positioned from the opposite side of the injured limb. Both the frontal and lateral views must be obtained for images of the hip.

## Reduction of Fractures

Closed reduction of the fractures is carried out before surgical procedures start. In most cases, reduction of the femoral shaft fracture takes priority. Procedures must be carried out carefully and meticulously to reduce femoral shaft fractures and hip fractures. The hip fracture usually remains undisplaced after the femoral shaft fracture is reduced (see Chap. 9 "Femoral Fractures," other volume).

As most of the hip fractures are relatively undisplaced, caution must be taken not to displace the hip fractures during the maneuver to reduce the femoral shaft fracture. The use of the Steinmann pin in the distal femur helps to control the reduction procedures. K-wires 2 mm in diameter may be inserted percutaneously to fix the hip fractures temporarily before the closed reduction of the femoral fractures is to done.

In case the hip fracture is markedly displaced as a result of the injury and cannot be reduced together with the femoral shaft fractures, the femoral shaft fracture may be reduced and fixed before closed reduction of the hip fractures. A fixed and stable femoral shaft fracture facilitates the reduction of the hip fractures.

## Operative Procedures

After the fractures are reduced by the closed method, the operative site is sterilized and draped. The regions to be exposed extend from the iliac crest to the distal femur with complete exposure of the femoral shaft.

### Long Gamma Nail

This nail is a cannulated unslotted stainless steel nail (Fig. 2.2). The proximal segment is the same as the gamma nail except there is a 5° anteversion built in for the lag screw. The distal part is of different lengths ranging from 320 to 440 mm. The diameter ranges from 11 to 12 mm. The radius of curvature for the anterior bowing is 3 m. There are two screw holes for distal locking with the 6.0-mm fully threaded screws. There are left and right versions.

#### *Incision*

The incision is similar to that for the gamma nail except it may need to be slightly longer to facilitate the insertion of a long and rigid nail (see Chap. 11 "Operative Technique for Peritrochanteric Fractures" in "Proximal Femoral Fractures," other volume) (Fig. 2.4).

A 50-mm horizontal incision is made on the lateral side of the greater trochanter. Two-thirds of the incision is proximal to the greater trochanter. The fascia latta is incised along the skin incision. The short abductor muscle is split longitudinally. Hemostasis is assured. The site of the entry point is located similarly to gamma nailing or femoral nailing (see Chap. 9 "Femoral Fractures" and Chap. 11 "Operative Technique for Peritrochanteric Fractures" in "Proximal Femoral Fractures," other volume).

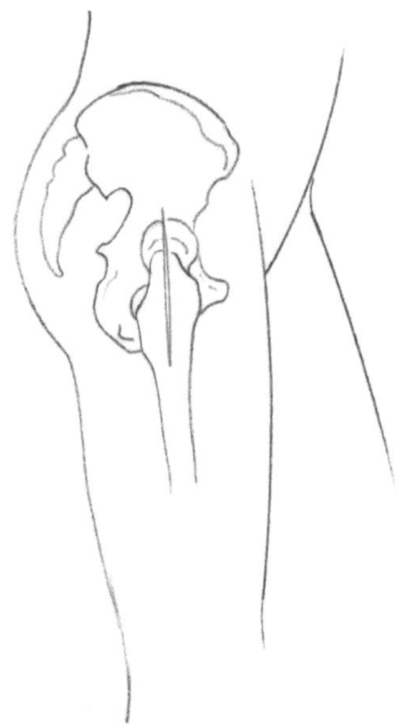

**Fig. 2.4.** Incision for the insertion of a long gamma nail

#### *Entry Point*

On the frontal plane, the entry point is at the tip of the greater trochanter. On the sagittal plane, the entry point is between the anterior third and the middle third of the greater trochanter (Fig. 2.5). The entry point can be accurately located with a straight and sharp awl, aided by X-ray control. However, in many instances, this point is represented by a small depression which can be felt with careful palpation.

After the entry point is accurately located and the site entered with the awl, the entry is gradually enlarged with a curved awl into the greater trochanter. Care must be taken not to use excessive force to displace the hip fracture. In cases with a trochanteric fracture, extra care must be taken not to displace the fracture medially and in the varus direction.

#### *Preparation of the Medullary Canal*

Reaming is required for the passage of the long and rigid nail. A reamer guide with the bent tip is passed through the entry point into the femoral canal. The tip of the guide must not impinge on the medial cortex in the subtrochanteric region.

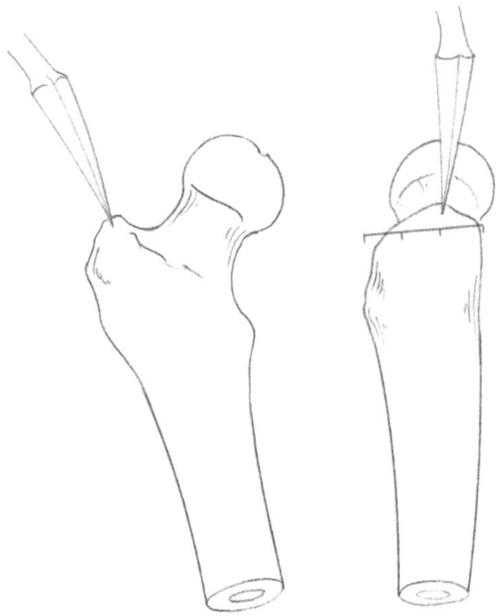

**Fig. 2.5.** Entry point in the greater trochanter. Tip of the greater trochanter on the frontal view and between the anterior 1/3 and the mid 1/3 on the trochanteric ridge in the sagittal plane

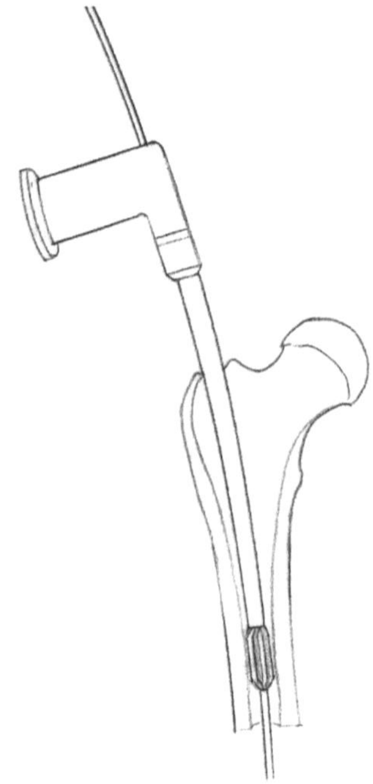

**Fig. 2.6.** Reaming must be adequate in the subtrochanteric region of the medullary canal

The same technique as described in Chap. 9 "Femoral Fractures", other volume, is used to pass the guide across the femoral shaft fractures. One must always try to feel the inner surface of the medullary canal with the tip of the guide while advancing the guide. The passage of the guide can be monitored occasionally with the C-arm and when the guide is inserted to the subchondral area in the distal femur. The final position of the guide is checked with the C-arm in the frontal and sagittal planes.

The length of the nail to be inserted is then estimated.

Reaming is started with the 9-mm reamer and increased stepwise in 0.5-mm increments. All precautions are observed during reaming. (see Chap. 4 "Intramedullary Fixation of Fractures", other volume). Special precaution is taken to ream the subtrochanteric area (Fig. 2.6). Reaming should always be done to 2 mm larger than the diameter of the nail to be inserted. The reamer guide is then exchanged with the nail guide with the help of a flexible Teflon tube.

### *Nail Insertion*

A long gamma nail of the correct diameter and length is mounted on the nail mount. The nail is inserted over the nail guide into the medullary canal. The tip of the nail should be monitored by the C-arm as the nail is passed into the medullary canal. Always insert the nail manually without using a mallet. The commonest obstacle for nail insertion is at the subtrochanteric region where the tip of the nail impinges onto the medial wall. In this case, the proximal end of the nail should be pushed towards the patient's trunk to release the impingement (Fig. 2.7).

The nail is inserted into the distal part of the femur and the nail guide is removed. Slight impaction of the nail may be needed at the final stage of insertion.

### *Lag Screw Targeting*

Targeting the lag screw follows the same standard procedure as for the gamma nail for trochanteric fractures (see Chap. 11 "Operative Technique for Peritrochanteric Fractures" in "Proximal Femoral Fractures", other volume). Again, the procedures should be carried out carefully so as not to displace the trochanteric fracture.

As most of these patients are young and the bone is of good quality, the use of the triple reamer to prepare the lag screw track requires particular care. Sometimes, with a very good bone quality, power-assisted reaming can be used to facilitate the procedure and avoid using undue force.

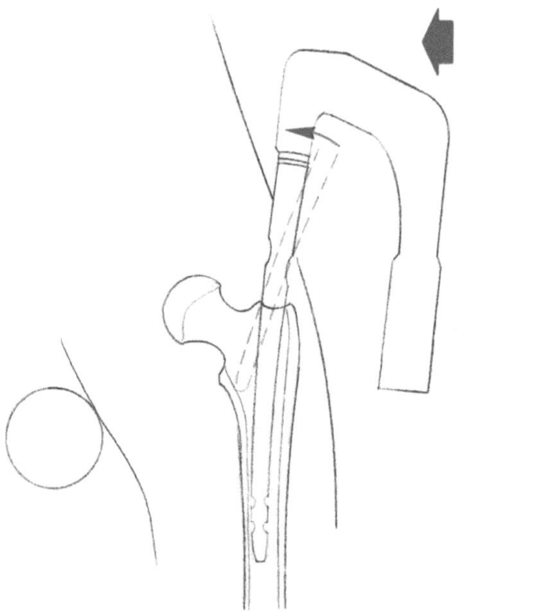

**Fig. 2.7.** The proximal end of the long gamma nail is pushed towards the patient's trunk to facilitate insertion

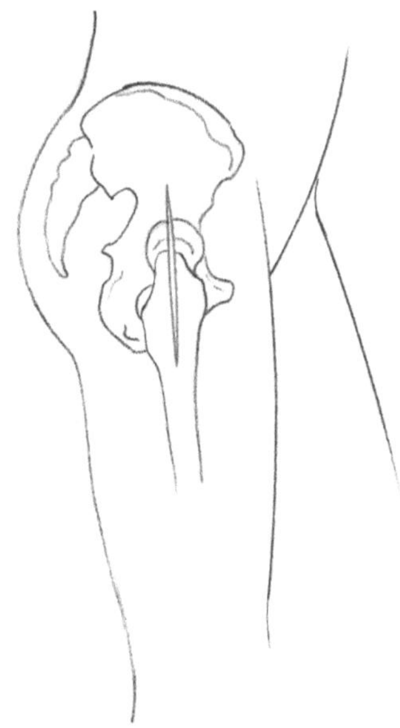

**Fig. 2.8.** Incision for the combining femoral locked nail and cannulated screw insertion. Note that the external surface of the greater trochanter is exposed

### *Distal Locking*

As most of the diaphyseal fractures are comminuted and unstable, distal locking should always be done with two fully threaded locked screws to achieve maximal stability.

The procedure for distal locking is exactly the same as the standard procedures in femoral locked nails (see Chap. 9 "Femoral Fractures", other volume).

### *Wound Closure*

All instruments are removed and the wounds are closed in layers. A suction drainage is inserted in the proximal wound only as deep as the tensor fascia muscle. Pressure bandage is used from the toes to the pelvis.

## Combination of Femoral Locked Nail and Cannulated Hip Screw Fixation

The first generation femoral locked nail, the Grosse-Kempf nail, is indicated in this technique. The diagonal proximal locking screw is particularly useful for secure locking in diaphyseal fractures with more proximal extension (Fig. 2.3).

Cannulated hip screws are used to fix hip fractures, particularly useful for intracapsular neck fractures. The use of the cannulated screw system helps to insert the screws in more precise position (Fig. 2.3).

Temporary fixation of the hip fracture may be considered if the hip fracture is minimally displaced and the fear of displacement during femoral nailing is substantial.

With X-ray monitoring, two 2-mm Kirschner wires can be inserted percutaneously into the femoral head and neck through the lateral cortex of the greater trochanter.

### *Incision*

A 100-mm incision is made on the midline of the outer surface of the proximal thigh with the tip of the greater trochanter as the center. Basically, this is the same as that in the femoral locked nail but with more distal extension. The tensor fascia muscle is split distally to expose the lateral surface of the trochanteric region so as to allow hip screw insertion at a later time (Fig. 2.8).

### *Entry Point to Medullary Canal*

The entry point to the medullary canal must be very exact. On the frontal plane, entry is at the tip of the greater trochanter. On the sagittal plane, the entry point is located slightly more posterior than the standard in the femoral locked nail procedure to make room for inserting the hip screw.

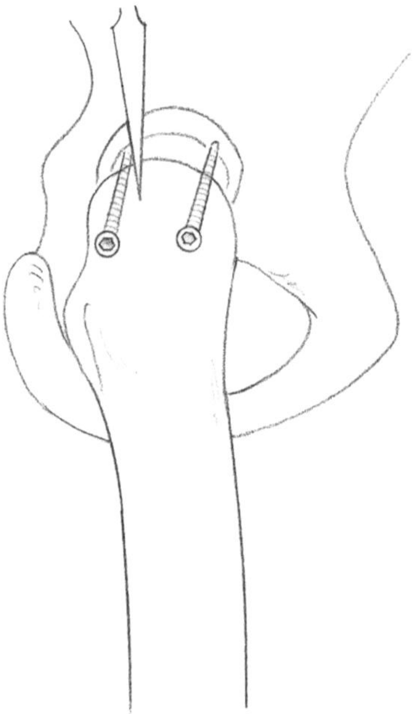

Fig. 2.9. Entry point for the insertion of femoral nail. Frontal plane, tip of the greater trochanter; sagittal plane, mid point on the trochanteric ridge, i.e., slightly more posterior than in standard femoral nailing

It is located in the mid point of the trochanteric ridge (Fig. 2.9).

### Preparation of the Medullary Canal

The standard procedure is carried out to prepare the medullary canal for the insertion of the femoral locked nail (see Chap. 9 "Femoral Fractures", other volume). The same principle as used with the canal should allow the insertion of the femoral nail with ease to prevent possible displacement of the hip fractures.

The medullary canal is reamed to at least 1.5 mm larger than the diameter of the nail to be inserted.

### Nail Length

The correct length of the nail is inserted and these nails are locked in the same way as standard femoral locked nails.

### Fixation of Hip Fractures

The position of hip fractures should always be checked before fixation starts. If the fracture is displaced, reduction of the fracture must be carried out. With the femoral fracture fixed by the

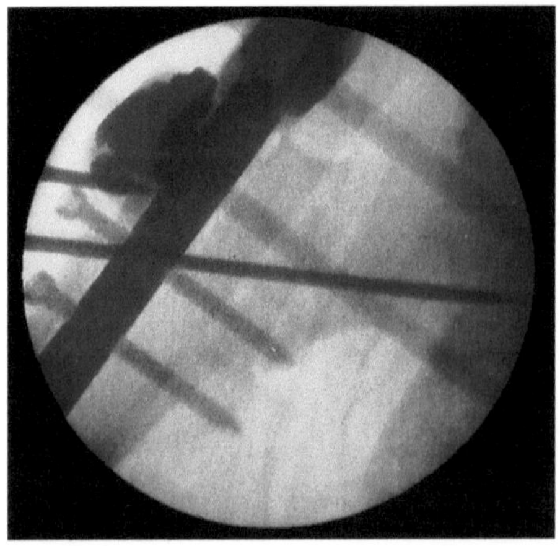

Fig. 2.10. The first guidewire is inserted anterior to the nail and in the inferior half of the femoral head and neck

intramedullary nail, hip fractures can be reduced in most cases.

The cannulated screws are to be inserted around the femoral nail to the femoral head. Both frontal and lateral views of the hip must be obtained by careful positioning of the C-arm.

Usually two screws are sufficient to fix the fracture. The screws inserted should be parallel to each other and are perpendicular to the fracture line. One of the screws should be in the inferior half of the femoral neck and head while the other should be inserted more superior but not to the superomedial quadrant of the femoral head.

Fixation should proceed as follows:

1. Guidewires are inserted with the C-arm positioned to give a frontal view of the hip. The entry point of the guidewire is determined so that the trajectory of the screw path is perpendicular to the fracture plane. The first screw should lie in the inferior half of the femoral neck and head (Fig. 2.10). With the C-arm positioned to give the lateral plane of the hip, the entry of the guidewire is determined anterior to the femoral nail. The first guidewire is inserted with a drive into the femoral head anterior to the femoral nail. The second guidewire is inserted similarly, either anterior or posterior to the femoral nail as judged by the space available (Fig. 2.11).
2. The length of the screws is then determined.
3. The path of the screws is then prepared by using the cannulated drill. In most cases, only the outer cortex should be tapped and the screws are inserted (Fig. 2.12).
4. In case of an intracapsular fracture, arthrotomy is done by inserting a pair of dissecting scissors anteriorly under X-ray monitoring into the hip joint. Arthrotomy is usually evident by the release of the intracapsular hematoma (Fig. 2.13).

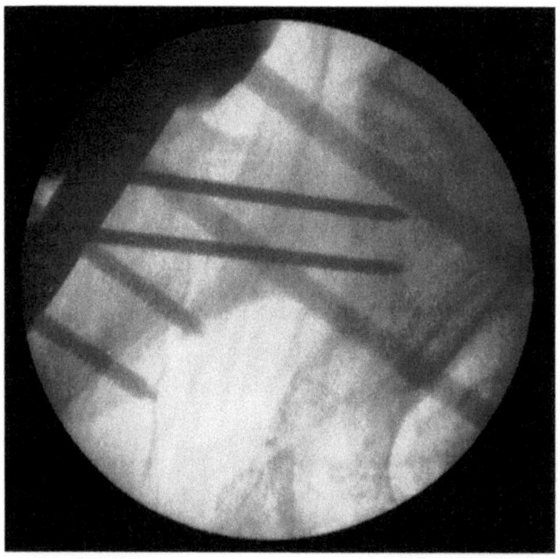

**Fig. 2.11.** The second guidewire is inserted more superior and posterior to the nail

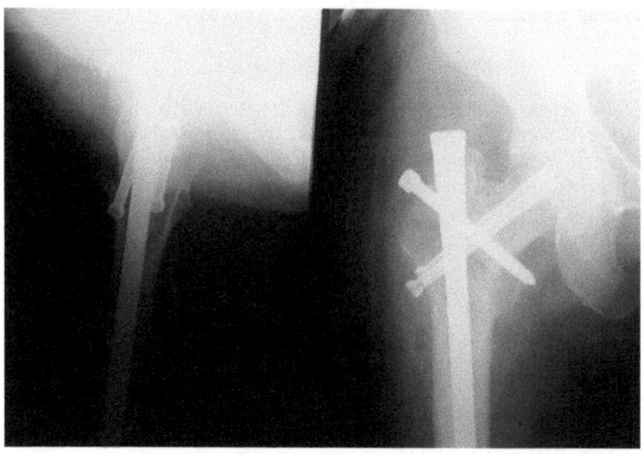

**Fig. 2.12.** Lateral X-ray showing the positions of the cannulated hip screws in relation to the femoral nail

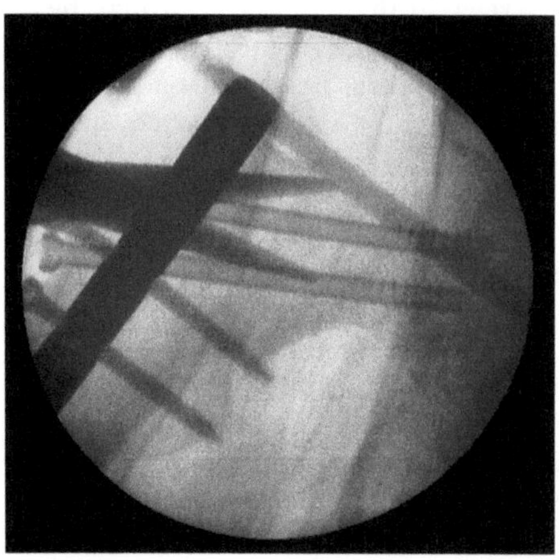

**Fig. 2.13.** Intraoperative X-ray showing arthrotomy through the anterior surface of the hip joint

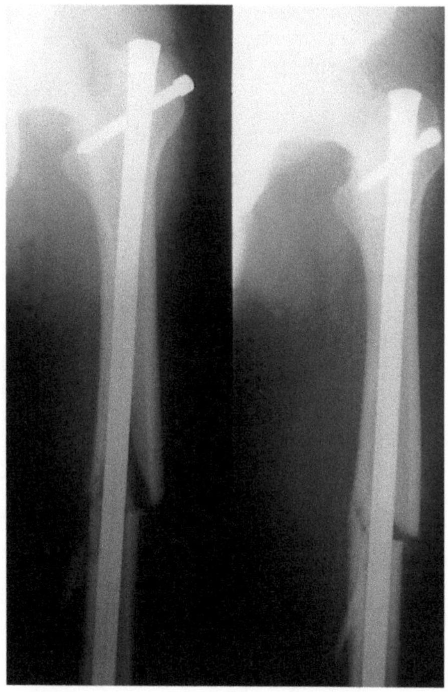

**Fig. 2.14.** A hip fracture was missed and became evident after nailing of the femoral diaphyseal fracture

5. The wound is closed in layers with a suction drainage inserted just beneath the tensor fascia latta. Pressure bandage is then used from the toes to the hip region.

## Postoperative Management

The injured limb is positioned in a 90/90 elevation. Early active movement is encouraged to prevent venous stasis. The drain can usually be removed after 48 h or until the drainage decreases. The pressure bandage is kept for at least 1 week, until the patient can be fully mobilized. Walking exercise is started according to the patient's general condition. The status of weight-bearing depends on the fracture configuration as well as the stability of fixation. Fractures fixed with a long gamma nail can be allowed to have weight-bearing as tolerated by the patient. In fractures fixed by the combined method, weight-bearing walking must be delayed for 4–6 weeks.

## Errors and Potential Hazards

The incidence of missed hip fractures with a diaphyseal fracture has decreased significantly in recent years due to the increase in awareness of the

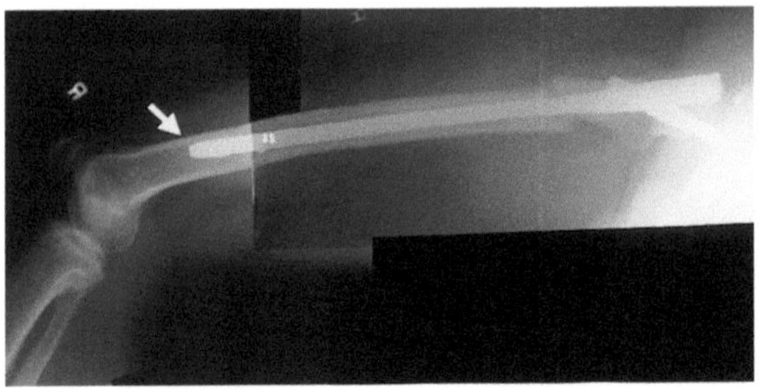

**Fig. 2.15.** Tip of the long gamma nail impinges on the anterior cortex of the distal femur

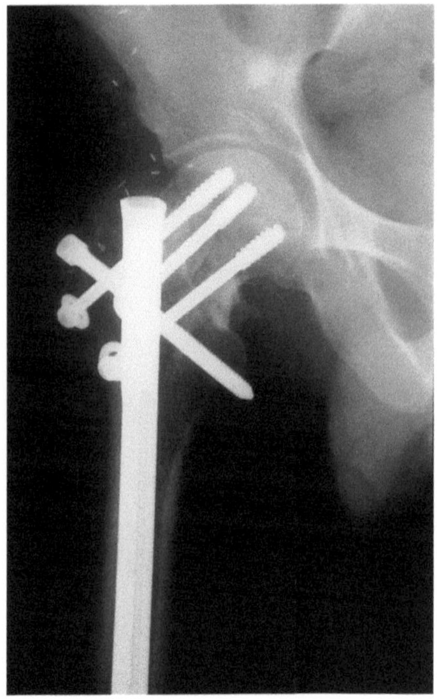

**Fig. 2.16.** A case presented late was treated with hip screw and locked nail. Revascularization of the femoral head was done with vascularized pedicled iliac crest bone graft on the anterior surface of the femoral neck

associated fractures resulting from high-energy trauma (Fig. 2.14). It is mandatory to check X-rays of the hip in *all* cases of femoral shaft fractures. One should always prepare to fix the hip fracture when the femoral shaft fracture is surgically fixed.

As most of the hip fractures in the combined fractures are minimally displaced, every effort should be taken not to displace the fracture during the preoperative preparation period and during the operation. Temporary fixation with K-wires during the nailing procedure may be useful to prevent displacing the hip fractures accidentally during operation.

Displaced hip fractures can usually be reduced in a closed procedure with the reduction procedure of the femoral fracture. However, if the hip fracture remains unreduced, a femoral shaft fracture should be fixed first so that a proper closed reduction maneuver can be undertaken with the stable femoral shaft.

All diaphyseal fractures should be treated with static locking to achieve stable fixation. Dynamization may be needed in fractures fixed with a long gamma nail to improve healing. This is particularly important when considering the removal of the implant in young patients. The fracture must be dynamized at least 6 months before the implants are completely removed. Dynamization is done by removing the distal two locking screws.

In fixing the combined fractures with a long gamma nail, special precautions should be taken for the fixation of the femoral neck fractures with the gamma lag screw. The risk of rotating the femoral head segment is substantial and this should be temporarily fixed with K-wires before the lag screw targeting is undertaken.

The insertion of the long gamma nail down the femoral shaft should always be done with minimal hammering as the nail is a rigid nail. The radius of the anterior bowing curvature may not fit elderly patients because they have a smaller radius of curvature in the bowing. The tip of the nail should always be monitored, especially at the distal third of the femur where the tip may impinge onto the anterior cortex (Fig. 2.15).

Arthrotomy should always be done after fixing the intracapsular hip fractures. This will minimize the risk of avascular necrosis of the femoral head. This can be done by a minimal invasive technique as described in "Operative Procedures."

Placing the screws in the femoral head may be affected by the proximal part of the femoral nail. The insertion of the femoral nail must be precise so as to allow room for the screws inserted anteriorly or posteriorly [10, 11].

## Complications

Avascular necrosis of the femoral head is not a common complication since most of the femoral neck fractures are undisplaced. Arthrotomy should always be done after internal fixation. In the case of delayed presentation of displaced femoral neck fractures, revascularization procedures should be done to prevent avascular necrosis, e.g., vascularized pedicled iliac crest bone graft (Fig. 2.16).

Nonunion of the fractures, more common in diaphyseal fracture, may need dynamization to promote healing.

## References


1. Alho A (1997) Concurrent ipsilateral fractures of the hip and shaft of the femur – a systematic review of 722 cases. Ann Chir Gynaecol 86:326–336
2. Alho A, Ekaland A, Grøgaard B, Dokke JR (1996) A locked hip screw-intramedullary nail (cephalomedullary nail) for the treatment of fractures of the proximal part of the femur combined with fractures of the femoral shaft. J Trauma 40:10–16
3. Bennett FS, Zinar DM, Kilgus DJ (1993) Ipsilateral hip and femoral shaft fractures. Clin Orthop Relat Res 296:168–177
4. Dümmer RE, Sanzana ES (1999) Hip dislocations associated with ipsilateral femoral neck fracture. Int Orthop SICOT 23:353–354
5. Gill SS, Nagi ON, Dhillon MS (1990) Ipsilateral fractures of femoral neck and shaft. J Orthop Trauma 4:293–298
6. Haas NP, Schütz M, Mauch C, Hoffmann R, Südkamp NP (1995) Versorgung ipsilateraler Frakturen des Femurschaftes und des proximalen Femurs – Therapieübersicht und aktuelles Management. Zentralbl Chir 120:856–861
7. Leung KS, So WS, Lam TP, Leung PC (1993) Treatment of ipsilateral femoral shaft fractures and hip fractures. Injury 24:41–45
8. Laporte C, Benazet JP, Scemama P, Castelain C, Saillant G (1999) Fractures homolatérales de la diaphyse et du col fémoral: éléments de choix thérapeutique. Rev Chir Orthop 85:24–32
9. Müller EJ, Siebenrock K, Ekkernkamp A, Ganz R, Muhr G (1999) Ipsilateral fractures of the pelvis and the femur – floating hip? A retrospective analysis of 42 cases. Arch Orthop Trauma Surg 119:179–182
10. Ostermann PA, Henry SL (1994) Die Behandlung ipsilateraler Femurschaft-und Schenkelhalsfrakturen mit dem Russell-Taylor-Rekonstruktionsnagel. Chirurg 65:1042–1045
11. Pietro R, Stefano L, Francesco F, Gregory KH, Massimo M (1999) Treatment of ipsilateral femoral neck and shaft fractures with the Russell-Taylor reconstructive nail. Orthopaedics 22:673–676
12. Rami M, David S, Ronit W, Shaul S, Meir L (1998) Midshaft femoral fracture, concomitant ipsilateral hip joint injury, and disruption of the knee extensor mechanism: a unique triad of dashboard injury. Am J Orthop (June):465–473
13. Richard HD, Barry LR, Spencer LB (1991) Ipsilateral femoral neck and shaft fractures: an overlooked association. Skeletal Radiol 20:251–254
14. Shuler TE, Gruen GS, DiTano O, Riemer BL (1997) Ipsilateral proximal and shaft femoral fractures: spectrum of injury involving the femoral neck. Injury 28:293–297
15. Simmermacher RKJ, Bosch AM (1999) The AO/ASIF-proximal femoral nail (PFN): a new device for the treatment of unstable proximal femoral fractures. Injury Int J Care Injured 30:327–332
16. Wu CC, Shih CH, Chen LH (1993) Femoral shaft fractures complicated by fracture – dislocations of the ipsilateral hip. J Trauma 34:70–75
17. Wu HJ, Cheng YM, Lin SY (1990) Ipsilateral hip and femoral shaft fractures treated with compression hip screw and long side-plate. Kaohsiung J Med Sci 6:251–256

CHAPTER 3

# Distal Femoral Fractures

K. S. Leung

The distal femoral fractures include supracondylar fractures, intercondylar fractures, and their combinations. As in most articular and juxta-articular fractures, operative treatment gives the best clinical result by achieving anatomical reduction of the articular fractures and providing early skeletal stability, which leads to early mobilization and return of joint function. The commonest method of treating these fractures is open reduction with internal fixation by plating [1–3, 8–10]. The open procedure requires a long incision with extensive dissection, which not infrequently results in devitalization of the fracture fragments. Bone grafting is required in fractures with comminution, which typically happens on the medial side of the distal femur where mechanical stability cannot be restored by lateral plating. This very often leads to delay in weight-bearing walking before the fracture consolidates and also leads to implant failure. The load-shielding biomechanical characteristic of the plates results in stress concentration proximal to the fixation, which can lead to fracturing of the femoral shaft proximal to the implant. This is particularly important in geriatric patients in whom these fractures occur quite frequently. The use of intramedullary implants had been advocated [4, 11, 13]. Most of them are open procedures and skeletal stability has to be augmented by additional fixations such as cerclage wires or bone grafting. The closed technique with intramedullary locked nails, as in the treatment of diaphyseal fractures, provides immediate skeletal stability irrespective of the fracture comminution. The extended use of the closed intramedullary fixation with these difficult fractures can certainly avoid many of the complications of the open procedures. In this chapter, the indications and surgical technique are described.

## Surgical Principles

The use of the intramedullary fixation for distal femoral fractures follows the principles of closed treatment of fractures. The fracture hematoma is not disturbed and the reamed material during the preparation of the medullary canal provides osteogenic material, which, dispersed into the fracture site, makes bone grafting unnecessary. The load-sharing biomechanical property of the intramedullary fixation also helps to prevent secondary fracture in the femoral shaft and the splintage effect reinforces the relatively weak femur in geriatric patients with osteoporotic bone.

As the fractures are very distal where the medullary canal flares, the use of the locked nails is mandatory. The nails must be inserted to the subchondral region. For very distal fractures, the distal part of the nail has to be removed just inferior to the distal locking screw hole.

Fractures with intercondylar elements that can be reduced with the closed method can also be treated with this method. The intercondylar fractures can be fixed with percutaneous lag screws inserted under fluoroscopic control with supplementary fixation using the distal locking screws of the intramedullary nail.

This technique cannot be applied to very distal fractures and condylar fractures that cannot be reduced by closed means. Fractures in the coronal plane may not be treated with this method.

## Indications

1. Supracondylar fractures of the femur irrespective of the comminution, AO classification [7] $A_1$, $A_2$, and $A_3$ (Fig. 3.1).
2. Supracondylar fractures with condylar extension, AO classification $C_1$ and $C_2$, which can be reduced anatomically by the closed method.

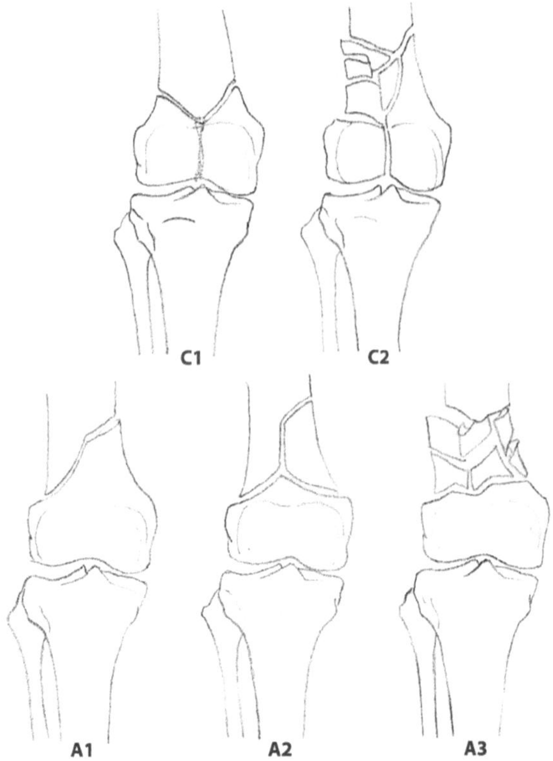


**Fig. 3.1.** Fractures classified according to the AO classification can be treated by intramedullary locked nails

## Preoperative Preparation

### Preoperative Immobilization

It is best done by skin traction as the distal fractures can usually be immobilized by a relatively smaller traction force as compared with that for the diaphyseal fracture. Skeletal traction, if required, should be applied through the tibial pin. Femoral pin traction should always be avoided in the preoperative period because it may increase the chance of infection as it is very near the operative site and accurate position of the femoral pin is required in case skeletal traction is used for closed reduction of the fracture during operation (see "Reduction" in "Operative Technique").

### Radiological Investigation

X-rays of the distal femur must be taken properly with good-quality films to delineate the pattern of the fractures and the extension of the fracture lines in distal and proximal directions.

X-rays of the entire length of the contralateral femur should also be taken to assess the length, the medullary diameter, and the degree of anterior bowing of the diaphysis, which may be excessive in geriatric patients. Determining the length of the femur before operation may preclude the need for cutting the distal end of the nail during operation. The nail can be modified before the operation with a better prepared tip for insertion. However, this is not always possible and intraoperative length estimation is usually more reliable in this operation.

## Special Instruments and Implants

Apart from the standard instrumentation for the intramedullary locked nail, the following equipment modification and instrumentation are required:

- A traction table with adjustable thigh support attached to the traction bar is essential for the reduction of the fracture in the sagittal plane (see "Closed Reduction") (Fig. 3.2). A sterile stirrup for traction may be helpful in case skeletal traction through the femoral condyle is required for fracture reduction.
- An extra long reamer guide (950 mm) is useful during the process of reaming. As the fractures are very distal, the use of the standard reamer guide (600 mm) may lead to frequent loss of the position of the reamer guide in the distal fragment when backing out the reamer for the change of the reamer heads during reaming.
- A sterile hack saw and an iron file should always be available so that the nail can be modified during the operation. The tip of the nail has to be cut and smoothened so that the most distal locking screw can be inserted in the subchondral area of the distal femur.
- A pair of large reduction forceps and the instruments for the insertion of the lag screws should also be available for fractures with condylar extension.

## Operative Technique

### Positioning and Anesthesia

The patient is positioned supine on a traction table (Fig. 3.3). The upper trunk is flexed towards the opposite side to have better exposure of the greater trochanter and facilitate the insertion of the nail. The lateral flexion of the trunk is maintained by using a proper guard. The opposite lower limb is flexed and elevated to make room for C-arm positioning, as in standard femoral nailing procedures.

The operation can be performed under either general or spinal anesthesia.

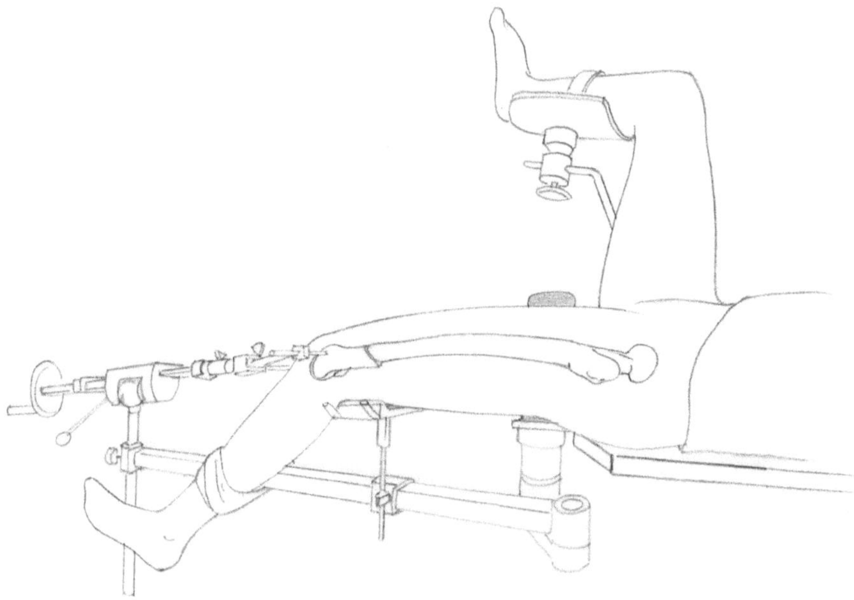

**Fig. 3.2.** The set-up of the traction table with the thigh support. The position of the thigh support should be adjusted to give the best reduction of the fractures in the sagittal plane

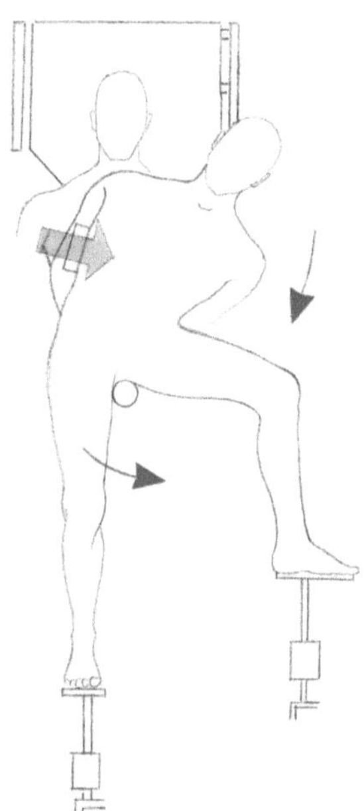

**Fig. 3.3.** Positioning of the patient on the traction table. Note the lateral flexion of the trunk to the opposite side and the substantial adduction of the distal fragment in achieving the reduction in the frontal plane

## Closed Reduction

This is the most important part of the operation. Apart from the common deformity of shortening, this fracture presents with some characteristic deformities that have to be corrected before fixation is undertaken. An understanding of the deforming forces caused by muscle pull of different types is essential in obtaining good reduction of the fractures.

### *Intercondylar Fracture Component*

Intercondylar fractures with minimal displacement can be treated with this method (Fig. 3.4). In the majority of these fractures, the displacements are caused by the vertical force that splits the condyles through the intercondylar notch and displacements occur in the frontal plane. The condyles are thus displaced sideways with the proximal ends separated.

Fractures can be reduced by longitudinal traction, which tightens the collateral ligaments of the knee; a similar mechanism is used in ligamentotaxis for the reduction of articular fractures. A minor degree of adjustment and manipulation with a pair of reduction forceps may be necessary during the process of temporary percutaneous stabilization. If reduction fails, the nailing procedure should be abandoned and open surgery should be carried out to achieve a congruent articular surface.

### *The Supracondylar Fracture Component*

Displacement in the frontal plane means that as the fractures occur distally, the tension in the adductor magnus always causes the proximal shaft to displace medially and results in a classical adducted position (Fig. 3.5). Displacement in sagittal plane means that the weight of the proximal long segment and the fracture in the distal femur with scanty muscle attachment results in the posterior sagging of the femur.

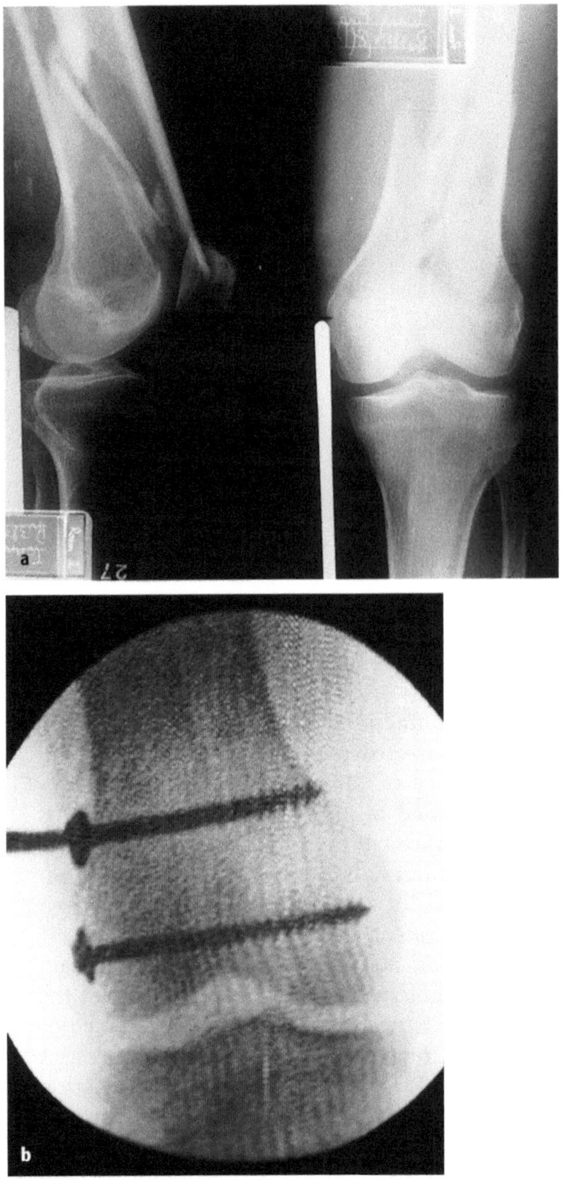

**Fig. 3.4 a, b.** X-ray film showing a minimally displaced intercondylar fracture (**a**) which is closely reduced and fixed by two percutaneous lag screws (**b**)

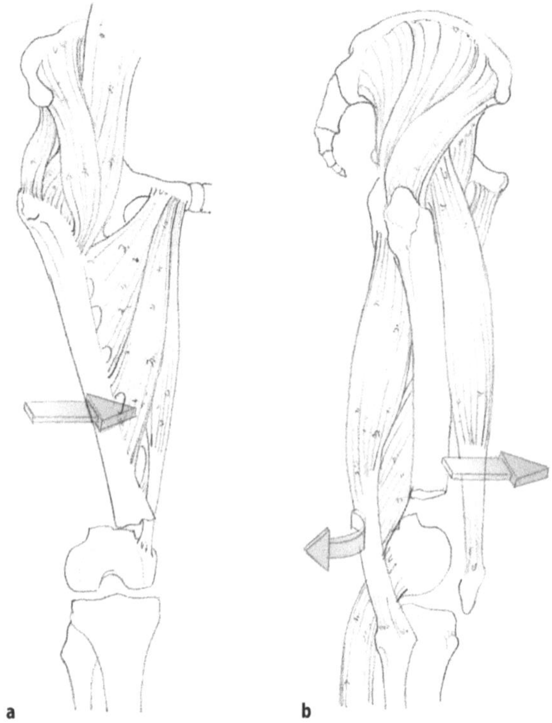

**Fig. 3.5 a, b.** Muscle actions that resulted in the displacement of the fractures in the frontal (**a**) and sagittal (**b**) planes

For the distal segment, the origins of the gastrocnemius muscles just proximal to the two femoral condyles lead to the rotation of the distal fragment in the sagittal plane and result in extension deformity of the distal fragment. There is usually a minimal rotational deformity along the longitudinal axis of the femur.

In diaphyseal fractures of the femur, reduction involves skeletal traction through the femoral condyles, giving a more effective force in correcting shortening and rotational deformities. In supracondylar fractures, as there is no strong proximal muscle acting across the fracture site, the length can be easily reduced by longitudinal traction using a foot piece (Fig. 3.6). In very muscular patients, skeletal traction with femoral pin traction may be necessary. In such a situation, special attention must be given to ensure the accurate position of the traction pin so as to facilitate reduction and prevent the blockage of nail passage.

To reduce the deformity in the frontal plane, the distal fragment should be adducted so as to realign it with the proximal fragment (Fig. 3.3). For the deformity in the sagittal plane, reduction can be achieved by flexing the knee to relax the gastrocnemius muscles. The use of the thigh support at the fracture site (Fig. 3.2) greatly facilitates reduction by correcting the posterior sagging and reducing the extended deformity of the distal fragment. This is by far the most effective means to reduce the rotatory displacement of the distal fragment and is strongly recommended.

If skeletal traction is required for the reduction, the traction pin should be inserted to the most anteroinferior region of the femoral condyle (Fig. 3.7), preferably under fluoroscopic control. This will help to reduce the extension deformity of the distal fragment when longitudinal traction is applied and will not block the passage of the nail to be inserted to the subchondral region of the femoral condyle. The use of a sterile stirrup

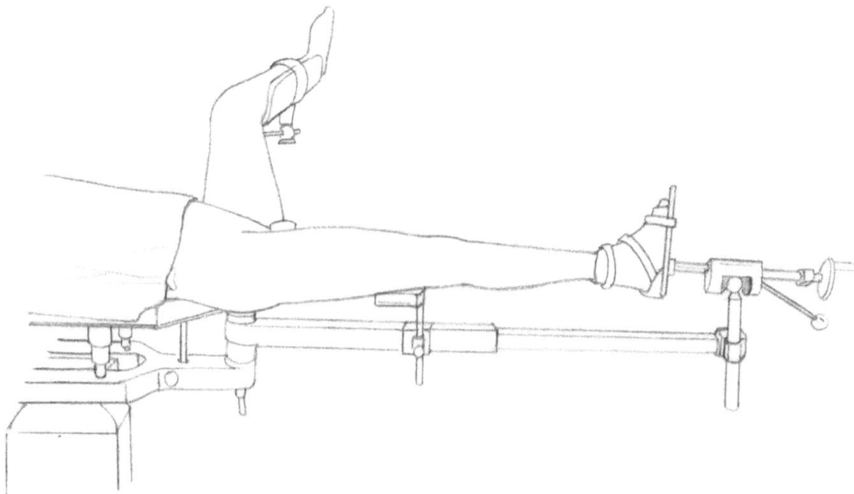

**Fig. 3.6.** Reduction of the fractures can be done with the traction through the foot-piece of the traction table with the use of the thigh support

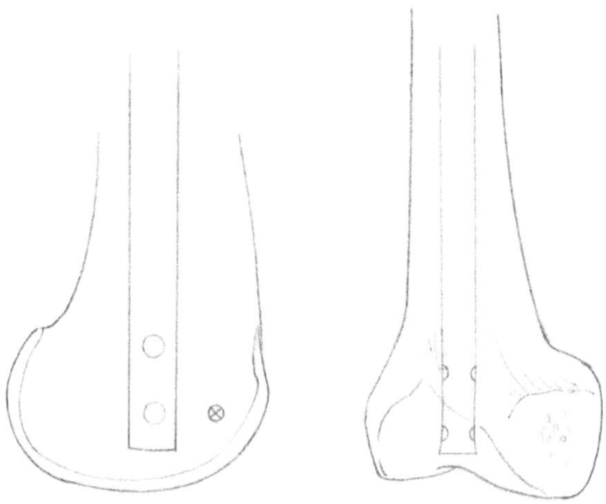

**Fig. 3.7.** The position of the Steinmann pin insertion in the distal femur. It should be inserted in the most distal and anterior part of the femur

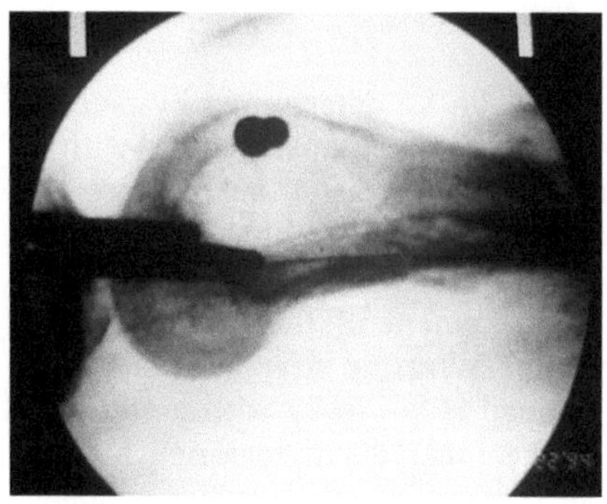

**Fig. 3.8.** X-ray film of the lateral view of the distal femur showing the positions of the two percutaneous lag screws fixing the intercondylar fractures

will also help provide a wider sterile field for the subsequent distal locking procedure.

After achieving satisfactory reduction of the fractures, the region from the iliac crest to the tibial tubercle is sterilized and draped. The thigh support is isolated from the surgical field with a waterproof sterile drape.

### Fixation of Condylar Fractures

This should be done before the standard nailing procedure is performed. After the condylar fractures are reduced and stabilized with a pair of reduction forceps used percutaneously, the fracture can then be fixed by lag screws inserted under fluoroscopic monitoring with small stab skin incisions. The screws should be accurately positioned so that they will not block the passage of the subsequent locked nail insertion. Two 6.5-mm lag screws should be inserted with one close to the anterior cortex and one close to the posterior cortex of the distal femur (Fig. 3.8). Care should be taken in determining the length of the lag screws by taking the trapezoidal shape of the distal femur into consideration.

### Preparation of the Medullary Canal

The medullary canal is prepared as in the standard technique of intramedullary nailing. The extra-long (900-mm) reamer guide is passed and centralized in the distal fragment both in the frontal and sagittal planes (Fig. 3.9). As the fracture is in the distal femur, the intact diaphysis should be reamed slowly and reamed to 2 mm larger than the diameter of the nail to be inserted.

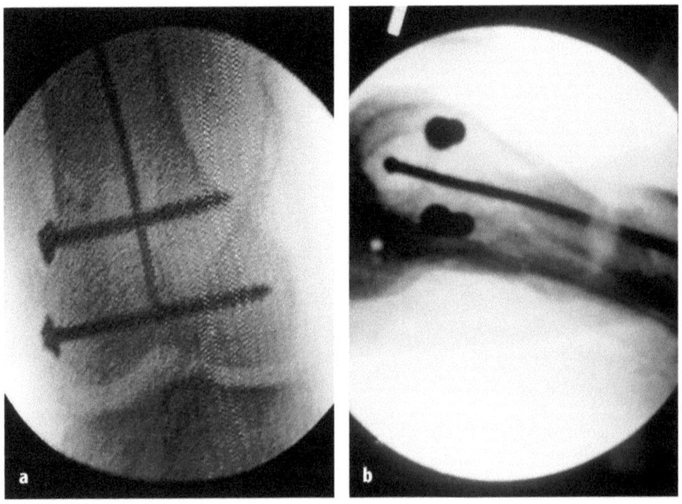

**Fig. 3.9 a, b.** Intraoperative fluoroscopic pictures showing the centralization of the reamer guide in both planes. The reamer passes between the two lag screws which fix the condylar fractures. **a** frontal view. **b** lateral view

## Preparation of the Nail

The length of the nail can be determined by placing the nail along the thigh and screening with fluoroscopy to ensure that the distal locking screw hole is as close to the subchondral bone as possible (Fig. 3.10). The nail selected should be 15 mm longer than the measurement of the total length of the medullary canal. With the selected nail, the distal 15 mm of the nail is cut away with a sterile hack saw close to the most distal locking screw hole. The cut edge is then rounded off by gentle hammering and filing so that the sharp edge of the cut end will not cut into the femoral cortex during insertion of the nail (Fig. 3.11).

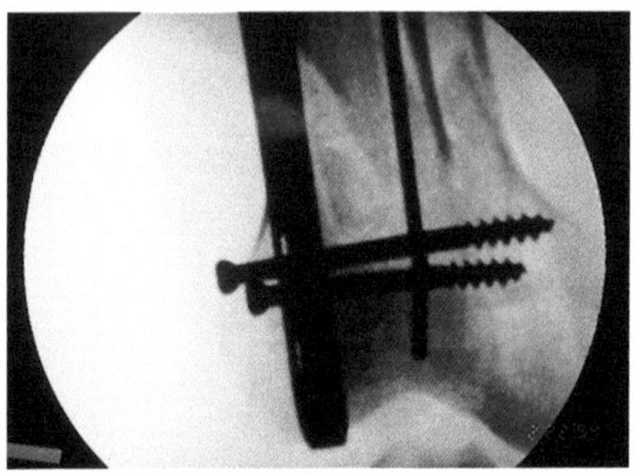

**Fig. 3.10.** The estimation of the length of the nail by placing the nail along the thigh so that the two locking screws can have optimal anchorage into the distal femur

## Nail Insertion

The reamer guide is then replaced by the nail guide which is again centralized in the distal fragment. The nail is then inserted manually over the nail guide. By gentle rotating the nail in a small arc, the nail can be inserted to the distal fragment with no difficulty. The advancement of the tip should be constantly monitored with the fluoroscope (Fig. 3.12). Minimal hammering should be used in order to avoid the nail tip cutting into the femoral cortex. The nail is then impacted into the subchondral bone of the distal femur (Fig. 3.13). The nail guide is then removed.

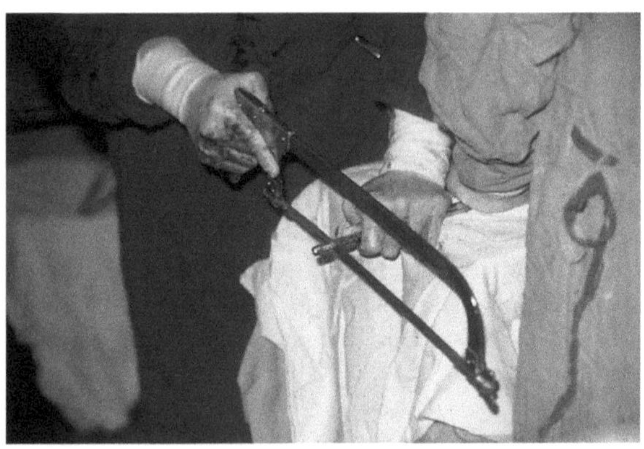

**Fig. 3.11.** The distal 15 mm of the nail is cut away with a sterile hack saw. The cut edges are rounded off by gentle hammering

## Locking

The indications for the locking of the nail are the same as those for diaphyseal fractures. Proximal locking is indicated in comminuted fractures. For

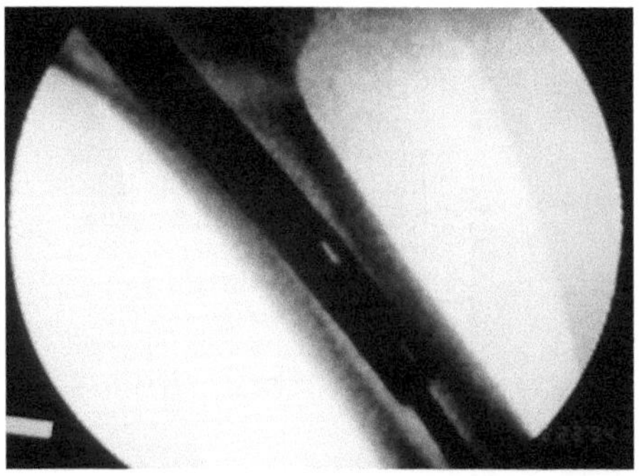

**Fig. 3.12.** The tip of the nail is monitored constantly with the image intensifier during insertion

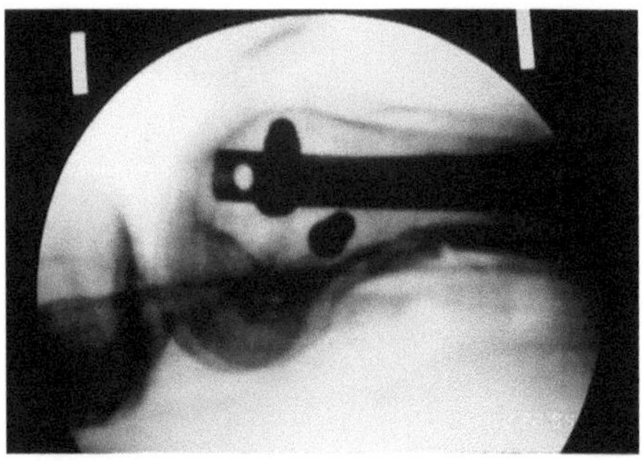

**Fig. 3.13.** The modified nail is inserted into the subchondral bone of the distal femur

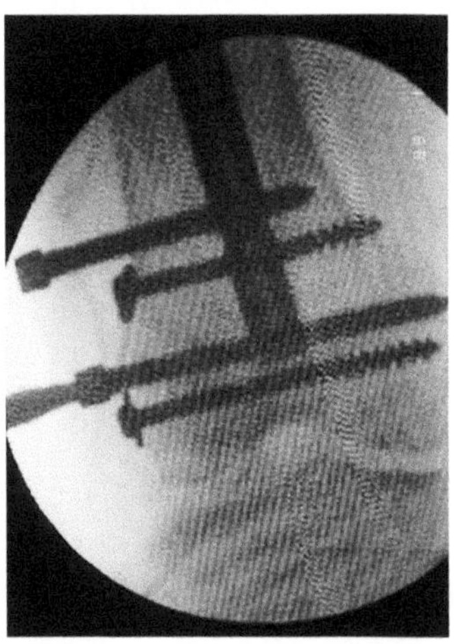

**Fig. 3.14.** The distal locking is done with two 6.35-mm fully threaded screws to give good longitudinal and rotatory stability

pure transverse fractures of the distal femur, only distal locking is indicated. Distal locking is done with the fully threaded 6.35-mm screws to improve the strength of purchase into the metaphyseal region in the distal femur (Fig. 3.14). Two locking screws must be used to provide rotational stability. Care should be given in measuring the

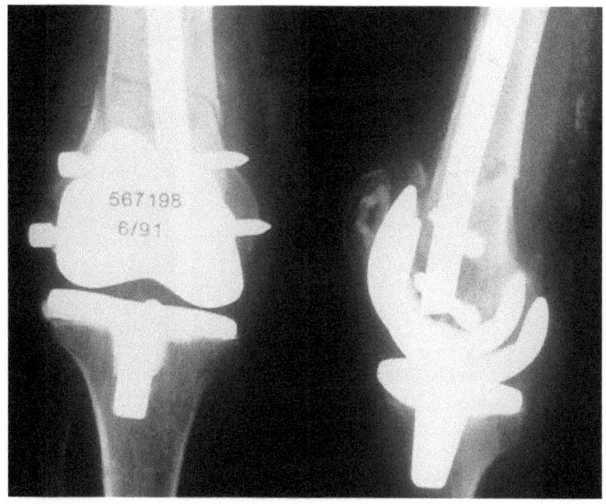


**Fig. 3.15.** Fixation of a supracondylar fracture in a patient with total knee replacement. (Courtesy of Dr. G. Taglang, CTO, Strasbourg)

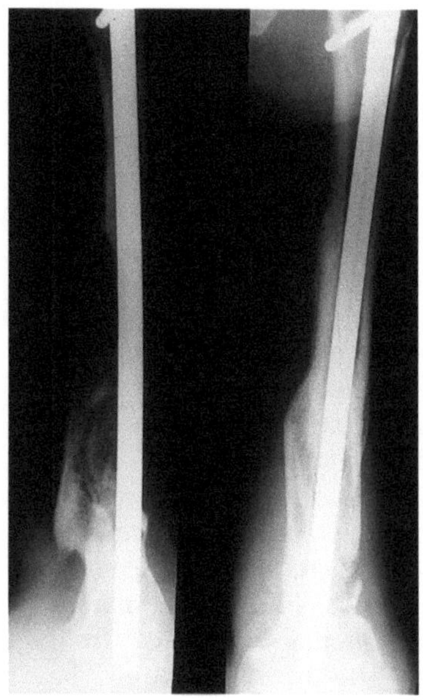

**Fig. 3.16.** Good corticalization of the callus 6 months after operation

length of the screws to avoid the screw protruding out the medial cortices of the distal femur. The use of the blunt tip screws will decrease the incidence of irritation on the medial side.

## Closure

The wounds are closed with a suction drain in the proximal wound. The lower limb is bandaged with the elastic bandage from the toes to the proximal thigh (Fig. 3.15).

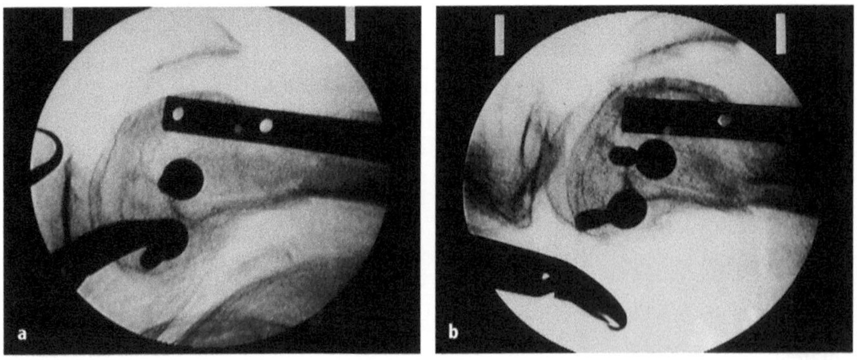

**Fig. 3.17 a, b.** The natural anterior bowing curvature of the femoral shaft may lead to the anterior protrusion of the nail through the fracture site (**a**). This is particularly common in geriatric patients. Anterior translation of the distal fragment will help to align the medullary canal so that the nail can be inserted properly (**b**)

### Special Indications

Special indications include supracondylar fracture in patients with total knee replacement, floating knee etc. (Fig. 3.15) (see chapter 7 this volume).

## Postoperative Management

The injured limb is elevated in a 90/90 position with both the hip and knee flexed to 90°. The suction drain is removed when the drainage fluid decreases, which usually can be done after 48 h. During this period, active and passive movement of the toes is encouraged.

The patient is allowed to sit out of bed once the drain is removed. Active and passive movement of the lower limb is started and continued throughout the rehabilitation period. For stable fractures, gradual weight-bearing walking can be started from the beginning. Full weight-bearing walking commences when there is callus observed on the X-ray films. For unstable fractures, non-weight-bearing walking should be started from the beginning. Weight-bearing should only be started when there is callus observed on the X-ray film and full weight-bearing walking is allowed when the callus corticalized (Fig. 3.16).

Dynamization of the fracture, which is seldom required, should be done 6 months after operation by removing the proximal locking screw. The distal locking screws should be removed after the fracture heals if they cause persistent irritation around the knees.

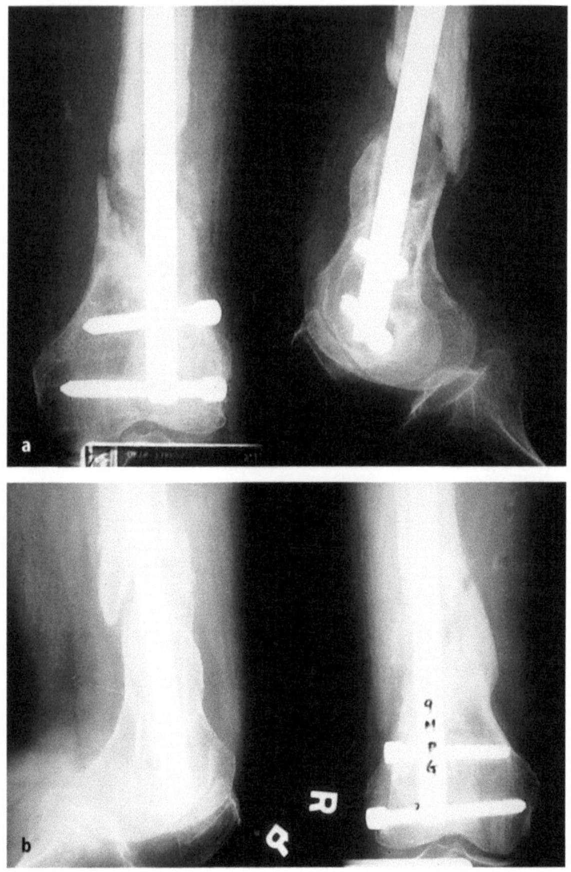

**Fig. 3.18 a, b.** Delayed union in a revision fixation after plate breakage in a 78-year-old female patient (**a**). Bone graft with cancellous allograft from femoral head was applied and resulted in union of the fractures 9 months afterwards (**b**)

## Errors and Potential Hazards

### Preoperative Radiological Assessment

Preoperative careful study of the fracture is important to delineate the exact fracture pattern and to detect the intercondylar fracture components. The measurement of the radius of curvature of the anterior bowing in the femoral shaft also helps estimate the difficulties that may be encountered when the nail is inserted. This is particularly important in geriatric patients in whom anterior bowing is usually increased.

### Reduction of Intercondylar Fractures

Intra-articular components should always be reduced anatomically. Failure in the reduction of the intra-articular components may lead to abandoning this technique, although the use of mini-arthrotomy to reduce the intra-articular components may be considered.

### Reduction of Supracondylar Fractures

In reducing the fractures in the sagittal plane, the conventional technique of flexing the knee to allow relaxation of the gastrocnemius muscles may not be necessary in all cases. Instead, correct use of the thigh support is essential for the closed reduction of the fractures in the sagittal plane. This support must be placed in a position that gives the best reduction of the fracture.

### Excessive Anterior Bowing in Femoral Shaft

In geriatric patients, the decrease in the radius curvature of the anterior bowing of the femoral shaft and the common occurrence of anterior comminution in the fracture site cause the frequent anterior protrusion of the reamer guide or the nail through the fracture site. Slight anterior translation of the distal fragment will align the passage of the medullary canal (Fig. 3.17). Gentle bending of the distal one-third of the nail with a bending press will also facilitate positioning the nail into the distal fragment.

### Preparation of Nail

As the distal 15 mm of the nail has been removed and the cut edge may be sharp, care must be taken to avoid the cut edge of the nail jamming into the cortex of the femur during the insertion of the nail. To avoid this three steps must be followed:

1. The medullary canal is reamed to 2 mm larger than the diameter of the nail.
2. The nail is inserted manually with minimal hammering.
3. The tip of the nail is monitored frequently with X-ray.

### Reaming

Reaming through the intact diaphysis of the femur should be slow and careful. Excessive force and reaming too rapidly may lead to jamming the reamer head.

### Postoperative Knee Pain

Postoperative lateral knee pain due to prominent screw heads of the distal locking screws is common [5, 6]. However, this usually should not interfere with knee movement. The irritation is due to the relatively large screw head of the 6.35-mm diagonal screws and the thin soft tissue layer in the lateral side of the distal femur. Patients should be reassured and the screws can be removed after the fracture heals.

### Implant Failure

Loosening and backing out of the distal locking screws may occur in geriatric patients with osteoporotic bone. The screws may be replaced by the Vecsei expansion screws. Implant failure in the form of fracture through the proximal screw hole, though uncommon, must be looked for in patients with delayed union (Fig. 3.18). Dynamization or bone graft should be done when delayed union happens. We do not find postoperative bracing [12] necessary.

## References

1. Giles JB, Delee JC, Heckman JD, Keever JE (1982) Supracondylar-intercondylar fractures of the femur treated with a supracondylar plate and lag screw. J Bone Joint Surg 64-A:864–810
2. Healy WL, Brooker AF Jr (1983) Distal femoral fractures. Comparison of open and closed methods of treatment. Clin Orthop 174:166–171
3. Johnson KD, Hicken G (1987) Distal femoral fractures. Orthop Clin North Am 18:115–139
4. Laros GS (1979) Supracondylar fractures of the femur: editorial comment and comparative results. Clin Orthop 138:9–12
5. Leung KS (1994) Intramedullary locked nailing for distal femoral fractures. Orthop Traumatol 3:260–266
6. Leung KS, Shen WY, So WS, Mui LT, Grosse A (1991) Interlocking intramedullary nailing for supracondylar and intercondylar fractures of the distal part of the femur. J Bone Joint Surg 73-A:332–340
7. Müller ME, Nazarian S, Koch P, Schatzker J (1990) The comprehensive classification of fractures of long bones. Springer, Berlin Heidelberg New York, pp 140–141
8. Pritchett JW (1984) Supracondylar fractures of the femur. Clin Orthop 184:173–177
9. Sanders R, Regazzoni P, Ruedi TP (1989) Treatment of supracondylar-intracondylar fractures of the femur

using the dynamic condylar screw. J Orthop Trauma 3:214–222
10. Schatzker J, Lambert DC (1979) Supracondylar fractures of the femur. Clin Orthop 138:77–83
11. Shelbourne KD, Brueckmann FR (1982) Rush-pin fixation of supracondylar and intercondylar fractures of the femur. J Bone Joint Surg 64-A:161–169
12. Wu CC, Shih CH (1992) Treatment of femoral supracondylar unstable comminuted fractures: comparisons between plating and Grosse-Kempf interlocking nailing techniques. Arch Orthop Trauma Surg 111:232–236
13. Zickel RE, Hobeika P, Robbins DS (1986) Zickel supracondylar nails for fractures of the distal end of the femur. Clin Orthop 212:79–88

CHAPTER 4

# Proximal and Distal Tibial Fractures

G. Taglang

## Surgical Principle

The proximal and distal fractures of the tibia are mostly treated by open reduction and plating techniques, especially when the articular surfaces are involved in the fracture.

But the fractures of the metaphyseal area of the tibia are also good indications for closed techniques such as intramedullary (IM) nails or external fixations techniques. The most important problems with conventional IM nails are rotational problems or telescoping problems in cases of comminuted fractures. The rotational problems in the proximal or in the distal areas of the tibia after conventional nailing can be controlled by using casts. The locking procedure is of course the best method to prevent rotational instability and telescoping. The indications for IM locking nails were extended in our unit to fractures with articular lines, but only if the articular fracture lines can be perfectly reduced.

In order to treat these fractures, a number of important rules of operative technique must be followed depending on the type and the pattern of the fractures.

## Indications

### Proximal Fractures

For the fractures situated in the proximal area of the tibia, the general rule in using locking nails is placing the two proximal locking screws optimally above the fracture line. We know, after biomechanical tests [1] and clinical experiments [2], that one screw alone is not sufficient to stabilize the proximal part of the tibia. This is particularly true in the antero-posterior plane in flexion and extension of the knee joint. In this situation, a single screw acts as an axis around which the proximal part of the tibia rotates.

Sometimes the fracture extends to the joint (tibia plateau). If this articular fracture can be easily reduced, we use the locking nail technique after perfectly reducing the joint and fixation is done mostly by percutaneous standard screws or cannulated screws. Positioning the screws in this area is very important so that the locking screws and the nail do not come in contact. For these reasons in these borderlines indications, we also use small-diameter nails (mostly 10 mm in diameter). With these small nails we systematically perform a static locking. When there is no need of percutaneous screwing, we prefer to use 11-mm nails with 4.6-mm screws, as we know that in very proximal fractures all stresses are supported by the locking screws. This explains the mechanical problems caused by other nail designs, which use small screws in this kind of fracture [3, 4].

### Distal Fractures

Distal tibia fractures can be easily treated with IM locking nails [5] because closed procedures are particularly indicated in this area for soft tissue reasons. We know that open procedures are riskier and that the complication rate is often high after plating techniques used in open fractures, for example.

When using locking nailing techniques in distal fractures, the two distal screws have to be inserted downstream of the fracture line. If this rule is not respected, the risk of secondary displacement of the fracture is very high. Distal tibia fractures are often associated with fibula fractures and malleolar fractures. These fractures, particularly when they are unstable, must be treated during the same procedure [6]. (For illustrations of distal fractures, see Chap. 12, "Atlas of Clinical Cases".)

## Preoperative Preparation

Before the procedure itself, a precise diagnosis of the proximal/distal tibia fractures must be made, meaning that all the fracture lines must be analyzed, particularly if the fracture lines extend to the knee or ankle joint. Our treatment policy in such fractures is to treat all fracture lines by a closed procedure. This means that the articular fracture lines must be controlled most of the time by percutaneous screws before the nailing procedure itself. This kind of screwing must be planned precisely, because if the screws are incorrectly positioned they can be an obstacle for the nail.

In cases of comminuted fractures, as for the femur, the correct length of the tibia has to be known before the beginning of the procedure. We currently use a CT scan examination of the opposite tibia (scout view). This technique is the most precise and avoids the parallax problems frequently observed with standard radiological techniques.

The skin is prepared just before the nailing procedure in the operating room by the nursing staff. In the case of an open fracture (see Chap. 5, "Intramedullary Nailing of Open Fractures" by C.M. Court-Brown), debridement, cleaning of the wound, and precise excision of soft tissues is a major step to achieving good long-term results for this kind of fracture. The use of a pulsed washing technique and a standard antibioprophylaxia have led to a decrease in the infection rate in our series. The antibioprophylaxia currently used in the unit consists of the administration of:

- Cephalosporins of the second generation (60 mg/kg per day)
- Ornidazole or metronidazole (40 mg/kg per day) for 48 h

The opening is graded according the Cauchoix [7] classification modified by Gustilo [8] for open Grade III fractures. Grading has to be done after the excision and the debridement steps.

## Special Instruments and Implants

With very proximal or very distal fractures, one of the main problems is perfect reduction before the skin incision, a result of positioning the patient on the table (see "Positioning"). However, in some cases, such as in nailing after a rather long period of conservative treatment, using an instrument for intraoperative reduction is necessary. We use a reduction instrument connected to a grip. This instrument was inspired by the small nail technique described by Küntscher. This technique is sometimes necessary in distal fractures to perfect positioning the reaming guidewire in the central part of the distal tibia epiphysis.

In some very rare cases, a percutaneous clamp can be used during the reaming/nailing procedure, especially in AP fracture lines without preliminary screwing. This technique has also to be used in case of segmental fractures.

With very distal tibia fractures, we have cut the distal tip of the nail (the last 12 mm) to be sure that the two distal screws are perfectly positioned distally from the fracture line. Given that in the new generation of nails, the distance between the holes and the distance between the last hole and the tip of the nail has decreased, this will be abandoned.

## Positioning

### Proximal Fractures

These fractures are the most difficult fractures to reduce.

As usual, the patient is placed in a supine position on the fracture table. Traction is applied by means of a sterile transcalcaneus Steinmann pin connected to a stirrup attached to the fracture table. The Steinmann pin is placed immediately before the procedure begins.

For proximal fractures, it is important to be able to perfectly monitor the reduction on the image intensifier in the AP plane and on the lateral view. For these reasons, the pieces of the fracture table must not be in superposition with the broken tibia, especially on the frontal view. Monitoring the lateral view on the image intensifier requires particular attention to the distance between the edge of the table and the tibia, so that it is not too great. If the distance is too great, displaying the image on the screen may prove difficult.

In normal conditions, a knee rest is fixed to the fracture table and the knee is flexed to 90°. However, in proximal fractures, the flexion of the knee can lead to a high level of extension force on the proximal fragment. Therefore we prefer, as do several other authors, positioning the patient with the knee joint in semiextension [9]. The most important point remains placing the knee rest under the posterior aspect of the thigh and not in the popliteal fossa. This is particularly important for three reasons:

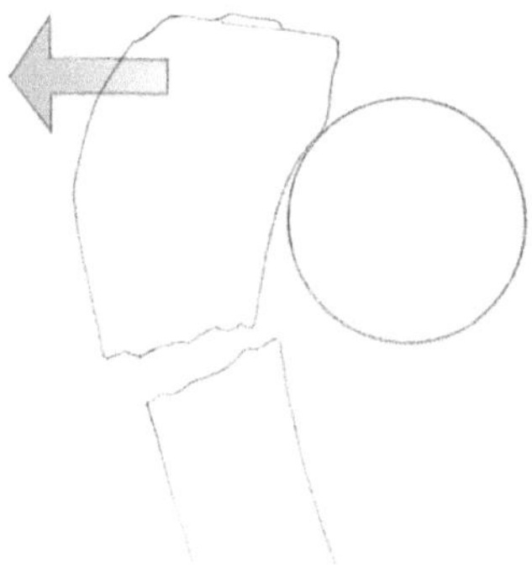

**Fig. 4.1.** The risk of pushing forward the proximal part of the tibia is high when the knee rest is positioned in the popliteal fossa

1. Avoiding vascular compression during the reduction. This situation can be dangerous during the proximal locking procedure, when the popliteal artery is just behind the posterior cortex of the tibia, in case the drill bit comes out.
2. Increasing the pressure in the compartments due to the compression of the venous popliteal system.
3. Pushing forward the proximal fragment, preventing a perfect reduction on the lateral view (Fig. 4.1).

To maintain the knee joint in an optimal position during the reduction and the nailing procedure, we have developed a holding system connected to the knee rest. This system consists in two parts situated laterally and holding the femoral condyles. With this system, the knee joint area can have no motion, especially in the frontal plane (Fig. 4.2). An anatomical reduction can be achieved with the stirrup, which is rigid and firmly connected to the fracture table.

### Distal Fractures

The Steinmann pin and the rigid stirrup are systematically used for the reduction of distal fractures.

Most of the distal fractures are reduced with adduction of the affected leg. Adduction allows the stretching of the muscular structures in the lateral compartment and thus the reduction of the fracture. No adduction in these fractures means systematically poor reduction with a valgus deformity.

With isolated tibia fractures having an intact fibula or a plastic deformation of the fibula, reduction is occasionally somewhat more difficult. We have never had to perform a fibula osteotomy to achieve reduction of the tibia, but we currently use the repositioning tube very frequently to manipulate the tibia from inside.

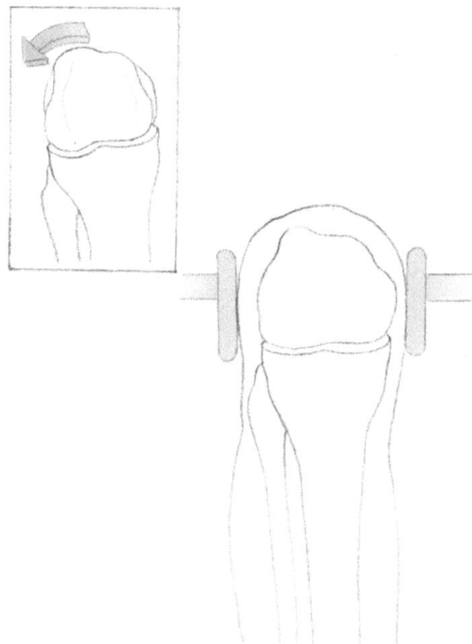

**Fig. 4.2.** The holding system is designed to maintain the femoral condyles

## Reduction

Reduction must be done before the skin incision. The following elements must be checked:

- Knee in flexion (90°)
- Knee rest under the posterior aspect of the thigh
- Lateral condyle supports in the proper position
- Position of the leg in adduction
- Opposite limb on a Köppel support with
- Flexion abduction of the hip joint
- Flexion of the knee joint to avoid conflicts with the image intensifier

The same steps must be followed for distal fractures, but it is particularly important to use the Steinmann pin and a rigid stirrup to perform an anatomical reduction.

It must be kept in mind that for the last centimeters of nailing, the nailing guidewire must be removed. In this situation, it is crucial to control the reduction on the C-frame to be sure there is no valgus deformity in the fracture site. If the fracture is again in valgus, the last centimeters of the bone must be nailed under control and a small drape around the leg will help to maintain the reduction.

## Operative Technique

In this chapter, we will consider the combination between epiphyseal fractures in the proximal or distal area and fractures involving the diaphyseal area. In most of the cases, the epiphyseal fractures have to be treated prior the nailing procedures. In fact, whatever the type of epiphyseal fracture, one must keep the final position of the locking nail in mind while inserting the different devices.

### Distal Fractures with Articular Fracture Line

#### *Medial Malleolar Fractures*

These fractures are mostly treated with the tension wire technique. The advantages of the system are clear. First, it is easy to put the pins in the anterior and the posterior parts of the epiphyseal end of the tibia after reduction. Thus there is room enough to put the nail in the right place. This is not possible if a compression screw is used, especially if the malleolar fracture is horizontal and the screw more or less vertical. With a vertical fracture, it is sometimes possible to use low horizontal screwing. The nail must stop before the screw. Second, the advantages of tension wiring from a biomechanical point of view are also clear compared with a screw that risks loosening. Each time the patient moves the ankle in flexion/extension, the tension wire acts as a "compression machine" on the fracture site.

#### *Lateral Malleolar Fractures*

These fractures can be treated by open procedures with plates or by closed procedures by IM pinning. The important point is to give the fibula the correct length and/or to repair the inferior tibiofibular joint.

#### *Posterior (or Third) Malleolar Fractures*

This fracture must be treated by an antero-posterior screw after reduction of the frontal fracture line. The reduction of this fracture is obtained by putting the ankle in the talus situation. Again, it is very important to place the screw as distal as possible to avoid any contact with the distal tip of the nail.

The use of a percutaneous clamp is sometimes necessary to fix the fracture temporarily before the fixation with a screw. Cannulated screws are very convenient for the fixation as they can be introduced by minimally invasive techniques. After placing a Kirschner wire, it is checked with the image intensifier. If the position of the K-wire is correct, the measurement is made and then the cannulated screw is inserted over the wire. The screws used are usually 5 mm in diameter.

### Proximal Fractures with Articular Fracture Line

The nailing technique can be used for the treatment of proximal tibia fractures with involvement of the joint in particular cases. The intra-articular fracture line is an extension of the metaphyseal fracture line and must be displaced only slightly.

In most cases, the fracture line comes on the lateral tibia plateaux area or is an antero-posterior fracture.

Before the nailing process begins, the articular fracture line must be reduced and fixed. This is done percutaneously if possible by using cannulated screws (most often two screws are used) inserted in the posterior part of the tibia epiphysis. These screws must not disrupt the nail insertion.

The nailing technique follows the basic principles. Two points are again important to check:

- Monitoring the reduction during nail insertion on the lateral view of the image intensifier. The tendency is always to the antecurvature in the fracture site (Fig. 4.3).
- Hitting the posterior cortex of the tibia with the tip of the nail and damaging it is a risk (Fig. 4.4).

### Proximal and Distal Extra-Articular Fractures

#### *Incision*

The incision is made in the same way as for conventional fractures treated with the locking nail. We prefer passing through the patellar tendon (more medially than laterally). After placing a self retractor, we open the canal by using the curved Küntscher awl. In proximal fractures, varus deformity must be monitored (Fig. 4.5).

#### *Guide Positioning*

The guide is passed through the hole made by the awl.

For proximal fractures, the risk of the guidewire coming out through the posterior fracture

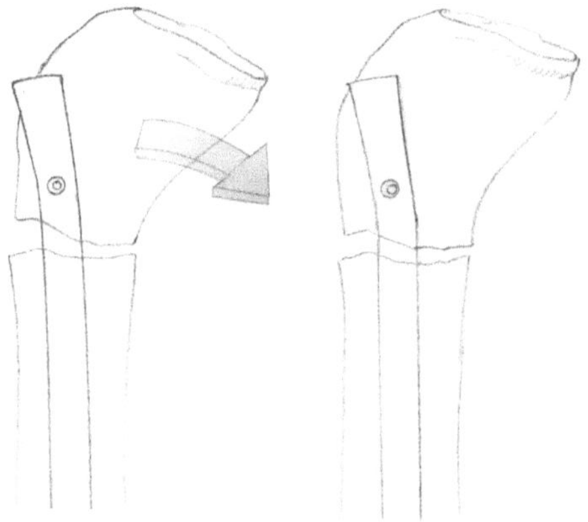

**Fig. 4.3.** The deformity with antecurvature is one of the difficulties in proximal tibia fractures

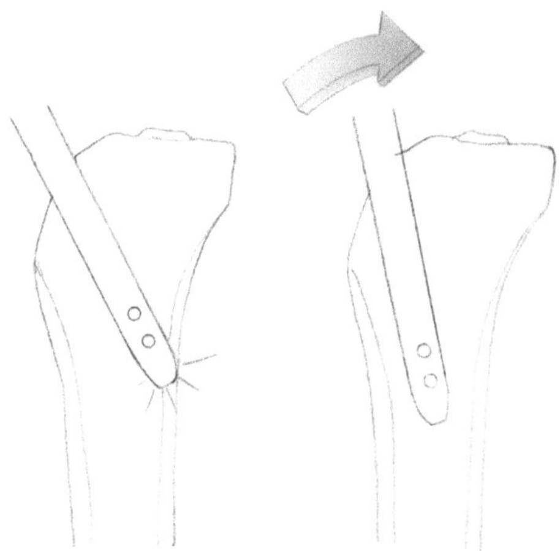

**Fig. 4.4.** To avoid the breakage of the posterior cortex during insertion of the nail, the surgeon has to push on the nailing device

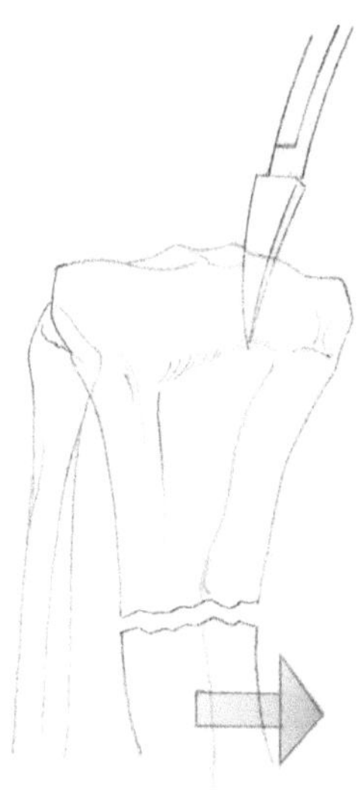

**Fig. 4.5.** Control of the varus deformity in proximal fractures is essential

lines is high. Prebending the tip of the guide easily prevents this type of complication.

Positioning the guidewire in the distal part of the tibia must be precise, especially for distal fractures. An incorrectly positioned guide will result in reaming in the wrong position and thus a valgus or varus deformity.

## *Reaming*

The use of reamed nails requires reaming step by step in 0.5-mm increments. As for other areas, reaming in a comminuted area could be dangerous and is forbidden. With segmental fractures, the intact fragment of bone must sometimes be stabilized to avoid any rotation during the reaming process.

In distal fractures, reaming must be done as distally as possible. If not, the introduction of the nail can create a gap in the fracture site (distraction by the nail penetrating in a dense bone area).

Inserting the nail without stress (especially on the posterior cortex) is the ideal method to use. Therefore, the medullary canal must be reamed up to a minimum of 1.5 mm beyond the diameter of the chosen nail.

Using a front-cutting reamer head with deep flutes is highly recommended to avoid pressure and heat problems.

## *Nail Insertion*

The nail is inserted after checking its length (determined by the difference method between 2 guidewires of identical length - one in the shaft and the other outside of the bone). The nail is introduced over a nailing guidewire; a Teflon tube is used to exchange the reaming guidewire.

The diameter is usually 11 mm, except in very narrow tibiae where 10-mm and even 9-mm nails can be used.

In proximal fractures, there is a risk of damaging the posterior cortex and/or displacing the fracture. The nail must therefore be introduced with no stress, slowly, and if possible without the use of the hammer.

For distal fractures, it is important to remember to remove the nailing guidewire when the nail penetrates in the final centimeters. Otherwise, the extraction of the guidewire can be difficult.

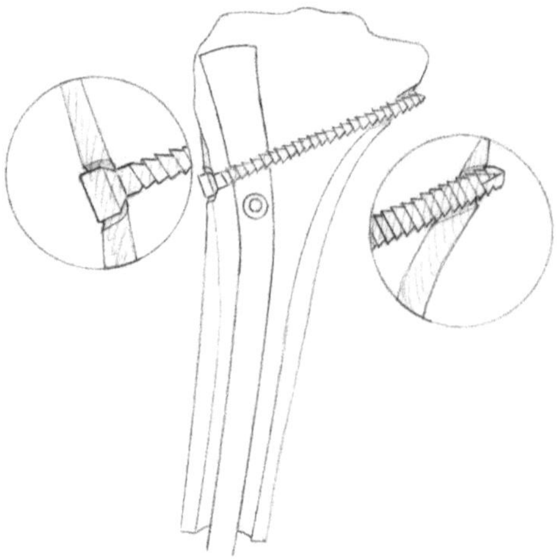

**Fig. 4.6.** The position of the AP screw is important in proximal fractures

#### *Locking Procedures*

For proximal fractures, the use of two proximal screws is mandatory. Again, this is to avoid secondary displacement of the fracture by monitoring the stability of the proximal part of the tibia in the AP and in the transversal plane. The position of the AP screw and the perfect grip of this screw in the posterior cortex of the tibia epiphysis are particularly important to ensure the stability of the implant (Fig. 4.6).

For distal fractures, the use of two screws distally is also very important to monitor the stability of the distal fragment perfectly (especially during flexion and extension of the ankle joint).

## Postoperative Management

The rehabilitation program varies depending on whether there is articular involvement of the fracture.

### Fractures Without Joint Involvement

In case of stable mounting, meaning with a good cortical contact (more than 50% of the circumference), full-weight bearing is possible in the first days after the procedure. In unstable situations such as comminuted fractures or fractures with a large third fragment, full weight-bearing is not allowed. Partial weight-bearing (30% of the body weight) is encouraged. Full weight-bearing is allowed after the sixth week.

### Fractures with Joint Involvement

Weight-bearing is usually delayed for the first 6 weeks. Mobilization of the ankle and the knee joints begins immediately.

Dynamization by removal of locking screws is not the rule. We recommend performing dynamization only in cases of delayed union.

Screws are removed proximally in distal fractures and distally in proximal fractures.

## References


1. Jaeger JH, Grosse A, Bouchet P, Kempf I (1975) Etude biomécanique de l'enclouage centro-médullaire verrouillé du tibia et du fémur. Geboas 4/5
2. Kempf I, Grosse A, Lafforgue D (1978) L'apport du verrouillage dans l'enclouage centro-médullaire des os longs. Rev Chir Orthop Reparatrice Appar Mot 74:635–651
3. Hutson J, Zych G, Cole J, Johnson KD, Ostermann P, Milne E, Latta L (1995) Mechanical failures of intramedullary tibial nails applied without reaming. Clin Orthop 315:129–137
4. Whittle AP, Wester W, Russell TA (1995) Fatigue failure in small diameter nails. Clin Orthop 315:119–128
5. Bonnevialle P, Savorit L, Combes JM, Rongieres M, Bellumore Y, Mansat M (1996) Value of intramedullary locked nailing in distal fractures of the tibia Rev Chir Orthop Reparatrice Appar Mot 82:428–36
6. Rzesacz EH, Konneker W, Reilmann H, Culemann U (1998) Combination of intramedullary nail and covered screw osteosynthesis for managing distal tibia fracture with ankle joint involvement. Unfallchirurg 101:907–913
7. Duparc J, Huten D (1981) Classification des fractures ouvertes. Cahiers d'Enseignement de la SFCO T 14:62–72
8. Gustilo RB, Mendoza RM, Wiliams DM (1984) Problems in the management of type III open fractures. A new classification. J Trauma 24:742–746
9. Tornetta P III, Collins E (1996) Semiextented position of intramedullary nailing of the proximal tibia. Clin Orthop 328:185–189

CHAPTER 5

# Open Fractures

C.M. Court-Brown, A.C. Masquelet, B. Schenck

Intramedullary Nailing of Open Fractures

C.M. Court-Brown

Principles of Management of Soft-Tissue Injury in Open Fractures

A.C. Masquelet and B. Schenck

## Intramedullary Nailing of Open Fractures

C.M. Court-Brown

The management of open fractures has changed dramatically over the last 15–20 years mainly as a result of improved plastic surgery techniques, but also because orthopedic surgeons have become more aware of the importance of debridement and early soft tissue cover and are now less absorbed by the minutiae of fracture fixation. It is interesting to note that the use of free flaps and local fasciocutaneous flaps only became widespread in the late 1970s and the early 1980s. Previously orthopedic surgeons had been more concerned with applying the perfect plate or debating the biomechanical aspects of external fixation than with treating the soft tissue injuries associated with fractures. Improved results in the management of open fractures have mainly arisen as a result of improved flap cover and the reemergence of intramedullary nailing as the preferred treatment option.

### History of Open Fracture Treatment

The concept of the open fracture was first documented by the author of the Edwin Smith Papyrus about 2800 BC [9]. This papyrus mentions a fractured humerus in which the fracture communicated with an overlying skin wound. The author of the papyrus states that this "ailment" should not be treated, presumably because of its severity and poor prognosis. Hippocrates also accepted that the prognosis of open fractures was poor but he did believe in treating them. He advocated the use of occlusive dressings using pitch or balsam and he felt strongly that delayed fracture reduction should be performed, usually between 7–10 days after the fracture, when the risk of purulent discharge was less. An analysis of the historical literature suggests that there does not seem to have been any significant change in the management of open fractures between the time of Hippocrates and the sixteenth century AD. At this time, Ambroise Paré challenged the view that open wounds should be treated by scalding oil or pitch. He suggested the use of soothing pastes containing oil of roses, turpentine, and egg yolk. He also advocated debridement by enlarging the wound to facilitate fracture reduction and removal of loose bone fragments.

Although Paré undoubtedly influenced his colleagues and successors, the concept of surgical wound cleansing was not accepted until the eighteenth century when Desault, and his pupil Larrey, popularized the procedure and introduced the term "debridement." The method of wound excision was probably first described by Milligan [58], a surgeon with the British Expeditionary Force in the First World War, but it was Trueta [85] who described the operation in detail.

As with orthopedic surgery, the origins of plastic surgery are ancient. Sushruta described operations for the reconstruction of the nose and earlobes about 600 BC. For the next 2500 years, most plastic surgery procedures appear to have been concerned with facial reconstruction and the use of plastic surgery techniques in the management of open fractures was not considered. This is not surprising when one considers that until recently, amputation was the main method of treating open fractures. Even when tubed pedical flaps were devised by Gilles during the First World War, their inherent problems meant that they had little use in the management of open fractures. The two major advances in plastic surgery which have improved treatment of open fractures are microsurgery, to allow the transfer of free flaps, and an improved understanding of the vascular supply of the skin and subcutaneous tissues. This has facilitated improved results from the use of local flaps. When one considers that the first successful free tissue transfer was performed in 1962 [52] and that fasciocutaneous flaps were only described in the early 1980s [68], it is obvious that the importance of plastic surgery in the management of open fractures is a relatively recent phenomenon.

The role of fixation in open fractures has also increased in recent years. The first book detailing the techniques of fracture fixation was published by Bérenger-Féraud in 1870 [1], but until Lister's work with antisepsis and the later introduction of antibiotics, the use of internal fixation in the management of open fractures was not widespread. Early fracture surgeons such as Arbuthnott Lane, Lambotte, and Sherman all used plates to fix open fractures but selected the method because of fracture instability rather than because the fracture was open. This was also true of the pioneers of intramedullary nailing, Hey Groves of England and Küntscher of Germany [48]. They both advocated secondary fracture fixation after the soft tissues had healed.

By the time of the Second World War, the introduction of better fixation techniques, improved asepsis, and antibiotics altered the whole picture. Surgeons such as Street [82], Bohler [4], and Lottes [51] showed that intramedullary nailing could give good results in open fractures. In addition, Bradford and Wilson [8] had reported good results with external fixation and Davis [26] had advocated primary plating. However, primary fixation of open fractures was not really accepted until the 1970s when Rhinelander [71] and other histologists showed that rigid fracture fixation promoted capillary ingrowth and facilitated bone union. At the same time, the AO group [60] provided an organized approach to fracture management and shortly thereafter the interlocking intramedullary nail was introduced [43, 47]. This technique revolutionized the management of long bone fractures and together with modern plastic surgery techniques, it has allowed surgeons to improve their treatment of open fractures.

The initial management of open fractures with unlocked Küntscher nails was reported by Zucman and Maurer [93] and Merle d'Aubigne et al. [57]. Zucman and Maurer [93] recorded an 8.1% infection rate with 0.7% aseptic nonunion and no malunions in 136 open fractures. However, only 15% of the open fractures were severe and the proportion of the more difficult distal third and comminuted fractures was low. Merle d'Aubigne et al. [57] had a 6.6% incidence of infection in 256 open fractures with a 2.4% incidence of nonunion. They compared their results with the use of plaster, traction, and plating and reported lower complication rates and reoperation rates using nailing. Lottes [51], using his unreamed nail, also reported relatively low complication rates in both closed and open tibial fractures. He had a 7.3% infection rate in open single tibial fractures and a 6.3% infection rate in open segmental tibial fractures. These early workers undoubtedly showed that unlocked nails could be used successfully in open tibial fractures and as these fractures are frequently comminuted and difficult to hold without an interlocking system, these early results of nailing open fractures were very encouraging.

## Epidemiology of Open Fractures

When discussing the use of intramedullary nailing in the management of open fractures, it is important to realize that the technique is only applicable to open fractures of the femur, tibia, humerus, and forearm diaphyses. Thus it is useful for surgeons to be aware of how common these fractures are and what types of open fractures they are likely to encounter and therefore have to treat. There is little information about the epidemiology of open fractures in the literature. However, an analysis of 515 consecutive open long bone fractures in the Orthopaedic Trauma Unit in Edinburgh, Scotland over a 6-year period between January 1988 and December 1993 has allowed epidemiological information to be collated [24]. The study collected information about both open metaphyseal and diaphyseal long bone fractures but as this chapter deals with intramedullary nailing, only the diaphyseal information will be presented.

The 515 open long bone fractures occurred in 474 patients. The distribution, descriptive indices, and causes of the different open diaphyseal fractures are shown in Fig. 5.1. Four hundred and thirty seven patients (92.2%) presented with one open long bone fracture and 34 (7.2%) had two open fractures. Of the remaining three patients, two presented with three open fractures and one patient had four open fractures. The average age of the entire group was 44.9 years and there were 312 (65.8%) males and 162 (34.2%) females. The average age of the males was 36.7 years and the females 61 years. Assessment of the soft tissue injury showed that 162 (31.4%) of the fractures

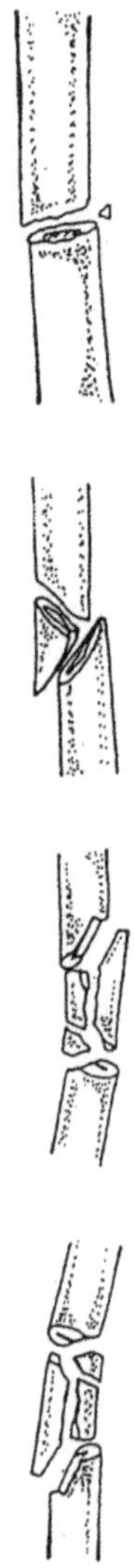

**Fig. 5.1.** The epidemiology of the different open diaphyseal fractures. The incidence is expressed as a percentage of all open fractures of the long bones, including proximal and distal metaphyseal fractures not shown here. (From [24] with permission)

Humeral diaphysis (AO-12)
n=16 (3.1%)
average age 48.4 years
56.2% male
AO Type A (50%), B (37.5%), C (12.5%)
Gustilo I (68.7%), II (18.7%), IIIa (6.2%), IIIb (6.2%)
RTA (50%), Fall (37.5%), Sport (6.2%), Blow (6.2%)
Average ISS 14
Other injuries 43.7%

Forearm diaphysis (AO-22)
n=34 (6.6%). Radius and Ulna (23), ulna (10), radius (1)
average age 34.8 years
70.6% male
AO Type A (32.4%), B (50%), C (17.6%)
Gustilo I (47.1%), II (29.4%), IIIa (8.8%), IIIb (14.7%)
RTA (44.1%), Fall (5.9%), Stairs (2.9%), Sport (17.6%)
Average ISS 12.2
Other injuries 50%

Femoral diaphysis (AO-32)
n=59 (11.4%)
average age 43 years
80.4% male
AO Type A (30.5%), B (37.3%), C (32.2%)
Gustilo I (20.3%), II (16.9%), IIIa (23.7%), IIIb (30.5%), IIIc (8.5%)
RTA (86.4%), Fall (1.7%), Height (8.5%), Blow (3.4%)
Average ISS 17
Other injuries 80.3%

Tibial diaphysis (AO-42)
n=230 (44.7%)
average age 42.8 years
76.2% male
AO Type A (40.2%), B (24.1%), C (35.7%)
Gustilo I (23.5%), II (19.6%), IIIa (23%), IIIb (29.6%), IIIc (4.3%)
RTA (62.2%), Fall (12.2%), Height (8.7%), Stairs (1.3%), Sport (7.4%), Blow (8.3%)
Average ISS 12.6
Other injuries 52.5%

were Gustilo type I, 128 (24.8%) were type II, and the remaining 225 (43.8%) were type III in severity. Of the type III fractures, 103 (45.8%) were type IIIA and 106 (47.1%) were Gustilo IIIB. The remaining 16 (7.1%) were Gustilo IIIC fractures. Examination of the morphology of the fractures showed that 185 (35.9%) fractures were AO type A with a further 148 (28.7%) being type B fractures. The remaining 182 (35.3%) fractures showed a type C morphology.

Of the open fractures, 297 (57.7%) occurred as a result of road traffic accidents with a further 98 (19%) following a simple fall. Fifty (9.7%) were caused by a fall from a height and 10 (1.9%) were caused by falls down stairs or embankments. A further 23 (4.5%) resulted from sporting accidents and of the remaining fractures, 32 (6.2%) occurred following a direct blow, assault, or crushing injury. The remaining 5 (1%) were caused by sharp objects including a dog bite, an explosion, and a shotgun injury. The average Injury Severity Score for the entire open fracture group was 12.9 and 109 (21.2%) of the patients presented with an ISS greater than 15. Two hundred and thirty one (44.8%) patients presented with musculo-skeletal injuries other than open long bone fractures. There was a direct relationship between the ISS and the number of open long bone fractures present at admission. In the 437 patients who had one open long bone fracture the average ISS was 12. The 34 patients with two open long bone fractures had an average ISS of 15.6. The two patients who presented with three open fractures had an average ISS of 27 and in the only patient who had four open long bone fractures the ISS was 4.

Extrapolation of the Edinburgh data allows surgeons to calculate how often they might have to decide on the suitability of a particular open diaphyseal fracture for nailing. The Edinburgh Orthopaedic Trauma Unit receives all fractures from a population of about 700,000 people. The British Orthopaedic Association [10] has estimated that in the United Kingdom the average Fracture Unit serves a population of about 241,000 people and if one assumes a rota of 1:5 surgeons on-call then an analysis of the figures in Fig. 5.1 indicates that the average United Kingdom Orthopaedic Surgeon treats 2.5 open tibial diaphyseal fractures per year. In addition, he or she is likely to treat 0.6 open femoral diaphyseal fractures, 0.4 open forearm diaphyseal fractures and 0.2 open humeral diaphyseal fractures each year. This illustrates the difficulty many surgeons face in deciding on a treatment method for fractures that they encounter relatively infrequently. Thus any surgeon contemplating locked intramedullary nailing of open fractures is probably going to be faced with nailing a severe fracture of the tibia or femur. Faced with this fact, it is advisable that surgeons learn the art of nailing on more straightforward closed fractures rather than embark on an ambitious undertaking with a severe open fracture in the middle of the night.

## Reamed or Unreamed Nailing in Open Fractures

In recent years there has been considerable debate on the role of reaming in intramedullary nailing. The debate has taken two forms. Firstly there is some evidence that reaming increases the incidence of adult respiratory distress syndrome in certain patients [67] and it is argued that other methods of management should be used, particularly in the seriously injured patient with conomitant chest injuries. This debate concerns the femur more than the tibia and is not specifically directed towards open fractures. However, the other area of contention is the effect reaming has on the vascularity of the bone. This debate concerns the tibia more than other bones and it is suggested by proponents of unreamed nailing that reaming damages the intramedullary vasculature in a tibia whose nutrient artery is already damaged by the effects of the open fracture. The resulting avascularity is said to increase the incidence of infection and nonunion as well as raise the intracompartmental pressure in the soft tissues, thereby inducing compartment syndrome. There is no clinical evidence for any of these observations and indeed there is no logical theoretical basis for them either. The fact that intramedullary vascularity is reduced after reaming and nailing has been known for a number of years. Klein et al. [45] have demonstrated that the use of reamed intramedullary nails reduces the cortical circulation of the canine tibia by about 70% whereas unreamed intramedullary nails reduce the circulation by only 31%. Schemitsch et al. [77] confirmed Klein's findings and estimated that cortical revascularization occurred about 6 weeks after unreamed nailing and 12 weeks after reamed nailing. However, in a recent paper Reichert et al. [69] showed that reaming the intact ovine tibia induced a sixfold increase in periosteal blood flow. The authors did not demonstrate a reduction in cortical flow and they suggested that the increase in periosteal flow compensated for the decrease in intramedullary blood flow. They also suggested that reaming by itself may be osteogenic, a theory proposed by Danckwardt-Lillestrom [25] and recently supported by Court-Brown et al. [23] with reference to exchange tibial nailing. It is likely that in open fractures there is little or no difference between reamed and unreamed nails. In severe open fractures, the prognosis is mainly determined by the severity of soft tissue damage and any vascular effect of reaming is probably negligible.

## Surgical Technique

A description of the technique of nailing diaphyseal fractures of the femur, tibia, humerus, and forearm has been given in Chapters 9, 10, 13, other volume. The technique of nailing open fractures does not vary much from that involved in the nailing of closed fractures, although there are a few minor variations that the surgeon should be aware of.

The most important point of any operation aiming to nail an open fracture is the debridement of the bone and soft tissues. A well-performed debridement is the key to surgical success and more skill and expertise is required to decide on the state of the soft tissues at the time of surgery than is required to position a nail in the intramedullary canal of the fractured bone. Surgeons debate whether the debridement should be done on a flat surgical table prior to the patient being transferred to a nailing table or it should be performed with the patient placed on a nailing table in the conventional manner. In reality, it probably does not matter and there is no evidence that in most cases an adequate debridement cannot be performed with the limb under a degree of traction on a nailing table. However, if there is severe contamination or soft tissue damage the surgeon may elect to use a conventional operating table to facilitate exposure and access to devitalized tissues. The patient is then subsequently transferred to a nailing table.

The purpose of debridement is to excise all dead or devitalized and contaminated tissue regardless of whether it is soft tissue or bone. Many surgeons make the mistake of retaining devitalized bone fragments in the mistaken belief that they will preserve bone continuity. In reality all they are doing is preserving dead tissue and thereby increasing the risk of osteomyelitis.

The operation of debridement has been described [85]. It consists of the surgical excision of all dead and devitalized tissues. It is important that the surgeon adequately extend the wound to allow all subcutaneous contamination to be recognized. Skin is resistant to crushing but susceptible to degloving, a particular problem in the elderly. Where degloving is not a problem, the surgeon should excise devitalized skin edges, but if degloving is present the skin should be resected until dermal bleeding is encountered.

All devitalized fat and muscle should be resected. It may well be very difficult to decide on the extent of muscle devitalization and where there is debate about muscle viability, a second debridement at 24–36 hours after the primary operation is mandatory. It is suggested that this be carried out for all Gustilo type III open fractures as a matter of routine. Similarly, all devitalized bone should be resected regardless of the length of the resulting bone defect. Once an adequate debridement has been performed, the fracture can be nailed. The technique of nailing Gustilo type I, II, and IIIA open fractures is exactly the same as the technique employed for closed fractures. Fracture reduction is usually straightforward and the reduced fracture can be held with a bone clamp. In Gustilo type IIIB fractures the situation is somewhat different. In these fractures there will often be significant bone loss and therefore in some Gustilo type IIIB fractures the surgeon may experience difficulty in assessing bone length. This is not often a problem in the tibia, as the length of the fibula can be used to assess the correct tibial length. In IIIB femoral fractures it may be difficult to assess bone length but the devitalized fragment or fragments may provide the surgeon with some useful information.

In Gustilo IIIB fractures associated with significant bone loss, the surgeon may also experience some difficulty in aligning the fracture correctly. This is usually straightforward in mid-diaphyseal fractures associated with bone loss, but if the area of bone loss is proximal or distal it may be difficult to adequately align the smaller fragment. If this is found to be the case and the surgeon cannot adequately align either the proximal or distal fragment, external skeletal fixation is probably a better method of treating the fracture.

When reaming an open diaphyseal fracture associated with a bone defect, the surgeon should be careful not to damage the soft tissues at the site of the bone defect. The reamers should be switched off when the bone defect is reached and restarted when the distal fragment is entered. The surgeon should obviously statically lock all open fractures associated with bone loss and it is in fact a sensible routine to statically lock all open fractures.

## Soft Tissue Cover

The techniques used to gain soft tissue closure in open fractures are described in "Principles of Management of Soft-Tissue Injury in Open Fractures". The soft tissue defect in open femoral fractures will usually heal either without plastic surgery or with a split skin graft. This is not the same in open tibial fractures, where soft tissue defects frequently require flap cover to achieve closure, particularly if the defect is over the subcutaneous border of the tibia. The usual options available to the plastic surgeon are a gastrocnemius flap, if the soft tissue defect is proximal in location, or a distally based fasciocutaneous flap. Alternatively, a free latissimus dorsi or rectus abdominus flap may be used if the defect is more distal. The decision between a local fasciocutaneous flap and a free flap is based on a number of factors such as size and location of the defect, the size and age of the patient, and the presence of other injuries. It is important, however, that the surgeon not use split skin grafts to cover a tissue defect on the subcutaneous border of the tibia, as this technique is bound to fail and osteomyelitis will ensue.

Early soft tissue cover is important if good results are to be obtained. Once the soft tissues have healed, the surgeon can consider the treatment of any residual bone defect, using either corticocancellous grafting techniques, free vascularized grafting, or segmental bone transport.

## Intramedullary Nailing of Open Femoral Fractures

The use of interlocking nails was popularized in the femur [44] and there is much less debate about their use in open femoral fractures (Fig. 5.2) than in open tibial fractures. The original papers on

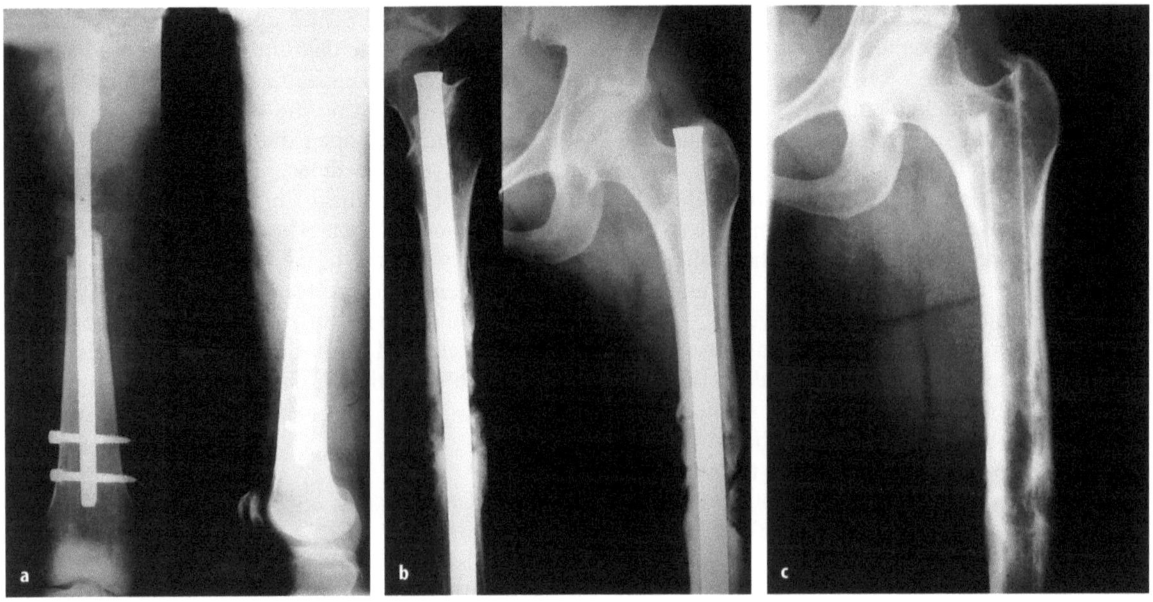


**Fig. 5.2a–c.** A Gustilo type 111B open femoral fracture associated with significant bone loss. This was treated by intramedullary nailing (**a**). The defect required two bone grafts to fill it successfully (**b**) and **c** shows that the final result was excellent

femoral nailing consisted of a mixed population of open and closed fractures and it is probable that the open fractures included in these series represented less severe fracture types. An analysis of some of the major papers dealing with mixed series of open and closed femoral fractures is presented in Table 5.1. It is clear that the results are satisfactory, although a relatively high incidence of malunion was quoted by Kempf et al. [44] and Søjbjerg et al. [81]. In particular, the infection rates are low. As confidence with femoral nailing grew, surgeons applied the technique to more severe open fractures and a number of surgeons documented the results of series consisting exclusively of open fractures (Table 5.2). Lhowe and Hansen [50] analyzed 42 patients with open fractures treated with both unlocked and locked reamed nails. Only 19% of the fractures were Gustilo type III and all fractures healed within 4 months, with excellent joint movement being noted. There was a 16% incidence of malunion, probably because of the use of thinner unreamed nails, and there was a low incidence of infection, nonunion,and nerve palsy.

Brumback et al. [12] analyzed 89 open femoral fractures of which 46 were type III in severity. They undertook primary nailing in those fractures in which surgery could be carried out within 8 h. In other cases, nailing was delayed for about 10 days. They only found infection in type IIIB open fractures and commented that two of their three infections occurred in delayed nailing procedures. They advocated the technique for all open femoral fractures where primary nailing could safely be undertaken.

Grosse et al. [32] published a combined open fracture series from Strasbourg, France, and Edinburgh, Scotland. One hundred and fifteen fractures were treated with the Grosse and Kempf intramedullary nail. Only three fractures required bone grafting and only three patients developed infection. Again the authors advocated primary interlocking nailing for all open femoral fractures regardless of the Gustilo fracture grading.

In the United States gunshot femoral fractures are a particular problem. The use of interlocking nails and the treatment of these particular fractures has been investigated by Wiss et al. [90] and by Nowatarski and Brumback [64]. Both papers detailed good results, which are summarized in Table 5.2. Infection rates were low and Nowatarski and Brumback [64] showed considerable financial savings in primary nailing compared with delayed nailing.

There now seems no doubt that intramedullary nailing of the femur using an interlocking nail is the treatment of choice for all open femoral fractures. Few surgeons disagree with this philosophy and it may be that nailing for open femoral fractures has been relatively rapidly accepted because the soft tissues rarely require anything more than split skin grafting to achieve closure. In the 59 open femoral diaphyseal fractures detailed in

**Table 5.1.** Results and complications of trials documenting both closed and open femoral fractures treated by reamed interlocking nailing

| Author | *n* | Malunion | Infection | Comminution | Neck fracture | Nonunion | Nerve palsy |
|---|---|---|---|---|---|---|---|
| Kempf et al. [44] | 52 | 21.1% | 2.1% | 3.8% | - | 7.6% | - |
| Wiss et al. [90] | 112 | 14.0% | 0% | - | 0.9% | 1.8% | - |
| Klemm and Borner [46] | 266 | 3.0% | 2.6% | - | - | 1.5% | 0.3% |
| Christie et al. [16] | 120 | 2.5% | 0% | 5% | 2.5% | 1.6% | 2.5% |
| Søjbjerg et al. [81] | 40 | 22.5% | 0% | - | - | 0% | - |

–, information not available from report.

**Table 5.2.** The results and incidence of complications of open fractures treated by reamed intramedullary nailing. The papers by Wiss et al. [91] and Nowatarski and Brumback [64] deal exclusively with the treatment of gunshot wounds

| Author | *n* | Malunion | Infection | Comminution | Neck fracture | Nonunion | Nerve palsy |
|---|---|---|---|---|---|---|---|
| Lhowe and Hansen [50] | 42 | 16% | 5% | - | - | 7% | 2% |
| Brumback et al. [12] | 89 | 2.2% | 3.4% | 2.2% | - | 0% | - |
| O'Brien et al. [65] | 63 | 12.7% | 4.8% | - | - | 4.8% | - |
| Grosse et al. [32] | 115 | 1.7% | 2.6% | - | 0.8% | 3.5% | 1.7% |
| Wiss et al. [91] | 56 | 10.7% | 0% | - | - | 3.6% | 8.9% |
| Nowotarski and Brumback [64] | 39 | 0% | 2.5% | - | - | 5.1% | 5.1% |

–, information not available from report.

Fig. 5.1, only 18 (30.5%) required split skin grafting with no fracture needing flap cover.

### Intramedullary Nailing of Open Tibial Fractures

Understandably surgeons have approached the fixation of open tibial fractures with some trepidation. Until recently the amputation rates associated with open tibial fractures were very high and surgical folklore certainly suggests that internal fixation of open tibial fractures is associated with poor results. This belief was confirmed in the minds of many surgeons when plating of open tibial fractures was popularized by the AO group [73]. The adoption of widespread tibial plating predated the evolution of modern plastic surgery techniques and therefore it frequently did not matter how well the surgeon plated the tibia, he or she found it impossible to close the skin defect and the results were often poor. It would be of interest to repeat the analyses of plate fixation of open tibial fractures using modern plastic techniques. The other feature of the use of plating for open tibial fractures is that plates cannot be used to span extensive areas of bone loss and it is therefore likely that the original papers tended to select less severe open tibial fractures. The use of plates in the 1970s and 1980s tended to make surgeons wary of the presence of exposed metal in the base of open tibial wounds and it is perhaps understandable that they tended to shy away from any form of internal fixation in severe open tibial fractures. Thus in the 1980s, external skeletal fixation came to dominate the scene, but as with all fracture treatment methods, complications were noted [3, 15, 20].

The initial papers dealing with nailing of open tibial fractures (Table 5.3) were published in the early 1990s. Court-Brown et al. [21] detailed the use of the reamed Grosse and Kempf nail in the management of 41 Gustilo type II and III fractures. The Edinburgh group had started reamed nailing of all open tibial diaphyseal fractures in 1987, regardless of severity, having previously used external skeletal fixation for type III open tibial fractures. Their results were excellent at the time, with an overall infection rate of 11.1% for the type III fractures. All of the infections were in type IIIB fractures and the infection rate in this subgroup was 23.1%. Nowadays, this result would be unacceptable, but it was certainly comparable to the results of external fixation at the time. However, Court-Brown et al. [19, 21] also demonstrated that in other respects, reamed intramedullary nailing was superior to external fixation with lower malunion and bone grafting rates and improved joint and patient mobility.

At about the same time, Whittle et al. [88] published the results of the use of the unreamed Russell-Taylor nail in the management of open tibial fractures. They examined the use of nailing in 50 open fractures, of which 34 were Gustilo type III. Their infection rate for the type III fractures was 12% with a 25% infection rate for the IIIB subgroup. These figures were virtually identical to those of Court-Brown et al. [21] when using a reamed nail. The disadvantages inherent in the use of the thinner unreamed nail were also pointed out by Whittle et al. [88]. They had a 10% screw breakage rate and a 6% incidence of nail breakage. In addition, many of their patients required supportive casts to facilitate postoperative mobilization.

Court-Brown [17] undertook a later analysis of the Edinburgh data. He extended the study period to 7 years and documented the results of 55 type III open tibial fractures treated by the Grosse and Kempf reamed nail. There were 27 type IIIA fractures (Fig. 5.3). All united with no infection or malunion encountered and no bone grafting required. In the 28 type IIIB fractures, there were the same three infections reported in 1991, but not more, giving an overall type III infection rate of 5.5% and a IIIB infection rate of 10.7%. These figures remain comparable with other units specializing in the management of open tibial fractures.

The other interesting facet of open fracture management noted by Court-Brown et al. [21] in 1991 was the relationship of bone loss to union time. The authors defined significant bone loss in relation to nailing as more than 2 cm and 50% of the bone circumference and demonstrated that open fractures associated with significant bone loss required open bone grafting whereas lesser amounts of bone loss usually did not. Once this definition had been formulated and applied, more IIIB open tibial fractures were treated with early bone grafting; it is interesting to note that the mean union time of Gustilo type IIIB fractures with significant bone loss had consequently fallen by 1994 [72].

The reason for the improvement in the Edinburgh results is undoubtedly due to a combination of three factors. Firstly, algorithms were introduced to guide surgeons (Figs. 5.4, 5.5). Secondly, open fractures became the domain of orthopedic traumatologists rather than surgeons who dealt with both elective and traumatic orthopedics, and thirdly, improved debridement and plastic surgery techniques were introduced into the unit. It is suggested that if a correct protocol is followed by experienced traumatologists good results will be obtained in open fractures, regardless of whether reamed or unreamed nails are used.

A number of surgeons reported negligible infection rates using the unreamed AO tibial nail. Haas et al. [35] examined the use of the AO nail in the treatment of severe open and closed tibial fractures. They reported on 30 open tibial fractures of which only 8 were type IIIB in severity. They had no infection but they had a 13.7% screw breakage rate and a 13.7% incidence of peroneal

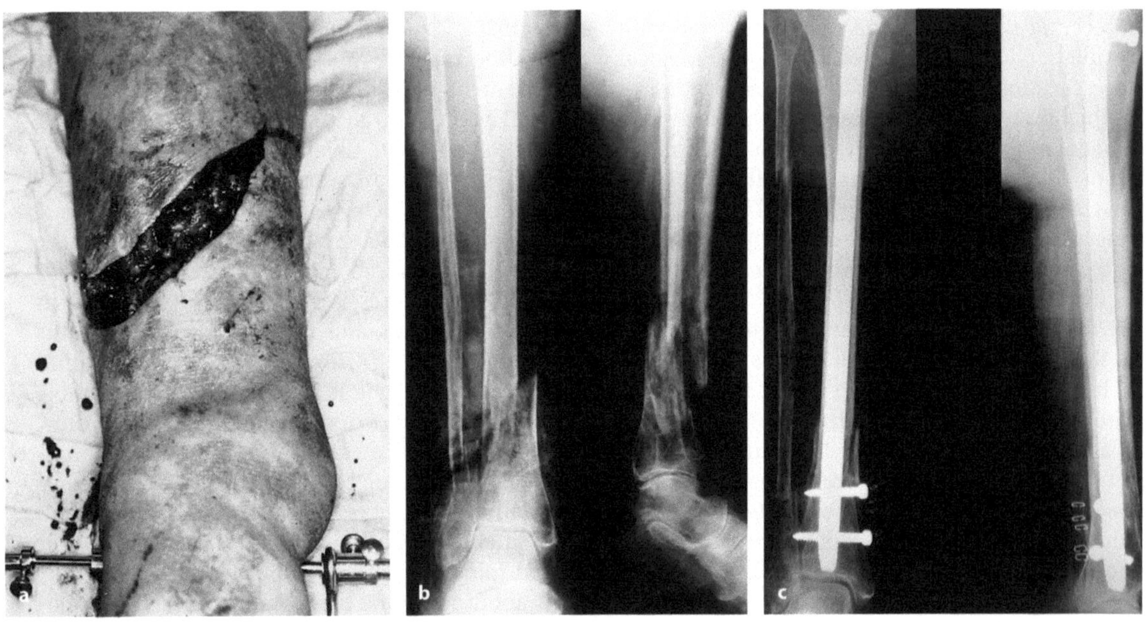


**Fig. 5.3 a–c.** A Gustilo 111A open tibial fracture in an elderly women. The skin wound was extensive (**a**) but the fracture morphology was straightforward (**b**). Nailing produced a good result (**c**)

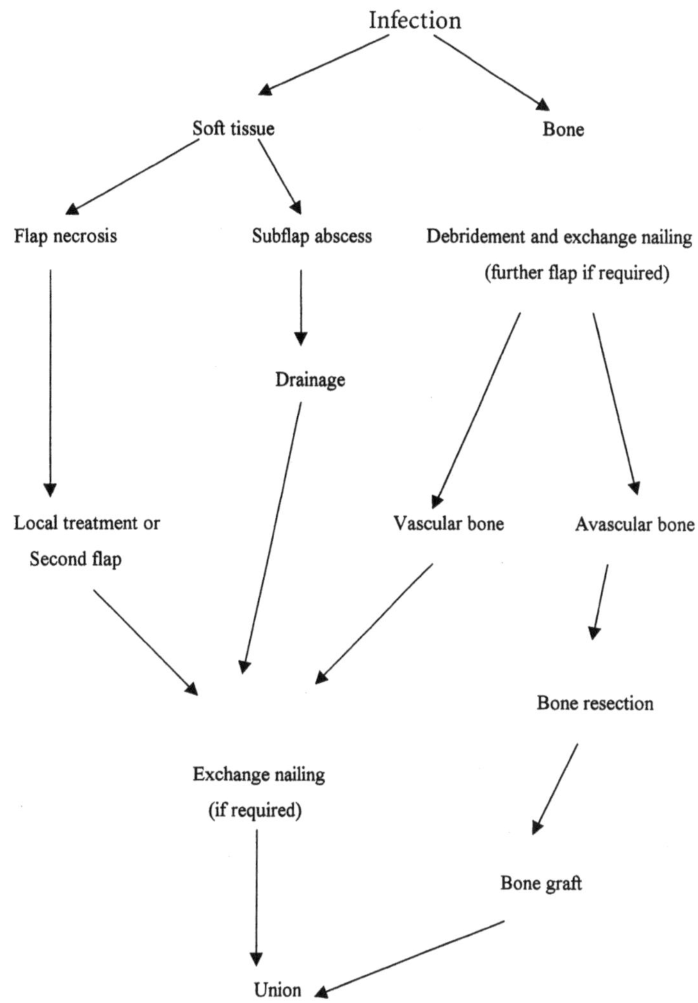


**Fig. 5.4.** An algorithm for the management of infection in severe open tibial fractures. (From [42] with permission)

nerve palsy. They also had a 42% incidence of compartment syndrome, although they did not state whether fasciotomy was performed for clinical reasons or because pressure monitoring had showed intracompartmental pressures to have reached a particular level. Oedekoven et al. [66] and Renner et al. [70] also reported no infection in open fractures but had a relatively high incidence of other complications.

Not all authors have reported insignificant infection rates using unreamed nails. Singer and Kellam [79] analyzed 43 open tibial diaphyseal fractures treated with the unreamed Russell-Taylor nail. Twenty six were type III fractures, with only nine IIIB fractures being analyzed. The overall infection rate for the type III open tibial fracture group was 12% with a 22.2% incidence in the IIIB subgroup. It is interesting to note that these figures are virtually identical to those of Court-Brown et al. [21] and Whittle et al. [88]. P. Whittle (1995, personal communication) later reported that her results dramatically improved as a result of improved soft tissue surgery and there is little doubt that soft tissue management is the key to success in the treatment of open tibial fractures.

Table 5.3 gives the results of a number of studies using both reamed and unreamed nails in the treatment of open tibial fractures. It actually shows that there is very little difference between the results of reamed and unreamed nailing. Keating et al. [40] analyzed 112 tibial diaphyseal fractures treated by reamed nailing, with the overall results very similar to those of Court-Brown et al. [21] 6 years earlier. The methodology was very similar in the two papers but Keating et al. made use of an antibiotic bead pouch technique and early bone grafting, which probably accounts for the slight improvement in infection rate and the incidence of nonunion. The only prospective study comparing reamed and unreamed nailing in the management of open tibial fractures was undertaken by Keating et al. [41]. The results are shown in Table 5.3. The authors found that the only statistically significant difference between reamed and unreamed nailing

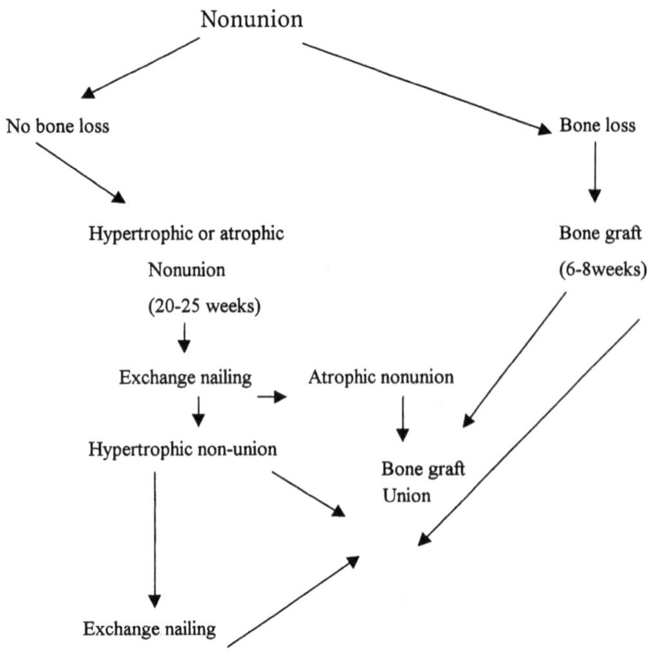


**Fig. 5.5.** An algorithm for the management of aseptic nonunion in severe open tibial fractures. (From [42] with permission)

**Table 5.3.** Results of studies using reamed and unreamed nails for open tibial fractures

| | *n* | Type (weeks) | Union (%) | Infection (%) | Nonunion (%) | Malunion (%) | Joint stiffness (%) | Compartment syndrome (%) |
|---|---|---|---|---|---|---|---|---|
| **Unreamed nails** | | | | | | | | |
| Whittle et al. [88] | 50 | GI–GIIIB | 30.3 | 8 | 4 | 2 | – | ? |
| Bone et al. [6] | 29 | GI–GIIIA | 28.9 | 6.9 | 48.3 | 0 | – | 0 |
| Sanders et al. [75] | 64 | GI–GIIIB | 31.1 | 4.0 | 17.1 | 0 | – | ? |
| Singer and Kellam [79] | 43 | GI–GIIIB | 26.4 | 12 | 47 | 49 | – | 20 |
| Bonatus et al. [5] | 72 | GI–GIIIB | – | 4 | 17 | 9.5 | – | 2.8 |
| Keating et al. [41] | 41 | GI–GIIIB | 28.8 | 2.4 | 12 | 2.4 | 38 | 4.9 |
| Henley et al. [37] | | GII–GIIIB | – | 6.7 | – | 8 | – | ? |
| **Reamed nails** | | | | | | | | |
| Court-Brown et al. [21] | 41 | GII–GIIIB | 33.2 | 9.7 | 36.3 | 4.9 | 36.6 | 0 |
| Keating et al. [40] | 47 | GI–GIIIB | 30.2 | 6.4 | 9 | 4.2 | 28 | 2.1 |
| Keating et al. [41] | 112 | GI–GIIIB | 32.8 | 5.4 | 8 | 6 | 14 | 7 |

G, Gustilo grade.
–, information not available from report.

was the increased screw breakage rate associated with unreamed nailing!

It is particularly useful to examine the Gustilo IIIB fractures treated by both reamed and unreamed nailing (Table 5.4), as these are the fractures which are associated with the worst prognoses. Court-Brown et al. [21] emphasized the difficulty of comparing Gustilo IIIB fractures. Seven of their fractures had bone loss of less than 2 cm and involving less than 50% of the circumference. These fractures united without open bone grafting in an average of 38 weeks compared with 78 weeks for the fractures with larger bone defects, which all required open bone grafting. They later documented that the average union time for the fractures associated with significant bone loss could be reduced to 56 weeks by early bone grafting [72] and the latest publication from the same unit has shown that the union time for Gustilo IIIB fractures associated with bone loss has been reduced to 45 weeks Keating et al. [42]. Table 5.4 shows a wide spectrum of results associated with the management of Gustilo IIIB open tibial fractures from the excellent results gained by Tornetta et al. [83] to the poorer results of Sanders et al. [75] and Court-Brown et al. [21]. The differences are much more likely to be due to definition than to technique and an overview of Table 5.4 actually

**Table 5.4.** Results of studies investigating the treatment of Gustilo type IIIb fractures with reamed and unreamed nails

| | *n* | Union (weeks) | Infection (%) | Nonunion (%) | Malunion (%) | Joint stiffness (%) | Compartment syndrome (%) |
|---|---|---|---|---|---|---|---|
| **Unreamed nails** | | | | | | | |
| Whittle et al. [88] | 12 | – | 25 | 0 | – | – | – |
| Tornetta et al. [83] | 15 | 23.0 | 6.6 | 0 | 0 | – | – |
| Sanders et al. [75] | 21 | 40.3 | 23.8 | 80 | 0 | – | – |
| Schandelmaier et al. [76] | 17 | 31 | 5.9 | 17.6 | 41.2 | 35.3 | – |
| **Reamed nails** | | | | | | | |
| Court-Brown et al. [21] | 13 | 50.1 | 23.1 | 69.2 | 15.4 | 84.6 | 0 |
| Keating et al. [41] | 20 | 39 | 11 | 17 | 5 | 32 | 6 |

–, information not available from report.

**Table 5.5.** Results of the use of external skeletal fixation in the treatment of Gustilo type III fractures

| | *n* | Type | Union time (weeks) | Nonunion (%) | Infection (%) | Pin complication (%) | Malunion (%) | Refracture |
|---|---|---|---|---|---|---|---|---|
| Chan et al. [15] | 17 | GIII | – | 60 | 38 | 100 | 41 | 0 |
| Edwards et al. [27] | 176 | GIII | 37.7 | 7 | 15 | 29 | 9 | ? |
| Court-Brown et al. [20] | 51 | GIII | 36.7 | – | 17.6 | 35 | 50 | 0 |
| Tu et al. [86] | 18 | GIII | 23.8 | 27.7 | 11.1 | ? | 16.6 | ? |
| Schandelmaier et al. [76] | 15 | GIIIB | 37 | 33.3 | 13.3 | 40 | 13.3 | 6.6 |
| Tornetta et al. [83] | 14 | GIIIB | 28.3 | 14.2 | 14.2 | 21.4 | 14.2 | 0 |

G, Gustilo grade.
–, information not available from report.

suggests that the results of reamed and unreamed nailing of Gustilo IIIB fractures are similar.

Over the last 20 years, there has been considerable interest in the use of external fixation in the management of severe open tibial fractures. The popularity of intramedullary nailing has resulted in many surgeons abandoning external fixation for closed and less severe open fractures. However, some surgeons still remain unsure of the role of intramedullary nailing in severe open fractures and still prefer external fixation. Table 5.5 shows the results of a number of papers dealing with the management of type III open fractures with external fixation. It shows that the complications associated with the use of external fixation of these fractures are considerable. Chan et al. [15] analyzed the results of 60 type III open tibial fractures. They were treated with three different types of fixator, although most were treated with a multiplanar device. The high complication rate may be partially accounted for by the fact that early bone grafting was not routinely employed and that 82% of the patients had the soft tissue defect closed with split skin grafts.

Edwards et al. [27] undertook a retrospective study of 176 patients admitted to a level 1 trauma centre, usually with multiple injuries. They used a multiplanar fixator. Because the patients were admitted between 1977 and 1982, 57% were treated with split skin grafts, although 32% had muscle or myocutaneous flap procedures. However, this group used early bone grafting and there is little doubt that their results are better.

Court-Brown et al. [20] examined two types of fixator in the treatment of type III open tibial fractures, demonstrating no difference between a uniplanar and multiplanar device. They analyzed the different type III subgroups separately and showed that the results of the IIIA fractures were much better than the IIIB and IIIC fractures. In their IIIA group, the infection rate was 5%, compared with 35.7% for the IIIB group. They noted an 85.7% amputation rate in the IIIC group. This study examined patient function. In the IIIA group, 55% of patients had returned to full function at 2 years, compared with 28.6% of the IIIB fractures. Return to work averaged 31.5 weeks in the IIIA patients and 63.7 weeks for those patients with IIIB fractures. In this study, early bone grafting was not routine but flap was more commonly performed with 57.1% of the type IIIB fractures receiving flaps.

All of the remaining three studies detailed in Table 5.5 carried out comparative studies examining unreamed nailing and external fixation. Tornetta et al. [83] examined IIIB fractures. They noted a similar spectrum of secondary procedures in both groups, but union was faster in the intramedullary nail group and joint motion uniformly better. They felt that intramedullary nailing was superior to external fixation in the management of these injuries. Tu et al. [86] looked at both IIIA and IIIB fractures. They also demonstrated improved rates of nonunion and malunion in reamed nailing, but the highest infection rate occurred in patients with IIIB fractures treated by unreamed nails, where they recorded 37.5% infection. They recommended unreamed nailing for type IIIA fractures and external fixation for IIIB fractures. Schandelmaier et al. [76] examined type IIIB fractures. They found a significantly shorter time to union with nailing but they could demonstrate no difference in the incidence of exchange nailing, infection, malunion, or refracture. The major difference between their two groups was in patient function, with the nailed patients demonstrating better hindfoot movement and walking distance. The unreamed nail group also had a significantly reduced time to full weight-bearing, less revision surgery, and easier access for plastic surgery.

Henley et al. [37] compared unreamed intramedullary nailing with external fixation in Gustilo type II, IIIA and IIIB fractures. They found that the intramedullary nailing group had significantly less malunion and that significantly fewer secondary procedures were required after the initial operation. Intramedullary nailing also resulted in fewer infections, but there was no significant difference found in the healing rates for the two implant groups. The authors concluded that it was the severity of the soft tissue injury rather than the choice of implant which affected bone healing and the incidence of infection. These studies have indicated that intramedullary nailing is preferable to external skeletal fixation for treating Gustilo IIIB open tibial fractures but it must be stated that information about these fractures remains scanty because of the small size of the studies.

Recently, however, Keating et al. [42] reported on the treatment of 57 Gustilo IIIB fractures treated in Edinburgh, Scotland and Vancouver, Canada. They found that the mean time to union was 43 weeks and that fracture with little or no bone loss united in a mean of 32 weeks. If there was significant bone loss the mean union time was 45 weeks and if there had been infection the mean time to union was 53 weeks. Aseptic nonunion developed in 24 (42%) fractures and in 15 (62.5%) of the fractures complicated by significant bone loss. Overall 10 (17.5%) fractures had infective complications. The authors distinguished between bone and soft tissue infection and devised algorithms for treating infection (Fig. 5.4) and aseptic nonunion (Fig. 5.5) associated with Gustilo IIIB open tibial fractures.

## The Requirement for Plastic Surgery in Open Tibial Fractures

An analysis of the requirement for plastic surgery in open tibial fractures shows that there is a quite different spectrum from that seen with open femoral fractures. Court-Brown and Quaba [18] analyzed the relationship between plastic surgery and orthopedic trauma surgery in 244 open tibial fractures. The results are shown in Table 5.6. One hundred and thirty-four of the 244 open tibial fractures required plastic surgery techniques to facilitate wound closure. Thus 54.5% of all open tibial fractures required plastic surgery. Fifty-five of the patients needed split skin grafting to close their wounds and a further 58 required local flaps, with 56 of these being proximally or distally based fasciocutaneous flaps. Ten local muscle flaps were used, of which nine were gastrocnemius flaps and the remaining 11 fractures were treated with distant free flaps. It is obvious that the successful management of open tibial fractures requires close collaboration between the orthopedic traumatologist and the plastic surgeon.

## Intramedullary Nailing of Open Humeral and Forearm Fractures

The status of intramedullary nailing of open humeral and forearm fractures is as yet undefined. Both humeral and forearm nailing are discussed in general terms in Chap. 12 and 13, other volume. With regard to the humerus, current debate centers around the usefulness of humeral nailing

**Table 5.6.** The use of plastic surgery techniques in the closure of open tibial fractures (from [18] with permission)

| | I | II | IIIA | IIIB |
|---|---|---|---|---|
| *n* | 59 | 53 | 55 | 68 |
| No. plastic surgery | 86.4% | 56.6% | 32.7% | 5.9% |
| Split-skin graft | 10.2% | 22.6% | 36.3% | 23.5% |
| Local flap | 3.4% | 17.0% | 27.3% | 45.6% |
| Local muscle flap | 0% | 1.9% | 3.6% | 10.3% |
| Distant flap | 0% | 1.9% | 0% | 14.7% |

compared to other treatment methods such as plating and external skeletal fixation. There are as yet no papers detailing the use of nailing in open humeral fractures, although there is no reason to believe that it should not be successful. The relative rarity of severe open humeral fractures, the fact that most are type I in severity, and the presence of good soft tissue cover around the humerus suggests that intramedullary nailing of open humeral fractures should be straightforward. The nailing of forearm fractures is as yet in its infancy and the use of this technique in the management of open forearm fractures has not yet been seriously investigated.

### Secondary Nailing of Open Fractures

With increased interest in the use of intramedullary nailing for the management of open fractures, it was only natural that surgeons would investigate the use of nailing in the management of some of the complications of fractures as well as the use of the technique in combination with other fracture management techniques. There are three situations where a surgeon might choose to use secondary intramedullary nailing in the management of open fractures. These are where there is infection around a primary intramedullary nail, where there is an aseptic nonunion after primary nailing, and where the surgeon wishes to change from primary external fixation to secondary intramedullary nailing.

Both the treatment of infection and aseptic nonunion in previously nailed fractures require the surgeon to make use of the technique of exchange nailing. This technique has been examined in depth by Court-Brown and his colleagues in Edinburgh [23]. The operative technique is simple. The patient is placed on a nailing table as for a primary nailing procedure and the original nail and cross screws are removed. The intramedullary canal is reamed, starting with a drill bit of the same size as the extracted nail. Successively larger bits, by 0.5 mm each time, are used to remove endosteal fibrous tissue until bone is seen on the end of the drill bit, usually at a diameter of about 1 mm above the original reaming. More reaming is required if the original nail had been of an inappropriately small diameter. The new nail is introduced. Locking screws are rarely needed unless the nonunion is very distal or proximal or very rarely when there is residual instability. This technique is used in infected cases to remove the infected pyogenic membrane from the intramedullary canal. This has been described in detail by Court-Brown et al. [22]. In this study the authors examined 12 infected tibiae which had been treated by a primary reamed intramedullary nail. Seven of these infections had occurred in closed and type I open fractures and five had occurred in Gustilo type II and III open fractures.

The authors divided the infected nailed tibiae into three groups depending on their presenting symptoms. Group 1 patients presented with pyrexia associated with local pain, erythema, and generalized swelling at the fracture site, but no clinical evidence of an abscess. These patients were treated by oral antibiotics without nail removal. In all cases the fractures healed in a time appropriate for their fracture grading and the nail was removed after union with reaming of the pyogenic membrane.

The Group 2 patients presented with signs similar to the Group 1 patients, but with evidence of a pyogenic collection. Where a pyogenic discharge became established, the authors found exchange nailing to be useful in managing the infection. Group 3 patients tended to present late with persistent pyogenic discharge and these patients were treated by exchange intramedullary nailing as well as resection of all devitalized bone and soft tissue. They were then treated by flap cover and later corticocancellous bone grafting.

The use of exchange intramedullary nailing in the management of aseptic tibial nonunion has proven to be a very useful technique. Court-Brown et al. [23] analyzed the rates of aseptic nonunion in a group of 547 tibial diaphyseal fractures, of which 109 were open fractures. Table 5.7 details the incidence of aseptic nonunion in the different Gustilo fracture types as well as the success of exchange nailing. It is clear that exchange nailing is an extremely useful technique and greatly reduces the requirement for open bone grafting in these patients. No open bone grafting was required in Gustilo type I, II, and IIIA fractures and only one of five exchange nailings failed to result in union in a Gustilo type IIIB fracture not associated with significant bone loss. In all fractures with significant bone loss of more than 2 cm and 50% of the circumference, bone grafting was required. Table 5.7 indicates that in four patients with significant bone loss, exchange nailing was attempted but was unsuccessful.

A review of exchange nailing in Edinburgh over a decade of use has indicated that it is a very useful technique. It has reduced the incidence of open bone grafting in closed tibial fractures to virtually zero and, as illustrated in Table 5.7, only Gustilo IIIB fractures with significant bone loss now require bone grafting (Fig. 5.2). There are,

**Table 5.7.** The requirement for exchange nailing and open bone grafting in the different Gustilo open fracture types (from [23] with permission)

| Fracture type | Total | Uninfected fractures | Aseptic number | Nonunions | Exchange nailings | Bone grafting |
|---|---|---|---|---|---|---|
| G I | 29 | 28 | 2 | 7.1% | 2 | 0 |
| G II | 30 | 27 | 2 | 7.4% | 2 | 0 |
| G IIIA | 23 | 23 | 5 | 21.7% | 5 | 0 |
| G $IIIB_i$ | 15 | 13 | 5 | 38.5% | 5 | 1 |
| G $IIIB_{ii}$ | 12 | 11 | 11 | 100% | 4 | 11 |

G, Gustilo; i, fractures without significant bone loss (less than 2 cms and 50% of the circumference; ii, fractures with significant bone loss.

however, two situations where exchange nailing is ineffective. It does not help to secure union in infected fractures although, as already detailed, it is useful in removing the pyogenic membrane from the bone. In addition, it will not facilitate union in tibiae where a tube of bone has been created with bone graft, as healed corticocancellous bone graft does not have the same properties as normally vascularized cortical bone. There are few complications of exchange nailing. The only complication that was specific to this technique was a relatively high incidence of infection of the proximal entry wound. The usual incidence of proximal entry wound superficial infection is about 1.6% [19], but after exchange nailing, it was found that the incidence rose to 12.1%. There seemed to be no obvious explanation for this, as there is excellent vascularity in the area, but the significance of the higher figure is that the surgeon must be aware of potential for superficial infection to become deep infection.

There are three possible reasons why exchange nailing may stimulate bone union. Müller and Thomas [59] demonstrated the positive effect of increasing fracture stability on bone union in hypertrophic nonunion of the tibia. It does, however, seem unlikely that the extra stability gained by increasing the nail diameter by 1 mm will significantly affect the healing of a nonunion. The second possible reason is that reaming products are osteoinductive. This may be true for primarily nailed fractures, but it would seem unlikely that the effect of bone reamings in fibrous nonunions will be significant and the most likely reason for the success of exchange nailing is that proposed by Reichert et al. [69], who have shown that reaming causes a significant increase in the periosteal blood flow.

## Sequential External Fixation and Intramedullary Nailing

The last potential use for secondary intramedullary nailing in the management of open fractures is where a surgeon has used an external fixator as primary management (Fig. 5.6). Many surgeons still use external skeletal fixation for the management of severe open tibial fractures and even surgeons who favor intramedullary nailing may occasionally use external fixation in the management of multiply injured patients, for logistic reasons. Thus surgeons will be faced from time to time with the prospect of having to change an external fixator to an intramedullary nail.

A number of studies have examined the use of sequential external fixation and intramedullary nailing. Table 5.8 summarizes the results of seven papers which have utilized this technique. There is clearly a difference of opinion, with four of the papers listed in Table 5.8 showing a low infection rate and the other three detailing a comparatively high incidence of infection. It is interesting to observe that the only obvious correlation is with the delay between the removal of the external fixator and subsequent nailing of the tibia. Where the delay is relatively short, perhaps less than 2 weeks, the infection rate is low. The longer the delay the greater the incidence of infection, with Tornquist [84] having a catastrophic infection rate after an average delay of 218 days. Wheelwright and Court-Brown [87] advocated waiting until the pin tracks had granulated after the removal of the external fixator before intramedullary nailing was carried out. By following this policy, the authors had a low infection rate.

Siebenrock et al. [78] examined three groups of patients. Group 1 used external fixation throughout the management of the tibial fracture. In Group 2, the patients were treated with primary external fixation and secondary plating, and in Group 3, the surgeons used sequential external fixation intramedullary nailing. The distribution

**Table 5.8.** Results from studies using the sequential technique of primary external fixation and secondary intramedullary nailing

| Authors | *n* | Duration of ex fix (days) | Time before nailing (days) | Pin track sepsis (%) | Infection rate (%) |
|---|---|---|---|---|---|
| McGraw and Lim [56] | 16 | 59.5 | 21 | 44 | 44 |
| Maurer et al. [55] | 24 | 52 | 65 | 29 | 25 |
| Johnson et al. [39] | 16 | 84 | 13 | 12.5 | 0 |
| Blachut et al. [2] | 41 | 17 | 9 | 5 | 5 |
| Tornquist [84] | 6 | 72 | 218 | 100 | 66 |
| Wheelwright and Court-Brown [87] | 21 | 57.4 | 11.7 | 33.3 | 4.8 |
| Siebenrock et al. [78] | 24 | 45 | ? | 0 | 4 |

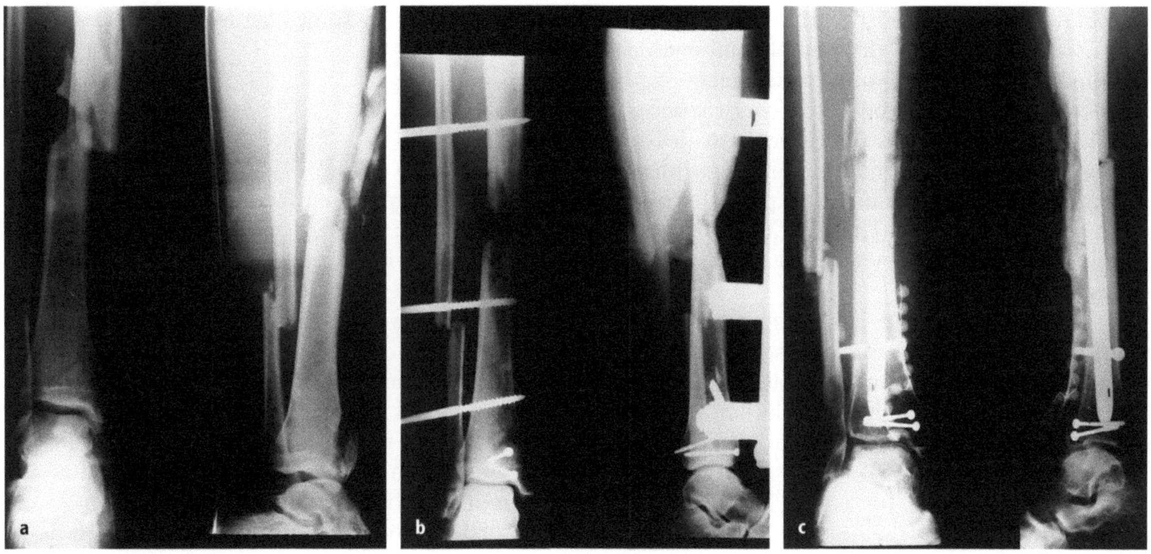


**Fig. 5.6.** A Gustilo 111B fracture (**a**) treated initially by external fixation (**b**). Union was achieved after intramedullary nailing (**c**)

of the different fracture types between the three groups is not known, but the authors stated that Group 3 patients had the lowest rate of infection, nonunion, and malunion as well as the shortest time to union. There is no obvious advantage to be gained in using primary external fixation and secondary intramedullary nailing now that studies have shown that primary intramedullary nailing is a satisfactory method of treating open tibial fractures. It would appear that if the delay between fixator removal and insertion of the intramedullary nail is kept to a reasonable minimum, good results can be achieved.

The results detailed in this chapter clearly show that there is a significant place for intramedullary nailing in the management of open diaphyseal fractures of the femur and tibia. Not only has primary nailing of open femoral fractures become routine, but it is likely that this technique will also become the routine method for treating open tibial fractures, provided the surgeons are aware of the importance of adequate debridement and rapid soft tissue closure. There is no reason to suppose that the results will not be equally effective in open fractures of the humerus and forearm, but more work is required to prove this.

## Principles of Management of Soft-Tissue Injury in Open Fractures

A. C. Masquelet and B. Schenck

### Introduction

Over the last 2 decades, considerable advances have taken place in the development of procedures for repairing soft-tissue defects. Until recently, the fracture was seen as the dominant element of these injuries, probably because trauma and orthopedic training was, by tradition, centered on the care of bone and joint injuries. Now, however, injury to the soft tissues has been accepted by the orthopedic and trauma surgeon as being the most important component of high-energy trauma, often dictating the initial, and sometimes the definitive, management of the injured extremity [49, 63].

Crucial questions have emerged about the assessment of the lesion, the proposed classification schemes, the predictive indices, the stabilization of the fracture, and the management of a large initial bone defect. Definitive answers to these questions should promote an optimal combination of techniques for soft-tissue management and bone reconstruction. However, the overwhelming variety of the lesions makes it difficult to devise any sort of standard decision-making algorithm, since every injury is unique and requires its own specific solution [54, 63]. Therefore, we will present only those principles which are valid for the majority of the cases.

The redefinition, in the last 2 decades, of the blood supply to the skin and muscles, with its clinical applications to wound coverage by the use of muscle or skin flaps, has revolutionized the treatment of complex musculoskeletal trauma.

## Why Close the Wound?

This question may seem ridiculous, but we should first be absolutely clear about the necessity to repair soft-tissue defects, based on a correct concept of soft tissues and soft-tissue defects.

Looking at the locomotor apparatus, the muscles, tendons, nerves, and vessels represent the motor's engine, which in turn drives the frame, made up of the bones and joints. The closing of a wound, i.e., the repair of the envelope, is essential for healing of the fracture and restoration of active motion [28, 38, 49].

The two main possibilities for treating a soft-tissue defect are promotion of spontaneous healing and surgical procedures.

If a soft-tissue defect is seen as a bowl, the various layers are its walls and the exposed deep structure its base. The possibility of spontaneous repair of the defect consists in the ingrowth of granulation tissue. In fact, is it desirable for this deep structure to be covered by granulation?

It is important to understand that in this situation granulation tissue is both good and bad: good because of the ability of the tissue to repair spontaneously by fibroblastic proliferation and bad because such tissue is always inflammatory and infected and healing leads to fibrous tissue. Thus, repair of the defect by granulation tissue implies two risks: an immediate risk of infection of the deep structure and, in the longer term, a retractile scar impeding the normal excursion of the underlying mobile structures.

### *Nerves and Vessels*

Nerves cannot remain exposed for long without definitive damage to their blood supply. They should be covered in some way by a surgical procedure.

### *Bone and Joints*

High-energy trauma often implies exposure of the skeletal frame. An exposed joint must be covered quickly to avoid infection. Fasciocutaneous flaps are preferable. They provide a supple tissue which is likely to preserve the motion of the joint, especially at the upper extremity. An exposed long bone requires precise assessment. If the vascularized periosteum is intact, without underlying fracture, as happens in a degloving injury, granulation tissue will provide excellent coverage. However, granulation tissue does not proliferate on denuded cortical bone unless the area exposed is quite small, when the defect is repaired from the surrounding tissues.

If there is a fracture the problem is quite different and repair of a soft-tissue defect by granulation is inappropriate. Granulation tissue is inflammatory and contaminated and leads to infection of the medullary canal through the fracture site [38]. One should remember that interrupted cortical bone, even without periosteum, can remain uncovered for a long time without being infected, unless the medullary canal is exposed. When this is the case, infection occurs very swiftly, so an open fracture should be rapidly covered using a surgical procedure, while a segment of healthy bone, with intact periosteum, can safely await coverage with granulation tissue.

It follows from these considerations that assessment of the tissue defect is crucial in selecting the repair procedure. Numerous factors should be taken into account, including the size of the defect, the nature of the surrounding tissues, their viability, the severity of any infection, the nature of the structure exposed, and the evaluation of how spontaneous repair of the defects might turn out. Successful wound closure implies removal of necrotic tissue, control of any infection, and the assurance of a good blood supply. Once decided, the management of tissue granulation is both technically demanding and time-consuming although trophicity and stiffness are often the price to pay. Ultimately, in the majority of cases, repair of a soft-tissue defect will be quickly obtained by a surgical procedure, using a flap.

## The Problem of Lesion Classification

Lesion classification provides a basis for determining treatment and estimating prognosis. Moreover, it is a tool for comparison of results. The classification of Cauchoix and Duparc [14] refers only to the external envelope without considering the deep lesions. Gustilo and Anderson [34] include the possibility of adequate bone coverage but do not detail the injuries to the soft tissues.

More recent attempts have sought to address the assessment of the soft-tissue injury in more detail. Tscherne's classification [61] refers to the overall severity of the soft-tissue lesion, whereas the AO scheme [61] seems to be the most accomplished attempt so far to evaluate soft-tissue injuries in specific terms. The progressive complexity of these classifications serves only to confirm that each major injury has its own specificity and that the initial major task for the surgeon is not so much to classify the injury but to describe, as well as possible, all of its components, bone and soft tissue alike, without forgetting the periosteum [11].

## The Assessment of the Patient and the Problem of an Early Amputation [7, 36, 49]

In complex injuries, one should determine whether limb salvage is possible and desirable.

Generally speaking, in the upper limb, there is no indication for amputation when reconstruction is feasible. Any function of the upper limb, however poor, is always preferable to a prosthesis. The dilemmas of amputation largely concern the lower extremity, since a well-fitted prosthesis below the knee should be seen as an excellent alternative option [29]. On the other hand, amputation at the level of the thigh should only be considered when salvage is impossible.

As a rule, amputation should not be performed in the emergency situation; it must be discussed with the patient. The only two elements which must be consistently and accurately assessed in decision-making are the posterior tibial nerve deficit, providing sensitivity to the plantar aspect of the foot, and the degree of muscle damage. These two factors correlate best with outcome in terms of initial and ultimate function.

## Bone Stabilization

Bone stabilization cannot be considered separately from soft-tissue reconstruction procedures, even if the latter are not be performed immediately. Internal fixation, whether by intramedullary nail or screws and plates, will, after debridement, require either a viable soft-tissue envelope or immediate coverage. If wound closure is not possible without using a flap, coverage and fixation should be undertaken in the same operation, as this will ensure an excellent and definitive debridement and the certitude that the surgical procedure employed will be viable [54].

It is of paramount importance to understand that there is a high risk of infection in leaving any fracture exposed after it has been stabilized by an internal fixation procedure, because this makes it difficult to carry out repeated debridement and cleaning of the fracture site.

In most situations, plating is recognized as inappropriate because it further damages the periosteum and the additional volume of material makes closure more difficult. Intramedullary nailing combined with immediate wound closure is now a widely accepted protocol in open fractures. But if the surgeon decides not to close the wound immediately because of infection, uncertain quality of debridement, or lack of expertise in flap procedures, he should apply an external fixator with a unilateral frame. This represents a safe, reliable, and reasonable solution which will provide effective stabilization of the fracture with easy access to the soft tissues.

Placement of the fixator pins must not impede the rotation of flaps; surgeons should calculate the main possibilities of coverage before placement of the pins [31]. This consideration must be strongly emphasized during specialist training and when using multispecialist teams.

Fixation of the fibula, which is best done using an intramedullary pin, considerably improves the rigidity of the skeletal frame and contributes to the stability of the soft-tissue envelope. In our opinion, a segmental fracture of the fibula should always be stabilized at both levels.

## Emergency Management

### *Debridement*

This stage is of crucial importance to obtain a clean wound. The principle is to evacuate the hematoma and to excise all nonviable tissue. The skin wound should be widely extended to permit exploration of the deep-tissue planes and the removal of nonviable muscle segments.

The current trend is to be less aggressive in skin excision and more aggressive in excising nonviable deep tissue [63]. Initial excision can be done under a tourniquet, which should then be deflated for the more detailed final stages. Extensive fasciotomies should be performed prophylactically, to prevent compartment syndrome.

Cleaning of the bone ends is essential to prevent medullary infection. A large, completely detached bone fragment should not be routinely discarded. If the wound is not obviously and massively infected, it is worth keeping the fragment and fixing it by minimal internal fixation, to improve the reduction and the stability of the fracture. Nonetheless, we emphasize that if this is to be done, immediate wound closure must be possible, which is not always the case.

It is acknowledged that irrigation lowers the risk of infection. However, we do not advocate pulsatile irrigation techniques. These may provoke additional trauma to soft tissue and instead of removing deeper particulate foreign matter, may drive it further in.

### *Revascularization*

If there has been prolonged ischemia it is advisable to revascularize the extremity as soon as possible. Before stabilization of the bone, a temporary shunt is employed to restore continuity of the main vascular axis and to supply the distal extremity. Then, after stabilization of the skeleton, vascular repair by a graft is usually carried out.

### *Bone Stabilization*

The following principles should be restated:

- If closure is delayed an external device is mandatory. Fixation of the fibula using an intramedullary pin in severe trauma improves the stability of the skeletal frame and the soft-tissue envelope.
- In cases of circumferential bone loss, a cement spacer or antibiotic-impregnated polymethylmethacrylate (PMMA) beads may be placed into the bone defect during closure. Major bone reconstruction is not advocated as an emergency procedure. The cement spacer will preserve space for secondary reconstruction [49, 54]. Moreover, the bone membrane induced by the foreign body promotes corticalization of a later cancellous bone autograft [54].

### *Wound Closure*

When should the wound be closed? After thorough debridement, followed by vascular repair and bone stabilization, closing the wound may be problematic. If vital structures such as nerve and vascular grafts have not been left exposed and the bone was stabilized by an external fixator, coverage can be delayed for 3–5 days. Godina [30] has shown that coverage within 72 h is effective and safe and decreases infection rates. Coverage should be done in the acute phase – the first 5 days according to Byrd et al. [13] and the first 17 days according to Yaremchuk et al. [92]. Most authors [28, 31, 74, 80] agree that coverage is required before the end of the first week.

The routine of performing immediate coverage in all cases [62] is not, in our opinion, a safe approach because of the difficulty and uncertainty of evaluating tissue viability in the emergency situation.

Schematically, one can consider several situations:

- Skin closure is achieved at the outset; indeed, this is the ideal solution, which corresponds to stages I and II of most classifications.
- Skin closure is not possible, but coverage of the vital underlying structures, tendons, neurovascular bundles, and fracture remains feasible by suturing vascularized subcutaneous tissue or muscle to the edges of the surrounding skin without using a flap.
- Some components remain exposed but they are covered with well-vascularized tissue. Granulation tissue will proliferate, but one should try to foresee the final functional outcome in order to estimate whether this process is desirable. For example, intact bone and tendons on the dorsum of the foot can, in functional terms, tolerate coverage by granulation tissue.
- Wound closure is impossible as a primary procedure. At the end of the debridement and stabilization, the fracture site remains exposed. Clinical assessment of tissue viability of the wound is crucial in determining which type of surgical procedure is needed to cover it. Here again, different scenarios must be considered:

- The debridement performed is judged as definitive: the remaining tissues are obviously healthy, well supplied, and noninfected, and a local rotational pedicle flap is feasible. Coverage must be done immediately because rotating a local flap will be more difficult a few days later, due to edema and the development of an inflammatory reaction which can impair the mobilization of the flap and its arc of rotation. When conditions for coverage are ideal but when a local flap is not possible, one can perform a free flap immediately, but this requires a very specialized environment and facilities.
- Debridement is uncertain, tissue viability is not well defined, and the wound is massively infected. Immediate coverage does not seem a reasonable option. All viable tissues should be retained and reassessed 1 day later. Repeated debridement is required until the wound is finally clean. Between surgical debridements, a temporary dressing should be applied and left in place. Dressings must prevent desiccation and infarction of vital exposed structures (nerves, arteries, tendons, and bones); so instead of packing the wound with wet gauze which dries in a few hours, an antibiotic bead pouch can be applied to maintain a physiologically moist environment. The dressing should promote neither the desiccation of the structures exposed nor the granulation process, which leads to infection. Proinflammatory dressings are contraindicated.
- The very similar wounds resulting from farmyard injuries, high-velocity gunshot injuries, or electrical injuries should be debrided a number of times before the definitive closure. It is important that delayed coverage be performed no more than 10 days after the initial injury, and preferably before the end of the first week. It must be done, in any event, before the development of granulation, which will affect all the tissues and particularly the venous return from the injured area.
- Delayed definitive coverage allows good assessment of the tissue by means of repeated debridement and gives time for arteriography, which will help in planning the coverage procedure. Indeed, this situation requires a coordinated plan for fracture stabilization and soft-tissue repair. At the time of coverage, the final debridement must be performed at the site of the fracture. The fracture must be inspected; the medullary canals of the two bone ends must be washed and cleared of hematoma and small particulate matter. This presumes the use of a very versatile external fixator, which allows opening the fracture itself and immediate retrieval of the reduction by locking the device.

## Soft-Tissue Repair: How to Do It [53]

### *Principles*

Soft-tissue repair should be conceived as a reconstructive ladder escalating from the simplest procedure to the most sophisticated. Each procedure has its own indication depending on the size and depth of the defect, the structures exposed, and local considerations such as vascular status and availability of regional flaps. In many cases, different solutions are theoretically possible but are restricted by the local conditions to a single procedure.

The suggested sequence of surgical procedures is as follows:

1. Spontaneous healing or vacuum-assisted closure
2. Local plasties (rhomboid flaps)
3. Skin graft
4. Local skin flap "at random" (rotation, translation, or advancement)
5. Local rotational axial skin flap (peninsular flaps)
6. Rotational muscle flaps
7. Local island pedicled skin or muscle flap
8. Distant pedicled flap (groin flaps or cross leg flap)
9. Free skin or muscle flap with vascular anastomosis in situ
10. Free skin or muscle flaps revascularized by vascular grafts

When a simple solution is not indicated (skin graft or rotation flap), we use an island pedicled flap as far as possible. This is a safe, reliable, and quick procedure if the vascular conditions have been well assessed. Exposed bone is covered with fasciocutaneous flaps.

Distant pedicled flaps such as the groin flap for upper limb reconstruction and cross leg flap for the lower limb are not advocated for emergency use, especially if there is an underlying fracture. They are not closed procedures and always lead to a local area of inflammation or infection. The immobilization of the limb required by these procedures generates edema and stiffness and one should remember the high risk of venous thrombosis associated with the cross leg flap. Moreover, the blood supply of these flaps will depend on the vascular conditions at the recipient site. For these reasons, groin and cross leg flaps should be reserved as secondary resurfacing procedures. Nonetheless, despite the numerous drawbacks, the pedicled groin flap remains a reliable procedure for reconstructive surgery of the hand. The major possibilities of cov-

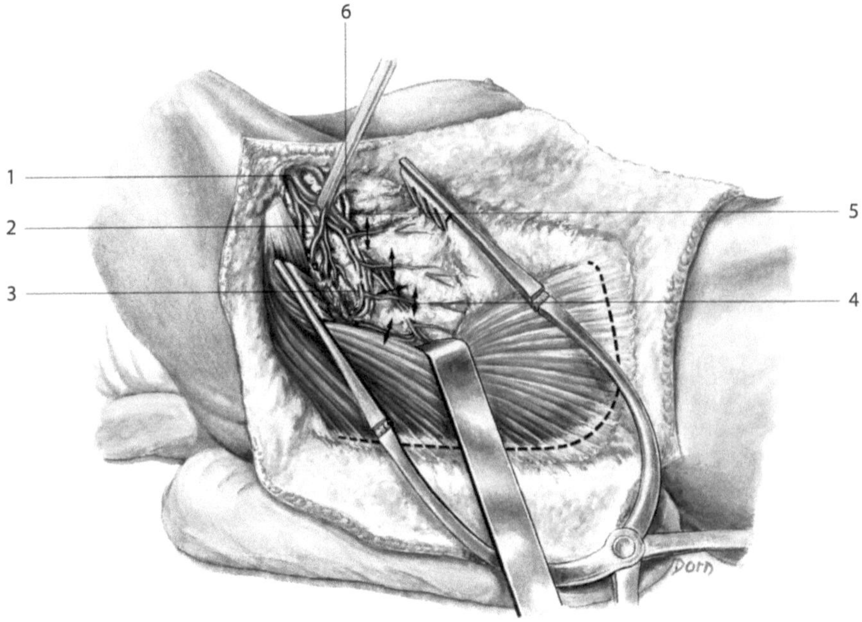


**Fig. 5.7.** The dissection of the latissimus dorsi muscle flap. The totality of the muscle flap can be raised on a patient lying supine with a carefully positioned sand bag. The anterior border of the muscle is slightly retracted in order to expose the vascular supply. The thoracic vessels should be ligated and divided to permit mobilization of the muscle. *1*, Subscapularis vessels; *2*, circumflex scapular vessels; *3* neurovascular pedicle; *4*, vascular pedicle to serratus anterior; *5*, thoracodorsal vessels; *6*, motor nerve to latissimus dorsi. *Arrows* indicate ligation of vessels needed to mobilize the muscle on its main proximal pedicle

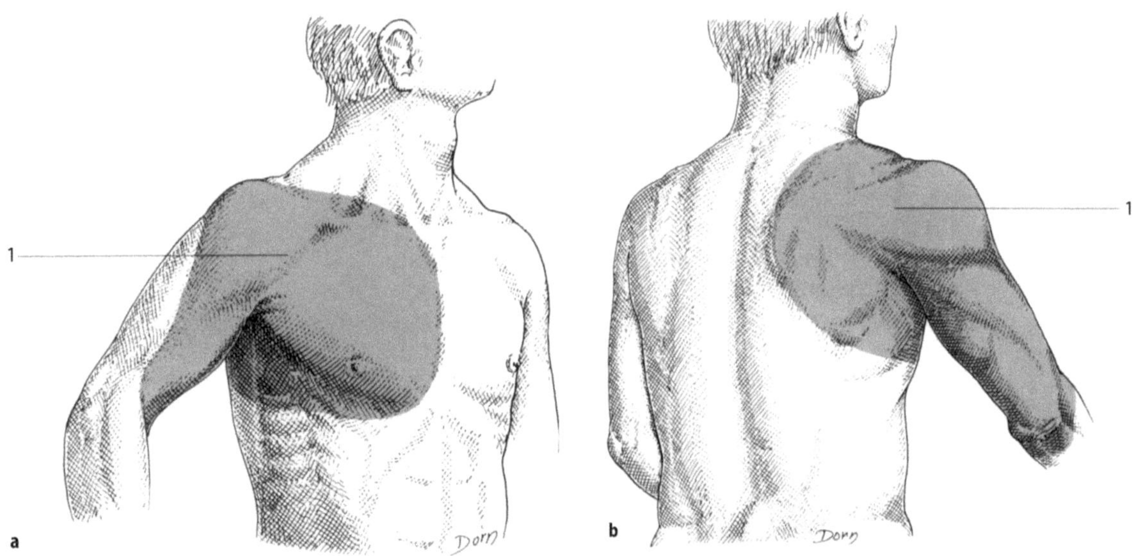


**Fig. 5.8 a, b.** Area of coverage of the pedicle latissimus dorsi flap. **a** Anterior aspect. **b** Posterior aspect. Note that the muscle can cover the posterior aspect of the elbow

erage by flap procedures depending on the site of the posttraumatic defect must now be explored.

### *Upper Limb*

Three areas should be differentiated: the upper arm, the forearm, and the hand and wrist.

#### Upper Arm

The upper arm includes the shoulder girdle and the elbow; there is no indication for a free flap at this level. Open fractures of the shoulder girdle, including the head of humerus, the acromioclavicular joint, and the clavicle can be covered to a limited extent by pedicled flaps of pectoralis minor muscle. Huge defects on the arm and the elbow can be safely reconstructed by the latissimus dorsi pedicled flap (Figs. 5.7, 5.8). Very large soft-tissue defects, which could compromise flexion of the elbow, are repaired by functional transfer of the latissimus dorsi using the Zancolli technique.

A latissimus dorsi muscle flap, later supplemented by a distal skin paddle, is a suitable and reliable technique for repairing open fractures of the elbow, which can encompass the distal humerus or proximal forearm.

Open injury of the proximal third of the arm, with associated soft-tissue and bone defects, can be treated in a one-stage reconstructive procedure by using a composite transfer that includes the latissimus dorsi muscle flap and a vascularized segment of the 9th or 10th rib.

#### Forearm

In the forearm, a fracture of the bone frame with a soft-tissue defect compromising the function of the hand is a forbidden area for pedicle flap procedures. A distant flap from the groin is always possible but its drawbacks are well known: the major risk is an infection of the fracture, which must remain partially exposed. More frequently, large defects of the forearm require a free flap. Primary repair of the envelope is of crucial importance, since reconstruction of tendon and bones can be performed in secondary procedures. Available flaps are latissimus dorsi, serratus anterior, and scapular muscle flaps. The so-called Chinese flap raised on the contralateral radial artery can be a good solution to restore both a tissue defect and the continuity of an interrupted artery giving rise to hand ischemia.

#### Hand and Wrist

The increasing number of pedicled flaps raised from the forearm has correspondingly reduced the indications for a free flap at this level. A Chinese flap, an interosseous posterior flap, or a pedicled fascial flap from the distal radial side or ulnar side of the wrist can solve practically all the problems. All of these generally require viable anastomoses between the vascular system at the palm or the dorsum of the wrist, since they are based on a distal pivot point and a retrograde arterial blood flow.

When no distally based pedicle flap is available, a free flap can come from the serratus anterior (coverage of the palm of the hand) or from the temporalis, dorsalis pedis fascia, or lateral brachial skin area for the dorsum of the hand.

### *Lower Limb*

Three areas should be differentiated: the pelvic ring and thigh, the knee and leg, and the ankle and foot. In fact, most open fractures occur in the lower limb including knee, leg, ankle, and foot.

#### Pelvic Ring and Thigh

Indications for soft-tissue repair following injury are very rare at the pelvic girdle and thigh. Limited defects exposing the anterior iliac crest are well covered by a pedicled rectus abdominis muscle flap distally based on the epigastric artery. Defects of the posterior aspect of the pelvis (posterior iliac crest, sacrum) can be covered with the gluteus maximus muscle flap. Combined trauma of the anterior part of the pelvic ring is a good indication for a proximally-based pedicled vastus lateralis muscle flap.

#### Knee and Proximal Third of the Leg

The two heads of gastrocnemius are suitable for covering the knee or proximal third of the leg. The area of coverage at the knee can be considerably increased by a large skin paddle overlapping the area of the muscle one and half times. A skin paddle supported by the distal part of the medial head of the gastrocnemius can cover defects at the junction of the proximal and middle thirds of the leg.

#### Middle Third of the Leg

This is the territory to be covered by the soleus muscle. Before using this muscle, one should assess the volume and the length of its muscle belly, which varies according to the size of the patient.

Wide short defects of the middle third are indications for a proximally based soleus muscle flap. Long and narrow defects over the medial or the anterior aspect of the tibia require a proximally based medial hemisoleus flap, which is more adaptable than using the whole muscle.

#### Distal Third of the Leg

Until recently, the distal third of the leg was a true forbidden area for local flaps. New advances have broadened the indications for a pedicled flap at this level.

- Small defects of the distal quarter of the leg are repaired by flexors of toes.
- The proximally based soleus flap generally covers the proximal part of the distal third. The area that can be covered depends on the morphology of the muscle.
- The distally based medial hemisoleus pedicled flap can cover nearly the entire distal third of the leg except for the supra malleolar region. The pivot point and blood supply are provided by a constant branch from the tibialis posterior artery at the middle of the leg (Fig. 5.9).
- Association of flaps can be an interesting procedure: proximally based soleus flaps and flaps from the flexors of the toes or soleus can be

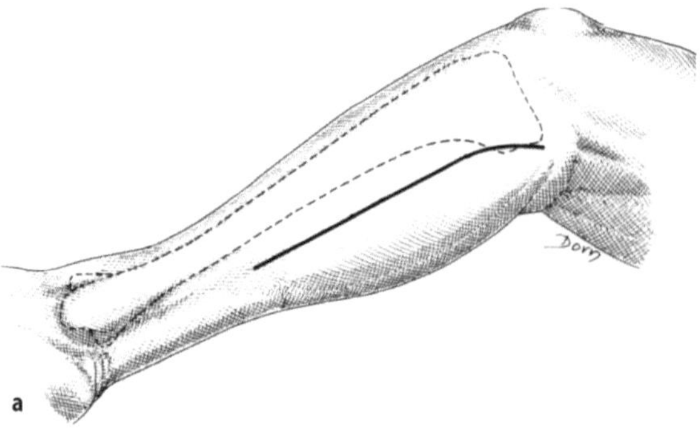


a

**Fig. 5.9 a–d.** The distally-based hemisoleus flap for covering the distal third of the leg. The flap is supplied by the mid-point branch that issues from the posterior tibial artery. **a** Incision. **b** The medial head of the gastrocnemius is retracted to expose the superficial aspect of the soleus. The proximal attachments are ligated and divided. The muscle is split along the vertical midline. *1*, Medial head of gastrocnemius; *2*, posterior tibial artery; *3*, medial hemisoleus; *4*, vascular pedicle, the pivot point of the flap; *5*, neurovascular axis in deep posterior compartment. **c** The medial hemisoleus is released as far as the secondary attachment, the pivot point of the flap. *1*, hemisoleus; *2*, vascular pedicle arising from the posterior tibial artery; *3*, vascular bundle to the skin; *4*, a distal hinge with the lateral portion of the muscle spared. **d** The muscle flap is rotated on its hinge. The flap is supplied by an arterial pedicle that is not located in the injured area

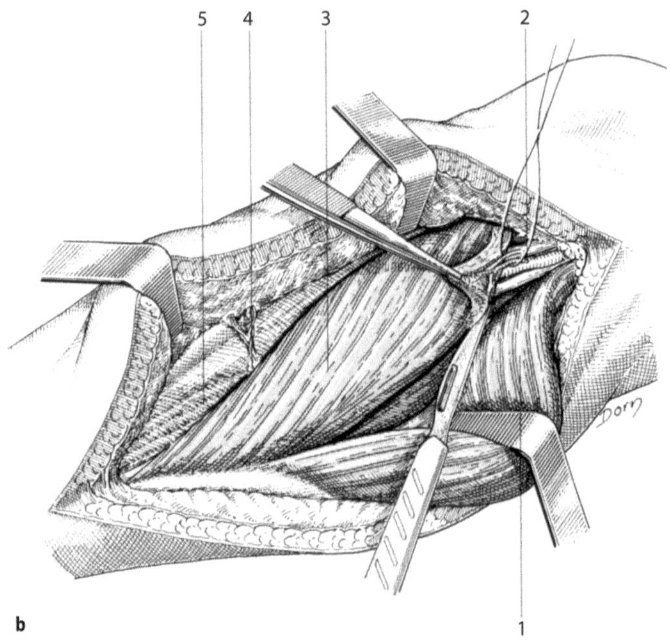


b

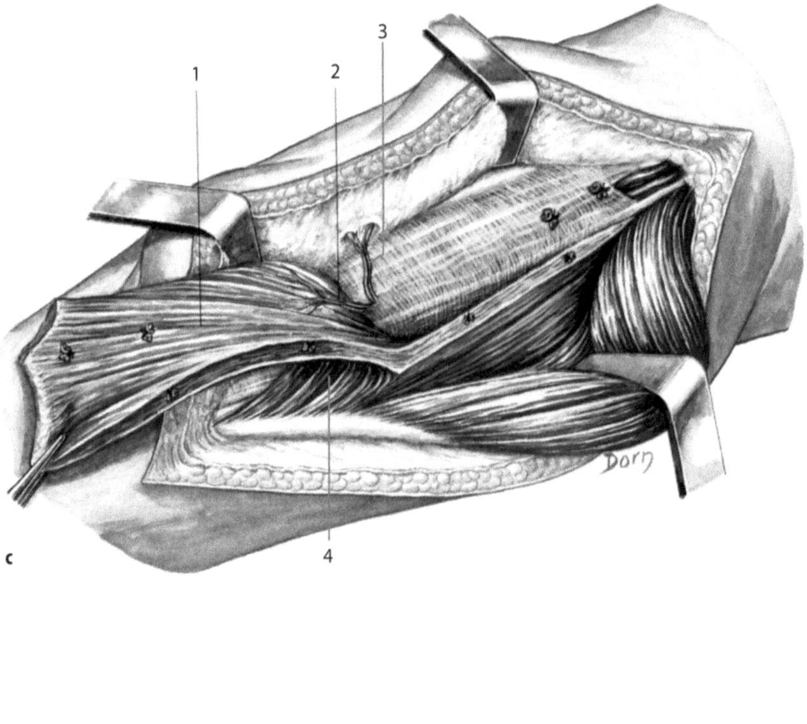


c

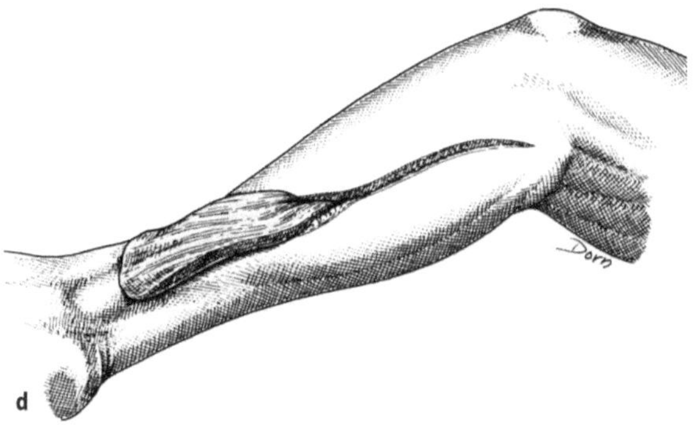


**Fig. 5.9 d.**

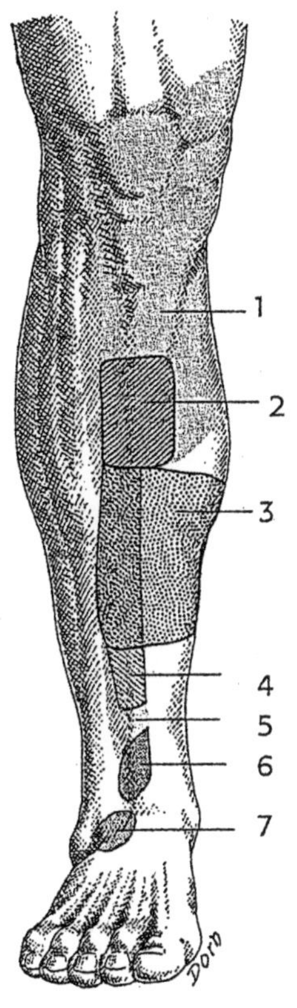


**Fig. 5.10.** Areas of coverage of pedicled flaps raised from the lower limb. Note that the areas of coverage of the soleus muscle and medial hemisoleus muscle are different. *1*, Medial head of gastrocnemius; *2*, proximally based hemisoleus (proximal third); *3*, soleus; *4*, distally-based hemisoleus (distal third); *5*, flexor digitorum longus; *6*, flexor hallucis longus; *7*, extensor digitorum brevis pedicled on the lateral tarsal artery (without interrupting the continuity of the dorsalis pedis artery)

combined with a subcutaneous fascial supramalleolar flap.

- The supramalleolar flap is a very quick and reliable procedure to repair a defect of the distal quarter of the leg (Fig. 5.11).
- The sural flap based on the vascular network of the sural nerve can also be used for the distal third.
- The indications for flaps according to the level of the defect are summarized in Fig. 5.10.

### Ankle and Foot

Soft-tissue defects of the foot are always challenging problems and we will give only the principles and the main procedures.

- Small defects of the hind foot may be covered by flaps from the abductor hallucis muscle on the medial side and from abductor digiti quinti on the lateral side. These procedures are rarely used in fresh fractures and should be reserved for secondary procedures.
- The extensor brevis muscle pedicled on its supplying lateral tarsal artery is suitable for covering a limited defect of the lateral aspect of the ankle. Continuity of the dorsalis pedis artery is not compromised (Fig. 5.10).
- The dorsum of the foot can be covered by a lateral supramalleolar flap (Fig. 5.11) and a distally based sural flap. Selection of the pivot point of the lateral supramalleolar flap is subject to a viable anastomosis. Fractures of the calcaneum rendered secondarily open by skin necrosis on the lateral aspect of the hind foot represent a good indication for a sural flap.
- The posterior aspect of the heel, including the distal insertion of an Achilles tendon, can be covered by supramalleolar or sural flaps (Figs. 5.12, 5.13). Large compound defects of the weight-bearing area on the heel remain an unsolved problem; repair usually requires a free flap; muscle flaps covered with skin are preferable as they are more adherent than a fasciocutaneous flap. Composite flaps including a piece of vascularized bone are difficult to match to the defect. Reconstruction of the bone is best performed secondarily, either by a bone graft or by a progressive bone transport.

The very last question is the most important of all: who should perform the soft-tissue repair?

The author believe that perfect cooperation between members of a plastic and trauma or orthopedic team is not always easy to achieve, even in highly specialized centers, and remain convinced that the best answer to the question lies in the training of specialized reconstructive surgeons capable of devising a coherent treatment strategy and of performing all the procedures, including bone stabilization, soft-tissue repair, and later, secondary procedures such as bone grafting. The complexity of the lesions produced by high-en-

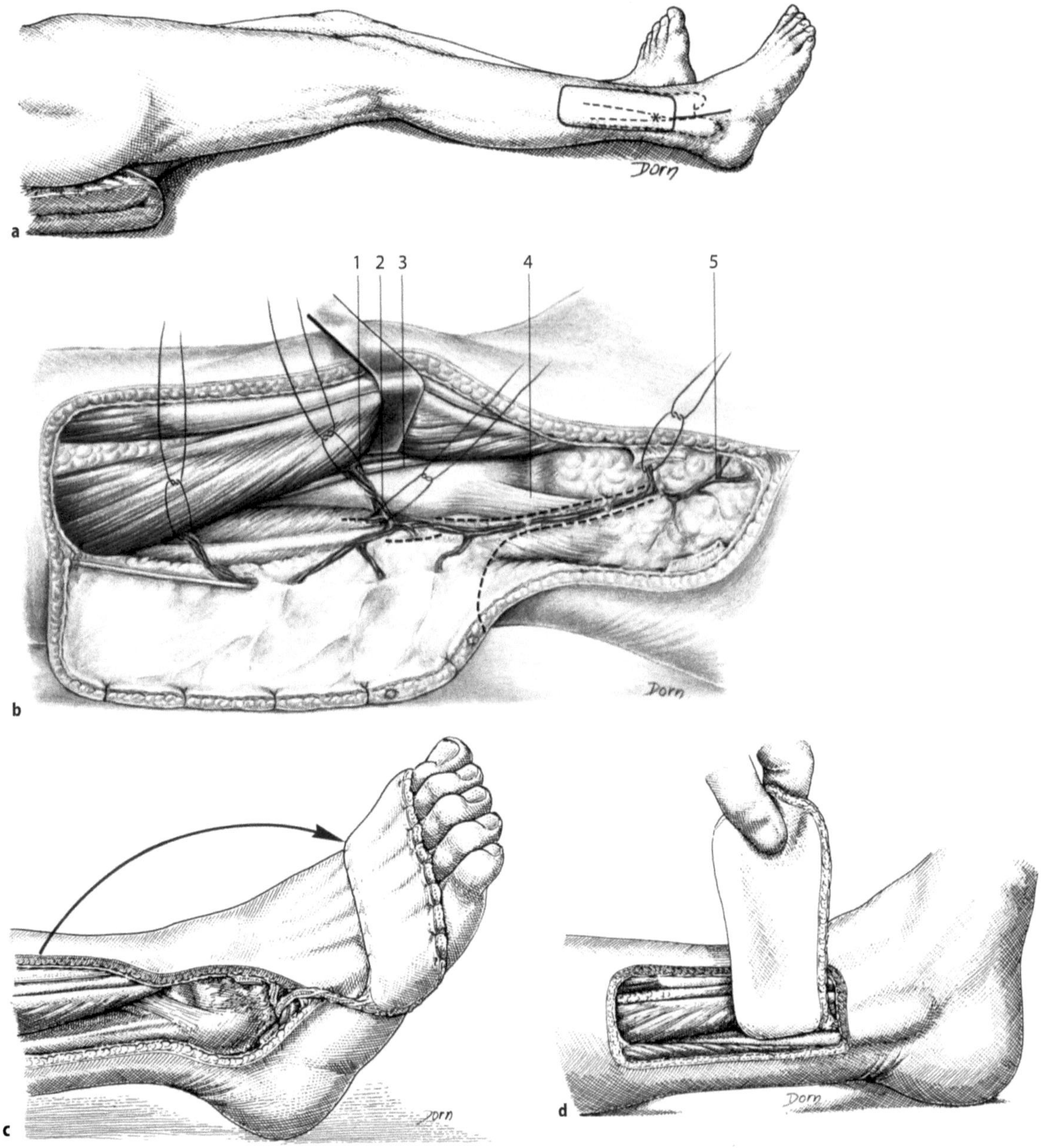


**Fig. 5.11 a–d.** The lateral supramalleolar flap is a very useful procedure for coverage of the distal quarter of the leg, the ankle, and foot. Nonetheless, it requires a good assessment of the vascular conditions of the injured area and special expertise in dissection. **a** Design of the flap. **b** Dissection of the flap. A posterior cutaneous hinge is maintained. Vascular pattern is identified to determine the pivot point of the flap, which is the sinus tarsi. At this point the perforating branch of the peroneal artery anastomoses with the lateral tarsal artery. The flap is supplied by one or two cutaneous branches that issue from the perforating branch very close to the interosseous membrane. *1*, Ligature of the anterior malleolar artery; *2*, anterior tibial artery; *3*, deep peroneal nerve; *4*, inferior tibiofibular ligament; *5*, anastomosis with the lateral tarsal artery. **c** The pedicle has been isolated and raised as far as the sinus tarsi. The arc of rotation provided by the pedicle allows coverage of all the areas of the dorsal aspect of the foot. **d** The lateral supramalleolar flap can be used as a rotational flap to cover the distal quarter of the medial aspect of the tibia

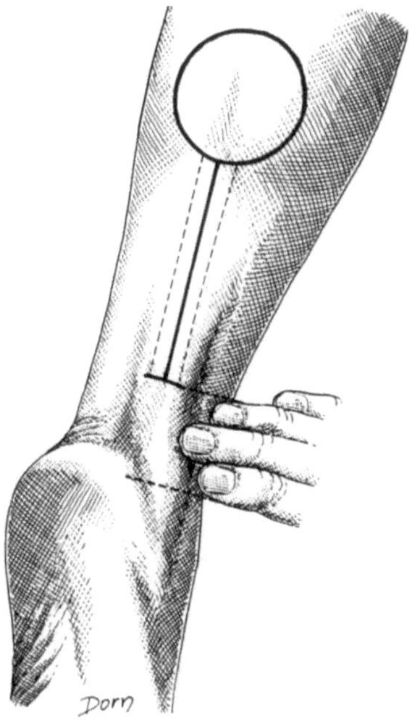

a

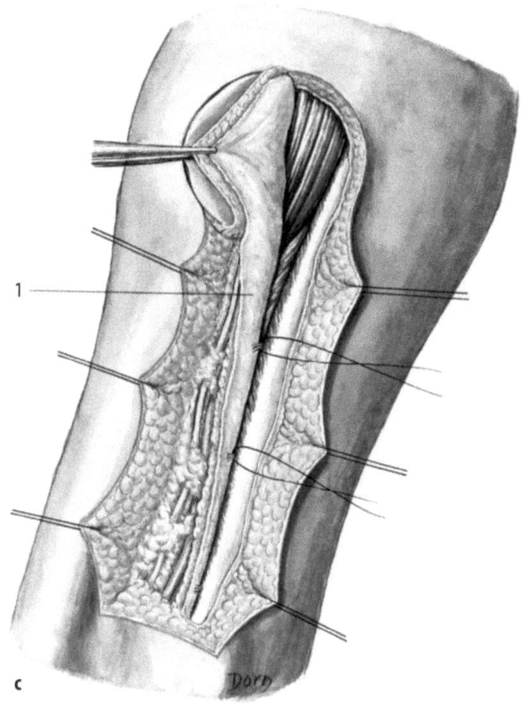


c

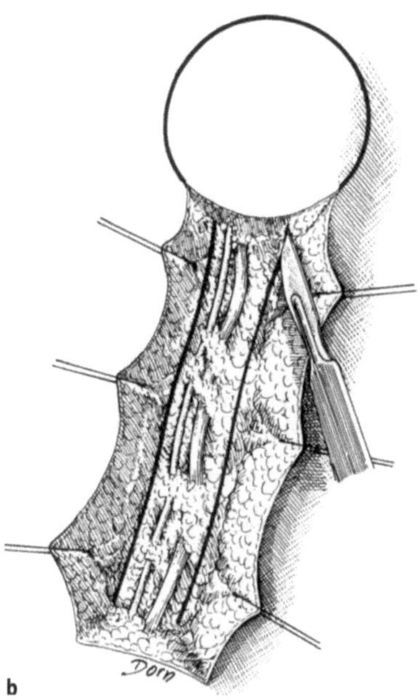

b

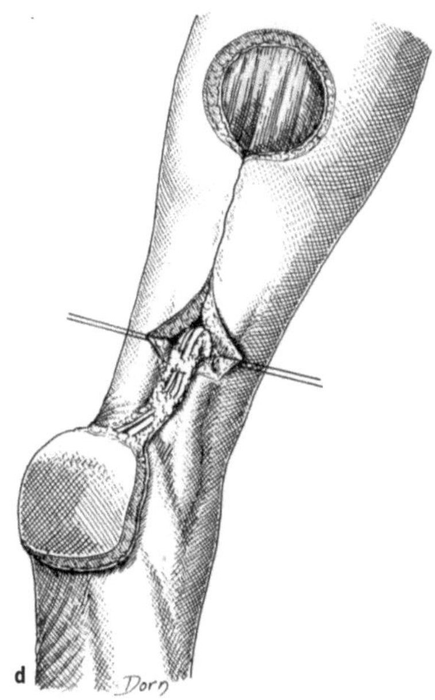

d

**Fig. 5.12 a–d.** The distally based neurocutaneous sural flap. The flap is supplied by the vascular axis of the sural nerve. The pivot point of the pedicle corresponds to a huge anastomosis of the vascular axis of the nerve with the peroneal artery. **a** Design of the flap. The pivot point of the pedicle is three finger's breadth proximal to the tip of the lateral malleolus. **b** Isolation of the subcutaneous fascial pedicle. **c** The flap and the pedicle are raised, fascia (*1*) included. **d** Arc of rotation allows coverage of the heel

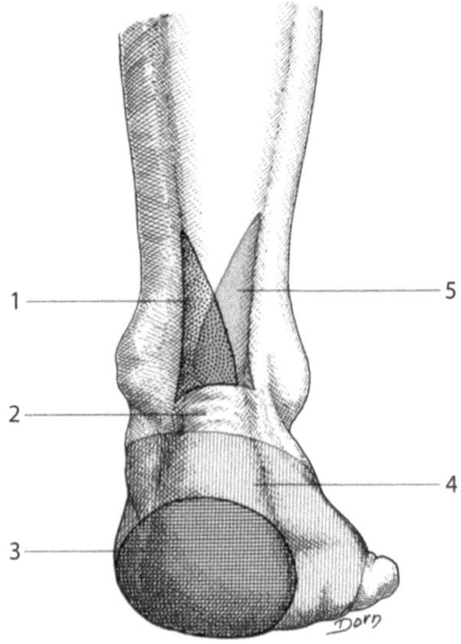


**Fig. 5.13.** Indications of flaps for coverage of the back of the foot. *1*, Flexor hallucis longus; *2*, medialis pedis flap, *3*, medial plantar flap; *4*, lateral supramalleolar flap and distally based sural flap; *5*, peroneus brevis

ergy trauma requires a holistic point of view rather than an aggregation of surgical procedures performed by various separate teams.

## References

1. Berenger-Feraud LJB (1870) Traite de l'immobilisation directe des fragments osseux dans les fractures. Delahaye, Paris
2. Blachut PA, Meek RN, O'Brien PJ (1990) External fixation and delayed intramedullary nailing of open fractures of the tibial shaft. A sequential practice. J Bone Joint Surg [Am] 72A:729–735
3. Blick SS, Brumback RJ, Lakatos R, Poka A, Burgess AR (1989) Early prophylactic bone grafting of high-energy tibial fractures. Clin Orthop 240:21–41
4. Bohler J (1951) Results in medullary nailing of 95 fresh fractures of the femur. J Bone Joint Surg [Am] 33A:670–678
5. Bonatus T, Olson SA, Lee S, Chapman MW (1997) Nonreamed locking intramedullary for open fractures of the tibia. Clin Orthop 339:58–64
6. Bone LB, Sucato D, Stegemann PM, Rohrbacher BJ (1997) Displaced isolated fractures of the tibial shaft treated with either a cast or intramedullary nailing. J Bone Joint Surg [Am] 79A:1336–1341
7. Bonanni F, Rhodes M, Lucke JF (1993) The futility of predictive scoring of mangled lower extremitities. J Trauma 34:99–104
8. Bradford C, Wilson P (1942) Mechanical skeletal fixation in war surgery: report of sixty-one cases. Surg Gynaecol Obstet 75:468–476
9. Breasted JH (1930) The Edwin Smith papyrus. University of Chicago Press, Chicago
10. British Orthopaedic Association (1992) The management of skeletal trauma in the United Kingdom. London
11. Brumback RJ, Jones AL (1994) Interobserver agreement in the classification of open fractures of the tibia. The results of a survey of two hundred and forty-five orthopaedic surgeons. J Bone Joint Surg [Am] 76:1162–1166
12. Brumback RJ, Ellison PS, Poka A, Lakatos R, Bathon GH, Burgess AR (1989) Intramedullary nailing of open fractures of the femoral shaft. J Bone Joing Surg [Am] 71A:1324–1331
13. Byrd HS, Spicer TE, Cierney G (1985) Management of open tibial fractures. Plast Reconstr Surg 76:719–730
14. Cauchoix J, Duparc J, Ducourtiaux JC (1957) Traitement des fractures ouvertes de jambe. Mem Acad Chir 83:811
15. Chan KM, Leung YK, Cheng JCY, Leung PC (1984) The management of type III open tibial fractures. Injury 16:157–165
16. Christie J, Court-Brown C, Kinninmonth AWG, Howie CR (1988) Intramedullary locking nails in the management of femoral shaft fractures. J Bone Joint Surg [Br] 70B:206–210
17. Court-Brown CM (1994) Reamed nailing in open tibial fractures. International Fracture Meeting, Strasbourg
18. Court-Brown CM, Quaba AA (1996) The relationship between plastic surgery and orthopaedic trauma surgery. In: Court-Brown CM, McQueen MM, Quaba AA (eds) Management of open fractures. Dunitz, London, pp 157–164
19. Court-Brown CM, Christie J, McQueen MM (1990a) Closed intramedullary tibial nailing. Its use in closed and type I open fractures. J Bone Joint Surg [Br] 72B:605–611
20. Court-Brown CM, Wheelwright EF, Christie J, McQueen MM (1990b) External fixation for type III open tibial fractures. J Bone Joint Surg [Br] 72B:801–804
21. Court-Brown CM, McQueen MM, Quaba AA, Christie J (1991) Locked intramedullary nailing of open tibial fractures. J Bone Joint Surg [Br] 73B:959–964
22. Court-Brown CM, Keating JF, McQueen MM (1992) Infection after intramedullary nailing of the tibia. Incidence and protocol for management. J Bone Joint Surg [Br] 74B:770–774
23. Court-Brown CM, Keating JF, Christie J, McQueen MM (1995) Exchange intramedullary nailing. Its use in aseptic tibial non-union. J Bone Joint Surg [Br] 77B:407–411
24. Court-Brown CM, Rimmer S, Prakash U, McQueen MM (1998) The epidemiology of open long bone fractures. Injury 29:529–534
25. Danckwardt-Lillieström G (1969) Reaming of the medullary cavity and its effect on diaphyseal bone. Acta Orthop Scand 28 [Suppl 1]:1–153
26. Davis AG (1948) Primary closure of compound fracture wounds. J Bone Joint Surg [Am] 30A:405–415
27. Edwards CC, Simmons SC, Browner BD, Weigel MC (1988) Severe open tibial fractures. Clin Orthop 230:98–115
28. Francel TJ, Vander Kolk CA, Hoopes JE et al (1992) Microvascular soft-tissue transplantation for reconstruction of acute open tibial fractures: timing of coverage and long-term functional results. Plast Reconstr Surg 89:478–487 ; discussion 488–497
29. Georgiadis GM, Behrens FF, Joyce MJ et al (1993) Open tibial fractures with severe soft-tissue loss. Limb salvage compared with below-the-knee amputation. J Bone Joint Surg [Am] 75:1431–1441
30. Godina M (1986) Early microsurgical reconstruction of complex trauma of the extremities. Plast Reconstr Surg 78:285–292
31. Gorman PW, Barnes CL, Fischer TJ et al (1989) Soft-tissue reconstruction in severe lower extremity trauma. A review. Clin Orthop 243:57–64
32. Grosse A, Christie J, Taglang G, Court-Brown C, McQueen M (1993) Open adult femoral shaft fracture treated by early intramedullary nailing. J Bone Joint Surg [Br] 75B:562–565
33. Gustilo RB, Anderson JT (1976) Prevention of infection in the treatment of 1025 open fractures of long bones. J Bone Joint Surg [Am] 58A:453–458
34. Gustilo RB, Mendoza RM, Williams DN (1984) Problems in the management of type III (severe) open frac-

tures: a new classification of type III open fractures. J Trauma 24:741–746
35. Haas N, Krettek C, Schandelmaier P, Frigg R, Tscherne H (1993) A new solid unreamed tibial nail for shaft fractures with severe soft tissue injury. Injury 24:49–54
36. Hansen ST Jr (1987) The type-IIIc tibial fracture. Salvage or amputation (editorial). J Bone Joint Surg [Am] 69A:799–800
37. Henley MB, Chapman JR, Agel J, Harvey EJ, Whorton AM, Swiontkowski MF (1998) Treatment of Type II, IIIa and IIIb open fractures of the tibial shaft: a prospective comparison of unreamed interlocking intramedullary nails and half-pin external fixators. J Orthop Trauma 12:1–7
38. Holden CE (1972) The role of the blood supply to soft tissue in the healing of diaphyseal fractures. An experimental study. J Bone Joint Surg [Am] 54:993–1000
39. Johnson EE, Simpson LA, Helfet DL (1990) Delayed intramedullary nailing after failed external fixation of the tibia. Clin Orthop 253:251–257
40. Keating JF, O'Brien PI, Blachut PA, Meek RN, Broekhuyse HM (1997 a) Reamed interlocking intramedullary nailing of open fractures of the tibia. Clin Orthop 338:182–191
41. Keating JF, O'Brien PI, Blachut PA, Meek RN, Broekhuyse HM (1997 b) Interlocking intramedullary nailing of open fractures of the tibia. A prospective randomised comparison of reamed and unreamed nails. J Bone Joint Surg [Am] 79A:334–341
42. Keating JF, Blachut PA, O'Brien PI, Court-Brown CM (2000) Reamed nailing of Gustilo grade-IIIB tibial fractures. J Bone Joint Surg [Br] 82B:1113–1116
43. Kempf I, Grosse A, Laffourge D (1978) L'apport du verouilage dans l'enclouge centromedullaire des os longs. Rev Chir Orthop 64:635
44. Kempf I, Grosse A, Beck G (1985) Closed locked intramedullary nailing. Its application to comminuted fractures of the femur. J Bone Joint Surg [Am] 67A:709–720
45. Klein MPM, Rahn BA, Frigg R, Kessler S, Perren SM (1990) Reaming versus non-reaming in medullary nailing: interference with control circulation of the canine tibia. Arch Orthop Trauma Surg 109:314–316
46. Klemm KW, Borner M (1986) Interlocking nailing of complex fractures of the femur and tibia. Clin Orthop 212:89–100
47. Klemm K, Schellmann WD (1972) Dynamische and statische verriegelung des marknagels. Monatsschr Unfallheilkd 75:568
48. Küntscher G (1945) Technik der Marknagelung. Thieme, Leipzig
49. Levin LS (1993) The reconstructive ladder. An orthoplastic approach. Orthop Clin North Am 24:393–409
50. Lhowe DW, Hansen ST (1988) Immediate nailing of open fractures of the femoral shaft. J Bone Jont Surg [Am] 70A:812–820
51. Lottes JO (1952) Intramedullary fixation for fractures of shaft of tibia. South Med J 45:407–414
52. Malt RA, McKhann CF (1964) Replantation of severed arms. JAMA 189:716–722
53. Masquelet AC, Gilbert A (2001) An atlas of flaps of the Musculoskeletal System. Dunitz, London
54. Masquelet AC, Begue T, Court C (1995) Fractures ouvertes de jambe. ENCYCL MED CHIR (Elsevier, Paris) Appareil Locomoteur 14·086·A·20
55. Maurer DJ, Merkow RC, Gustilo RB (1989) Infection after intramedullary nailing of severe open tibial fractures initially treated with external fixation. J Bone Joint Surg [Am] 71:835–838
56. McGraw JM, Lim EVA (1988) Treatment of open tibial shaft fractures. External fixation and secondary intramedullary nailing. J Bone Joint Surg [Am] 70A:900–911
57. Merle d'Aubigne R, Maurer P, Zucman P, Masse Y (1974) Blind intramedullary nailing for tibial fractures. Clin Orthop 105:267–275
58. Milligan ETC (1915) The early treatment of projectile wounds by excision of the damaged tissues. BMJ 1:1081
59. Müller ME, Thomas RJ (1979) Treatment of non-union in fractures of long bones. Clin Orthop 138:141–153
60. Müller ME, Allgower M, Willenegger H (1965) Technique of internal fixation of fractures. Springer, Berlin Heidelberg New York
61. Müller ME, Allgöwer M, Schneider R (1991) Manual of internal fixation. Springer, Berlin Heidelberg New York
62. Najean D, Tropet Y, Brientini JM et al (1994) Emergency cover of open fractures of the leg. Apropos of a series of 24 clinical cases. Ann Chir Plast Esthet 39:473–479; discussion 480–471
63. Norris BL, Kellam JF (1997) Soft-tissue injuries associated with high-energy extremity trauma: principles of management. J Am Acad Orthop Surg 5(1):37–46
64. Nowotarski P, Brumback RJ (1994) Immediate locking nailing of fractures of the femur caused by low- to mid-velocity gunshots. J Orthop Trauma 8:134–141
65. O'Brien J, Meek RN, Powell JN, Blachut PA (1991) Primary intramedullary nailing of open femoral shaft fractures. J Trauma 31:113–116
66. Oedekoven G, Claudi B, Frigg R (1993) Treatment of open and closed tibial fractures with unreamed interlocking tibial nails. Orthop Traumatol 2:115–128
67. Pape MC, Regel G, Dwenger A, Sturm JA, Tscherne M (1993) Influence of thoracic trauma and primary femoral intramedullary nailing on the incidence of ARDS in multiple trauma patients. Injury 24:S82–S103
68. Ponten B (1981) The fasciocutaneous flap. Its use in soft tissue defects of the lower leg. Br J Plast Surg 34:215–220
69. Reichert ILH, McCarthy ID, Hughes SPF (1995) The acute vascular response to intramedullary nailing. J Bone Joint Surg [Br] 77B:490–493
70. Renner N, Regazzoni P, Babst R, Rosso R (1993) Initial experiences with the unreamed tibial nail. Helv Chir Acta 59:665–668
71. Rhinelander FW (1974) Tibial blood supply in relation to fracture healing. Clin Orthop 105:34–81
72. Rose C, Court-Brown CM (1995) Reamed nailing of open tibial fractures. Osteosynthese 3:178–182
73. Ruedi T, Webb JK, Allgower M (1976) Experience with the dynamic compression plate (DCP) in 418 recent fractures of the tibial shaft. Injury 7:252–257
74. Sanders R, Swiontkowski M, Nunley J et al (1993) The management of fractures with soft-tissue disruptions. J Bone Joint Surg [Am] 75:778–789
75. Sanders R, Jersinovich I, Anglen J, DiPasquale T, Herscovici D (1994) The treatment of open tibial shaft fractures using an interlocked intramedullary nail without reaming. J Orthop Trauma 8:504–510
76. Schandelmaier P, Krettek C, Rudolf J, Kohl A, Katz BE, Tscherne H (1997) Superior results of tibial rodding versus external fixation in grade 3b fractures. Clin Orthop 342:164–172
77. Schemitsch EH, Kowalski MJ, Swiontkowski MF, Senft D (1994) Cortical bone blood flow in reamed and unreamed locked intramedullary nailing. A fractured tibial model in sheep. J Orthop Trauma 8:373–382
78. Siebenrock KA, Schillig B, Jakob RP (1993) Treatment of complex tibial shaft fractures: arguments for early secondary intramedullary nailing. Clin Orthop 290:269–274
79. Singer RW, Kellar JF (1995) Open tibial diaphyseal fractures: results of unreamed locked intramedullary nailing. Clin Orthop 315:114–118
80. Small JO, Mollan RA (1992) Management of the soft tissues in open tibial fractures. Br J Plast Surg 45:571–577
81. Søjbjerg JO, Eiskjaer S and Møller-Larsen F (1990) Locked nailing of comminuted and unstable fractures of the femur. J Bone Joint Surg [Br] 72B:23–25

82. Street DM (1951) One hundred fractures of the femur treated by means of the diamond-shaped medullary nail. J Bone Joint Surg [Am] 33A:659–669
83. Tornetta P, Bergman M, Watnik N, Berkowitz G, Steuer J (1994) Treatment of grade IIIB open tibial fractures. A prospective randomised comparison of external fixation and non-reamed locked nailing. J Bone Joint Surg [Br] 76B:13–19
84. Tornquist H (1990) Tibia non-unions treated by interlocking nailing: Increased risk of infection after previous external fixation. J Orthop Trauma 4:109–114
85. Trueta J (1944) The principles and practice of war surgery, 2nd edn. Hamish Hamilton, London
86. Tu YK, Lin CH, Su JI, Hsu DT, Chen RJ (1995) Unreamed intramedullary nail versus external fixator for open type III tibial fractures. J Trauma 39:361–367
87. Wheelwright EF and Court-Brown CM (1992) Primary external fixation and secondary intramedullary nailing in the treatment of tibial fractures. Injury 23:373–376
88. Whittle AP, Russell TA, Taylor JC, Lavelle DG (1992) Treatment of open fractures of the tibial shaft with the use of interlocking nailing without reaming. J Bone Joint Surg [Am] 74A:1162–1171
89. Wiss DA (1986) Flexible medullary nailing of acute tibial shaft fractures. Clin Orthop 212:122–132
90. Wiss DA, Fleming CH, Matta JM, Clark D (1987) Comminuted and rotationally instable fractures of the femur treated with an interlocking nail. Clin Orthop 212:35–47
91. Wiss DA, Brien WW, Becker V (1991) Interlocking nailing for the treatment of femoral fractures due to gunshot wounds. J Bone Joint Surg [Am] 73A:598–601
92. Yaremchuck MJ, Brumback RJ, Manson PN et al (1987) Acute and definitive management of traumatic osteocutaneous defects of the lower extremity. Plast Reconstr Surg 80:1–14
93. Zucman J, Maurer P (1970) Primary medullary nailing of the tibia for fractures of the shaft in adults. Injury 2:84–92

# CHAPTER 6

# Treatment of Nonunions

D. Dagrenat and I. Kempf

Pseudarthrosis of femoral and tibial fractures is a serious complication of diaphyseal fractures of the lower limb. It prolongs patient morbidity, the time lost from work, and therefore economic hardship.

We can define nonunion as follows: a definitive nonconsolidation of the fracture site, with a delay over 8 months generally admitted for nonunions. In these cases, only a change in treatment can lead to bone fusion. However, it is not necessary to wait 8 months to change the treatment when it is obvious that the fracture site will inevitably progress to pseudarthrosis in cases where treatment has initially failed.

Many methods of treatment have been proposed to solve this problem, with different fixation methods such as plates and screws, IM nailing, and external fixator and enhancement of the consolidation process using bone graft, electrical stimulation, and even ultrasound at the fracture site [1, 5, 7]. Conventional nailing with reaming using the closed procedure is an excellent method for femoral and tibial midshaft nonunions, as described by Küntscher, and the locking system has expanded the indications to proximal and distal nonunions.

Remember that a very simple and elegant method not only to prevent but also to treat confirmed nonunions in selected cases is dynamization by simply removing the proximal or distal locking screws (Fig. 6.1).

## Etiology and Indications for Locked Nailing

Nonunion generally follows a failure in the initial treatment, often of iatrogenic origin (poor fixation, extensive stripping of the fragments), or the patient misunderstanding or not respecting the follow-up instructions (period of discharge).

There are three different consolidation types often associated during the process of consolidation, whatever technique has been used initially:

- Endosteal, with a callus within the medullary canal
- Direct or primary consolidation obtained with strong fixation, which allows no movement at the fracture site [5]
- Periosteal callus, the natural mode, with an external callus whose size depends on the stability of the fixation: the less the fixation is stable the larger the callus is.

Nonunion occurs when the process of healing is interrupted, often because of iatrogenic causes.

Poor internal fixation, because of insufficient resistance of the implant or insufficient immobilization with an external brace or cast, leads to breakage of the osteosynthesis material.

Open procedures eliminate the periosteal process of healing.

There are many types of nonunions [7] of different origins, which require different kinds of treatment (Fig. 6.2).

Hypertrophic pseudarthrosis, with a very large callus that is unable to stabilize the fragments, is generally the result of an orthopedic treatment or of an insufficient fixation with an intramedullary (IM) nonlocking nail or too little plate. The hypertrophic aspect of the callus suggests that the periosteal process is still active and these types of pseudarthrosis are the indication of choice for IM locked nailing.

Atrophic pseudarthrosis suggests that the natural processes of healing have been compromised because of too much stripping of the periosteum during an open procedure or because of bone loss. These types of nonunions are generally the result of extensive plate fixation, either an IM nail with large bone loss or placed with an open procedure, or pseudarthrosis following multiple failed procedures. Treatment is more difficult in these cases, which can also require stimulation of osteogenesis at the nonunion site.

Two conditions must be satisfied to obtain bony fusion using IM locked nailing:

1. Good immobilization of the fracture fragments, which can be obtained with the intramedullary locking nail. The proximal and distal limits of

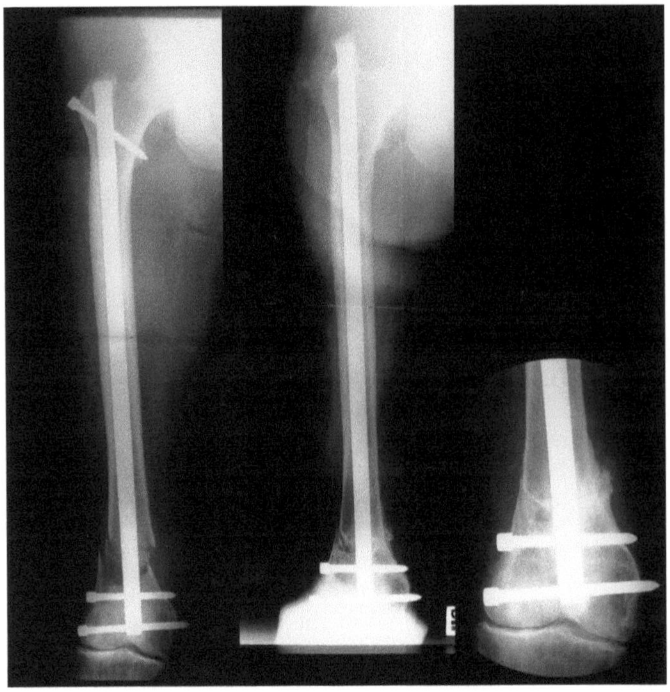

**Fig. 6.1.** Distal fracture with large gap. Risk of pseudarthrosis. Consolidation after dynamization

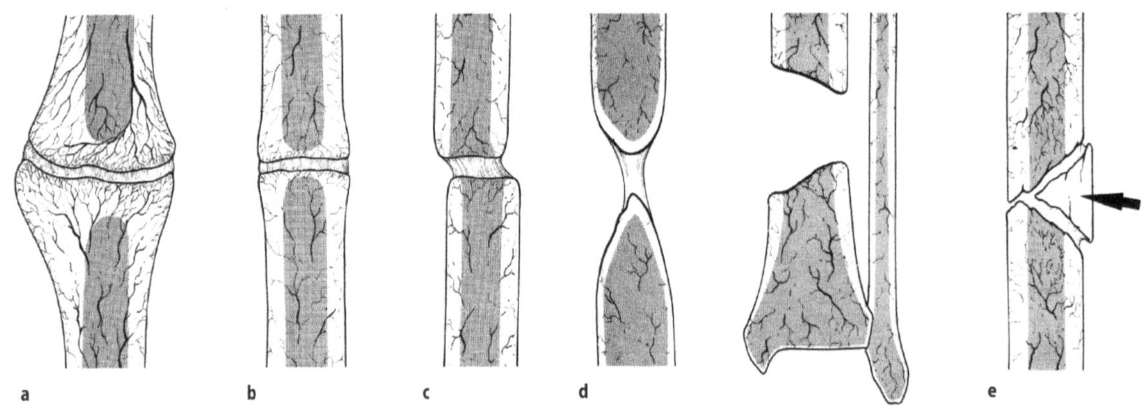


**Fig. 6.2a–e.** Different types of nonunions. **a** Hypertrophic. **b** Eutrophic. **c** Hypotrophic. **d** With bone loss. **e** Avascular third fragment

locked nailing are the same as those in fresh fractures.

2. Good stimulation of the natural process of healing, either mechanically with good dynamization to enhance external periosteal callus formation (dynamic systems with immediate mobilization and weight-bearing are advocated to obtain compression and closure of the fracture site [5]) (Fig. 6.3) or biologically with the reaming process, which brings healing factors and bone graft to the fracture site.

## Technical Aspects

Each case of pseudarthrosis is a particular case in and of itself, calling for rigorous analysis and understanding of why the initial treatment failed.

The limits of the indications are the same as those in fresh fractures, meaning that locked nailing is indicated for nonunions at the femur, 1–2 cm below the lesser trochanter or above the femoral condyles, and at the tibia, 5 cm below the tibial tubercle and 7.5 cm above the ankle joint.

The patient is placed on a fracture table, as for a fresh fracture.

The operation starts with the removal of the osteosynthesis implants. If a plate has been used, it must be removed using a minimal and direct

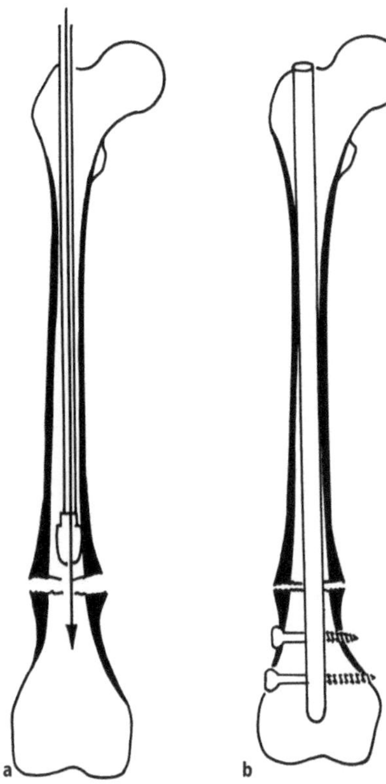


**Fig. 6.3 a, b.** Treatment of hypertrophic distal nonunion. **a** Reaming on a special sharp guidewire. **b** Dynamic locked intramedullary nailing. Immediate weight-bearing

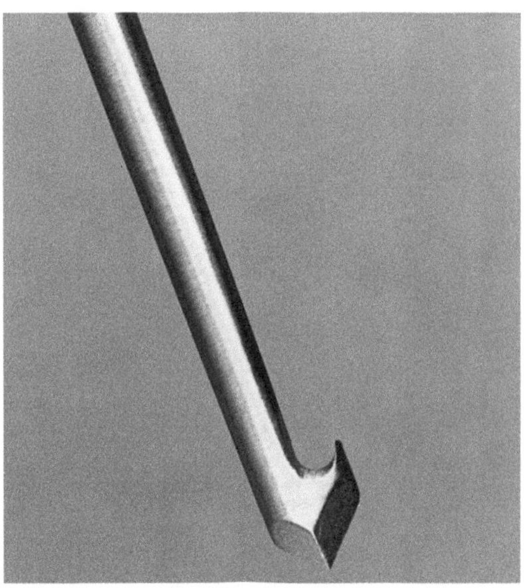

**Fig. 6.4.** Extraction hook for distal part of broken nail

approach, with particular care taken to prevent any periosteal damage. The nonunion site must not be resected and it is not necessary to add bone graft or perform bone resection. The site is simply closed over a Redon drainage.

If a nail is present, removal can be easily carried out through the insertion hole with the extraction ancillary.

If the nail is broken, the proximal part can be removed classically and the distal part removed with a special extraction hook, which must be slid in to the tip of the nail using fluoroscopic monitoring; the nail is removed from the bottom to the top (Fig. 6.4).

The nonunion site is then reduced as well as possible using the fracture table.

The nailing procedure is then carried out as for fracture treatment, using the fracture table and fluoroscopy. It is important to ream properly, in order to stimulate the nonunion site and implant a nail that is as large as possible, and therefore to increase the stability of the osteosynthesis.

For mediodiaphyseal pseudarthrosis, simple intramedullary nailing is adequate (Fig. 6.5). For proximal or distal nonunions, the locking procedure of choice uses dynamic systems, either proximal or distal, depending on the site of pseudarthrosis, to provide stimulating compression by immediate weight-bearing authorized after operation (Fig. 6.3).

Except for the minimal approach to remove the previous implants, the procedure is considered as a closed procedure, with no other intervention at the nonunion site. This closed procedure is very important and part of the success of the method.

Postoperative care is classic: Redon drainage, soft bandage of the incisions, preventive anticoagulation, and pain control.

Postoperative physical therapy involves positioning the patient in a chair the day after the operation and actively and passively mobilizing the articulations, often stiff after a long period of immobilization, using immediate passive motion. Weight-bearing is authorized as soon as possible, generally on the second or third day after operation, after the removal of the suction drains. Full weight-bearing with two crutches is encouraged and generally obtained within 1–2 weeks. It must be remembered that this weight-bearing is part of the treatment as it provides dynamic compression of the nonunion site [4, 6].

### Tricks and Pitfalls for Specific Cases

In supracondylar pseudarthrosis, the indication for the femur can be extended to very low nonunions, using a nail from which the tip has been sawn. To increase the stability of the distal lock-

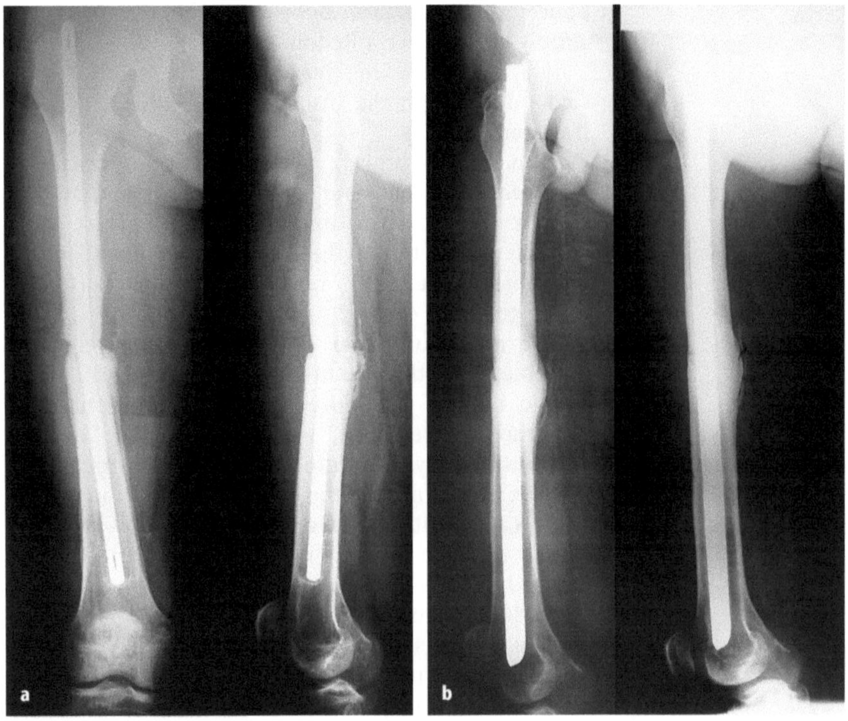

**Fig. 6.5.** **a** Mediodiaphyseal femoral nonunion with small curved nail. **b** Consolidation after renailing with reaming and thicker nail

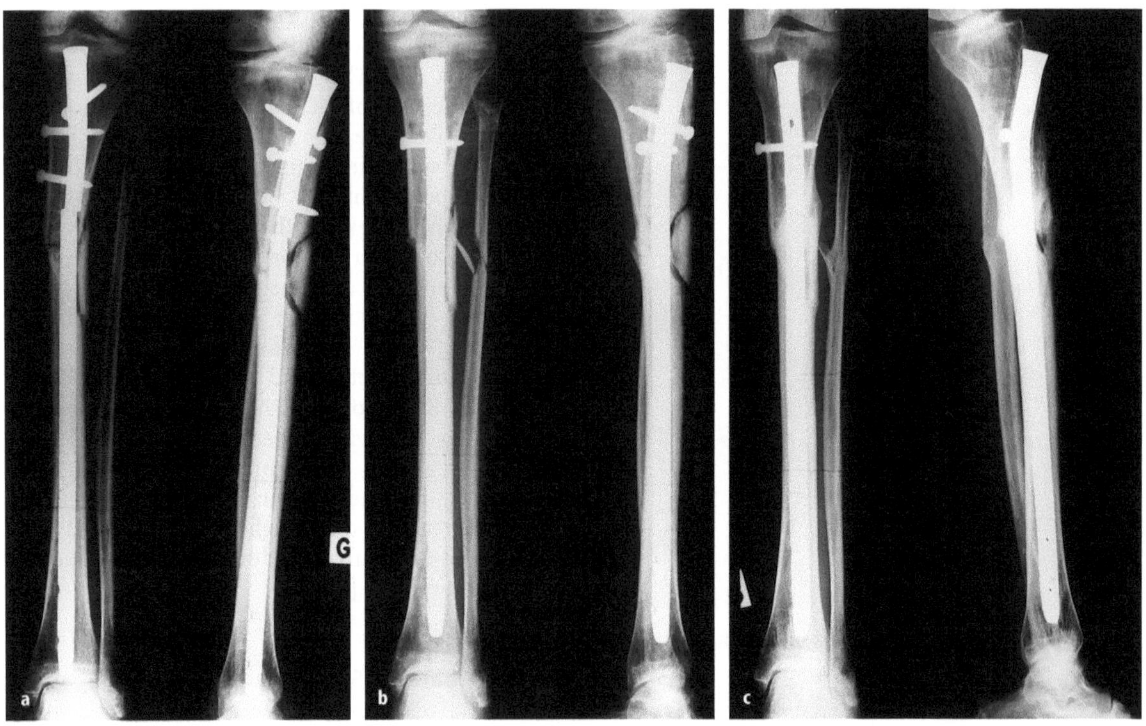

**Fig. 6.6.** **a** Proximal tibial nonunion. Nail was too long and consequently broke. Third fragment. **b** Dynamic locked renailing with shorter nail. Fibula osteotomy. **c** Consolidation with integration of third fragment

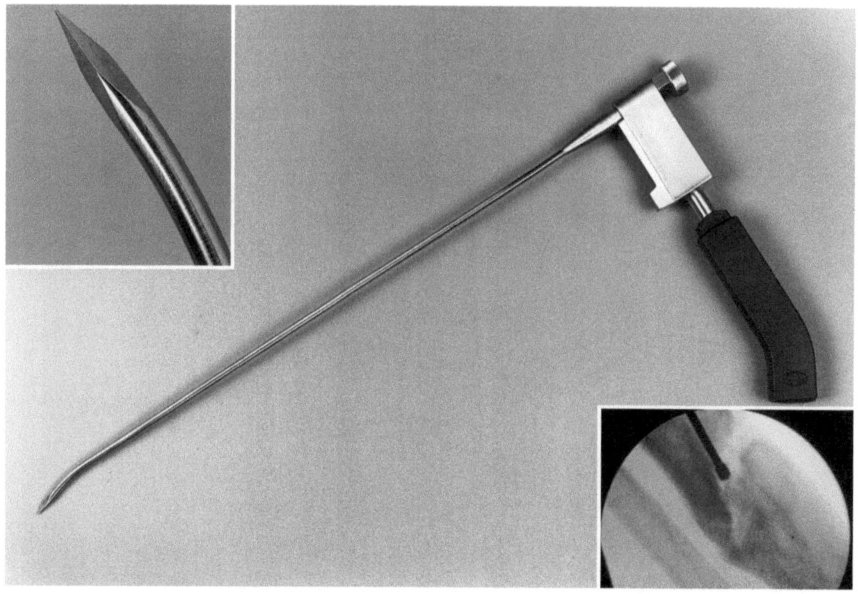

**Fig. 6.7.** Special very sharp guide to pass the obturated medullary canal. *Top left*, the tip of the guide; *bottom right*, Küntscher's sharp guidewire in situ

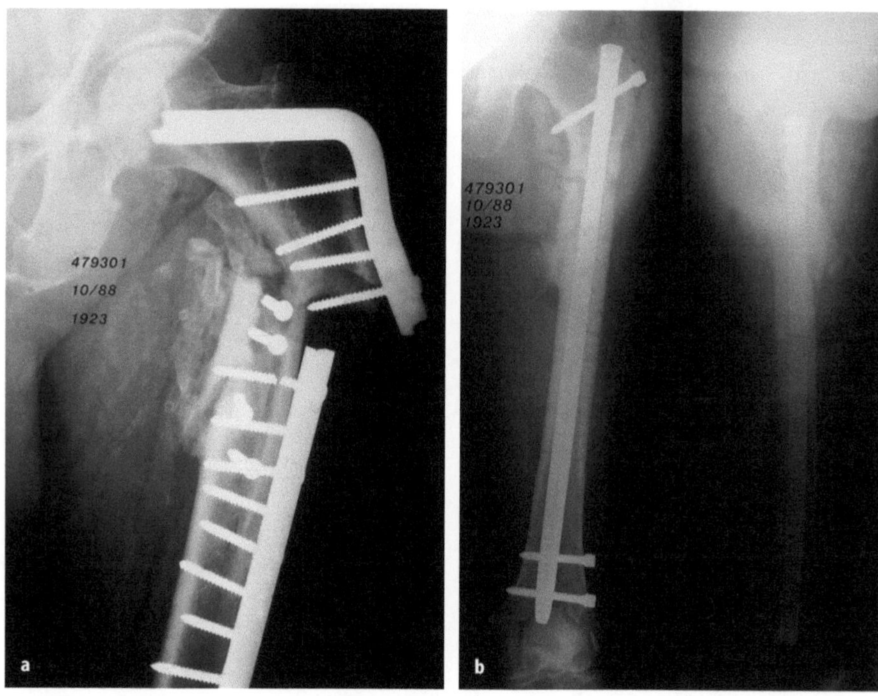


**Fig. 6.8.** **a** Proximal femoral nonunion after a plate osteosynthesis. **b** Consolidation after proximal dynamic locked nailing

ing screws, we advocate using fully threaded screws or Vécsei expansion screws, particularly when the distal femoral epiphysis is osteoporotic.

In cases of pseudarthrosis of the tibia caused by an early consolidation of the fibula fracture or no fracture of the fibula, we recommend an oblique osteotomy of the fibula or a minimal resection. This additional procedure is essential to allow effective compression of the nonunion site at the tibia during the weight-bearing (Fig. 6.6).

With malaligned pseudarthrosis, the closed method is still possible and generally re-establishes the sagittal and frontal axis of the bone when external handling on the fracture table is used to achieve the reduction. In some cases where the malunion cannot be reduced because of very hypertrophic

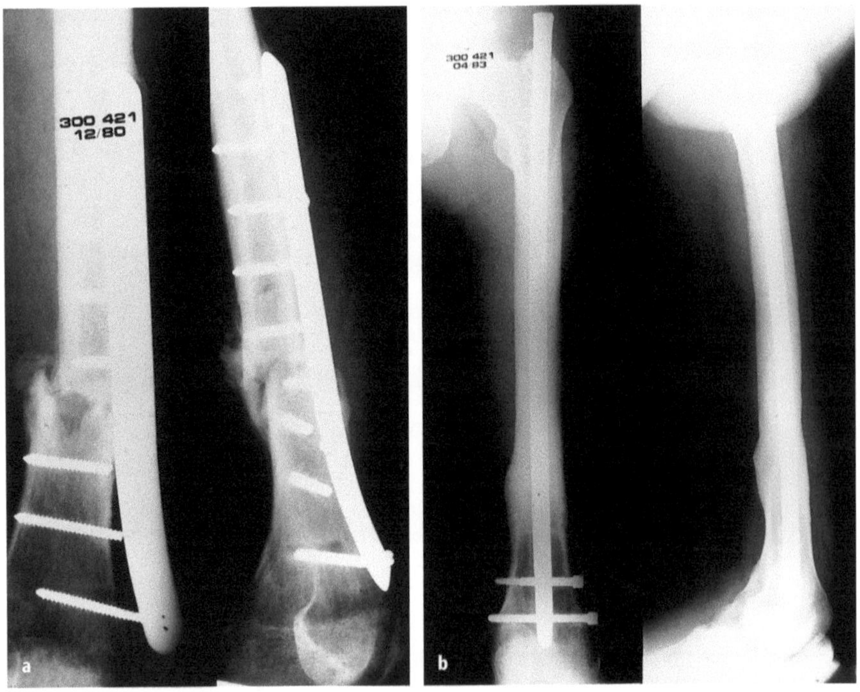

**Fig. 6.9. a** Distal femoral nonunion after a plate osteosynthesis. **b** Consolidation after distal dynamic locked nailing

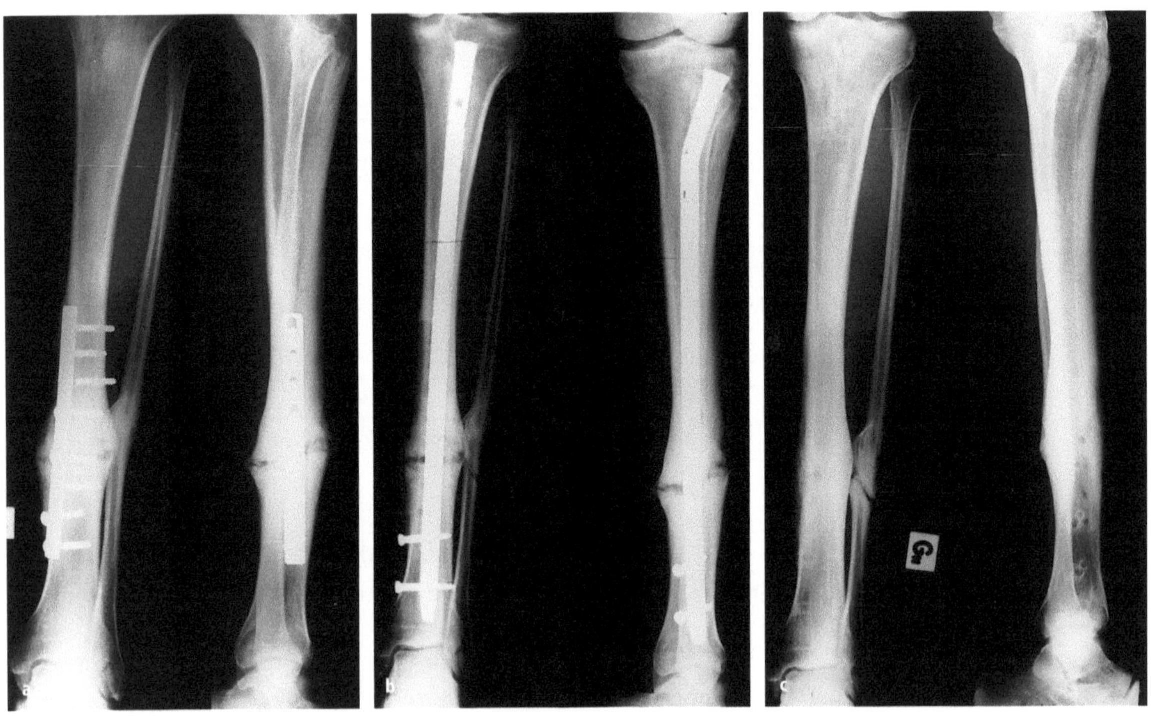

**Fig. 6.10. a** Distal tibial hypertrophic nonunion. Plate osteosynthesis. **b** Distal dynamic locked nailing. Oblique fibula osteotomy. **c** Late result after material removal

callus, especially in very old nonunions, we propose a closed approach using the intramedullary saw to perform a corrective osteotomy to achieve the reduction. On rare occasions, it is necessary to do an open osteotomy, using a minimal skin incision (1–2 cm) and a small chisel to cut the bone, aided by fluoroscopic monitoring. Again, the approach must be as minimal as possible, to respect closed procedure principles.

It is also very important to carry out reduction before reaming and nailing to avoid fixing a malunion permanently.

At times old pseudarthrosis will have a closed medullary canal at the fracture ends caused by endosteal consolidation, sometimes with very hard bone. For these cases, we use a special large curved guide, with a very sharp point at the end, which is inserted using a mallet, guided by fluoroscopic monitoring, thus reopening the medullary canal. The original Küntscher sharp guidewire can also been used (Fig. 6.7).

Small reamers (8 mm) are then utilized to progressively enlarge the medullary canal of the proximal fragment. This procedure is repeated as many times as necessary, in order to remove the sclerotic bone from the obstructed canal, which is then enlarged with the classic reaming procedure.

For atrophic pseudarthrosis, the problem is more complex. This is pseudarthrosis with a bone defect or is encountered after multiple nailings with the open procedure at the fracture site. The fracture fragments are like necrotic avascular bone, with no healing capacities. In these very particular and rare cases, a new nailing, even with reaming, is not sufficient to obtain consolidation. These are the only cases for which we advocate an open procedure, with the Judet technique [2], consisting in a gentle osteomuscular decortication, fresh autologous cancellous graft, and a certain amount of necrotic bone resection leading, unfortunately, to some shortening to obtain union of pseudarthrosis.

## Discussion and Conclusion

Interlocking nailing for aseptic nonunions of the femur and the tibia, especially proximal and distal nonunions, which are more difficult to treat with other methods, is an excellent method of treatment (Figs. 6.8–6.10), as long as the method is respected, a method based essentially on the closed procedure of reaming and nailing, proper alignment of the bone fragments, and a correct dynamic system based on early rehabilitation and weight-bearing. This method has led to healing nonunions at a success rate of 92%–95% in a series of 27 femurs and 39 tibias, with a low rate of morbidity, at times in very difficult cases [3].

Borderline indications remain atrophic pseudarthrosis with or without bone defect, where it can be necessary to open the nonunion site to add cancellous grafting.

## References

1. Basset A, Mitchel S, Schink M (1982) Treatment of therapeutically resistant non unions with bone graft and pulsing electromagnetic fields. J Bone Joint Surg 64A:1214
2. Judet J, Judet R (1965) La décortication ostéopériostée. Principe, technique, indications et résultats. Mem Acad Chir 91:463
3. Kempf I, Grosse A, Rigaut P (1986) The treatment of non infected pseudarthrosis of the femur and tibia with locked intramedullary nailing. Clin Orthop Relat Res 212:142–154
4. Kempf I, Grosse A, Karger C (1990) Traitement des pseudarthroses aseptiques du fémur et du tibia par l'enclouage centro-medullaire: apport du verrouillage, cahiers d'enseignement de la SOFCOT (Vol 36), Paris, Expansion Scientifique Française
5. Muller ME, Thomas JR (1979) Treatment of nonunion in fractures of long bones. Clin Orthop 138:141
6. Rosen H (1980) Compression treatment of long bone pseudarthrosis. Clin Orthop 148:117
7. Weber BG, Chech O (1976) Pseudarthrosis. Huber, Bern

# CHAPTER 7

# Retrograde Nailing of Fractures

P.H. Breedveld, J.P.A.M. Verbruggen, J.W.J.L. Stapert

In the contemporary operative technique of intramedullary (IM) nailing for the treatment of injuries of the humerus, femur, and tibia, as a standard the medullar canal is opened somewhere in the proximal part of the shaft. In selected cases, however, the patient can benefit from a retrograde introduction of IM nails.

## Femoral Fractures

Since the work of Seligson [6], who introduced a retrograde nail for the treatment of supracondylar femoral fractures, it is clear that there are only very few consequences for a healthy knee joint if the joint is opened to insert a retrograde nail [7, 9] (Figs. 7.1, 7.2).

Also, so-called normal femoral nails can be inserted retrograde through the knee joint [11]. In general, the procedure takes less time than the orthograde approach because the reduction of the fractures is easier. At this time, several indications for retrograde nailing are recognized.

## Indications for Retrograde Nailing

Several indications are suitable for retrograde nailing.

1. Multiple-trauma patients with femoral fractures to avoid the need to reposition the patient (Fig. 7.3).
2. A combination of a displaced acetabular fracture or a pelvic fracture component and a homolateral fracture of the femoral shaft to avoid an incision in the region of the pelvis in order not to compromise delayed repair of the pelvic or acetabular fracture.
3. Bilateral femoral fractures where the procedure can be shortened essentially because there is no need to place the patient in traction.
4. Femoral shaft fractures in patients with morbid obesity where orthograde nailing is more difficult due to the fat around the hip joint.
5. Patients with femoral shaft fractures below a prosthesis, osteosynthesis, or arthrodesis in the proximal femur or hip joint [5] and fractures proximal to a knee prosthesis [2].
6. Floating knee: a combination of homolateral femoral and tibial fractures. Osteosynthesis can be performed through one incision. Problems with the positioning of the patient with this combination of fractures [1] on the traction table are avoided (Fig. 7.5).
7. Nailing of femoral shaft fractures in children [3, 4, 8], in order not to damage the growth plate of the greater trochanter.

## Operative Technique and Tips

### Positioning the Patient

In most cases, a traction table is used with only the central post in position. It is not necessary to use the traction capabilities of the table.

The patient is positioned supine on the table. If there are no injuries to the pelvis a post is placed between the legs to counteract the manual traction during the reduction of the fracture. The injured leg is supported by a role or pad in order to ensure that the knee joint is flexed to about 30°–45° (Fig. 7.3).

If there is a combination with an unstable pelvic fracture, the pelvis is stabilized first with an external fixator. This fixator can be attached to the traction table.

Before the sterile part of the operation is started, the position of the image intensifier is checked to ensure that the entire femur can be seen.

### Entry Point

It is not necessary to make a large incision in the skin or patella tendon.

A 1-in. vertical incision will be enough to perform the reaming and insert the nail. If the knee joint is flexed to about 30°–45° the incision will be just distal to the apex of the patella. The patella tendon is split longitudinally to gain access to the knee.

In the adult patient, the entry point of the medullar canal is chosen with the help of the image intensifier. In AP and lateral views, the entry point should be exactly in the anatomical length axis of the femoral shaft. This point lies approximately 1 cm above the intracondylar notch (Fig. 7.4). If this spot is used, there is no interference with the fibers of the posterior cruciate ligament or with the weight-bearing cartilage of the knee joint or patellar femoral joint.

## Reduction of the Fracture

It is usually very easy to obtain good reduction of the fracture by simple traction on the knee with the leg flexed at 30°–45° [12]. Sometimes external manipulations are necessary to bring the fracture elements into line. After reduction, the reamer guide is passed along the fracture and reaming is started.

The reaming procedure should be performed as is done in the orthograde procedure. Care should be taken not to damage the patellar tendon with the reamer.

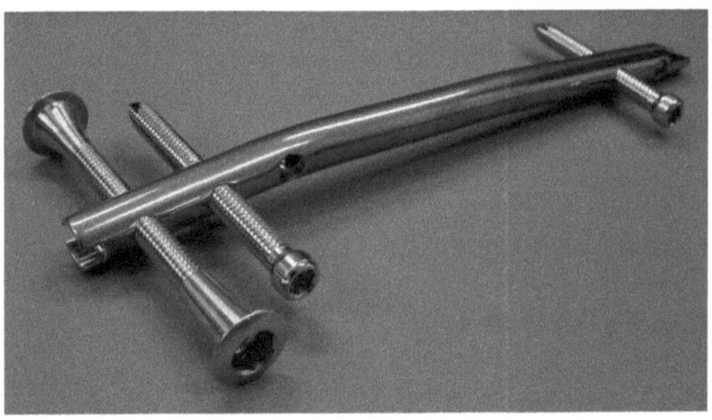

**Fig. 7.1.** Example of a supracondylar nail

## Inserting the Nail

Before the operation is started, one must determine whether the available target device has the right shape for the retrograde technique. If not, distal locking must also be performed with a freehand technique.

In some nail systems it is possible to perform the proximal and distal locking in the AP direction. At all times, care must be taken to ensure that image intensifier monitoring of the locking screw position is possible. This is easier when locking can be performed in the AP direction. While locking in the AP direction, care should be taken to avoid injury to the neurovascular system of the leg. It must be remembered that the sciatic nerve runs very close to the posterior aspect of the proximal femur.

After inserting the nail and locking, some surgeons irrigate the knee joint in order to remove drilling debris. We have never done so without adverse effects to the knee joint. In selected cases, if there is so-called back bleeding through the nail, a 24-h Redon drainage can be left in the knee.

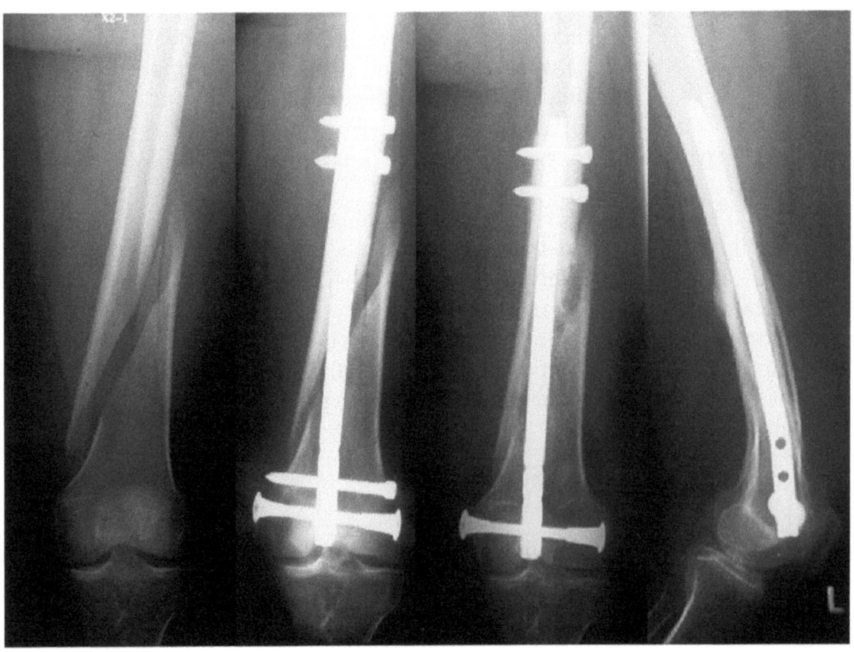

**Fig. 7.2.** Distal femur shaft fracture in a 58-year-old female patient treated with supracondylar nail. Pre- and postoperative image and image after 8 months

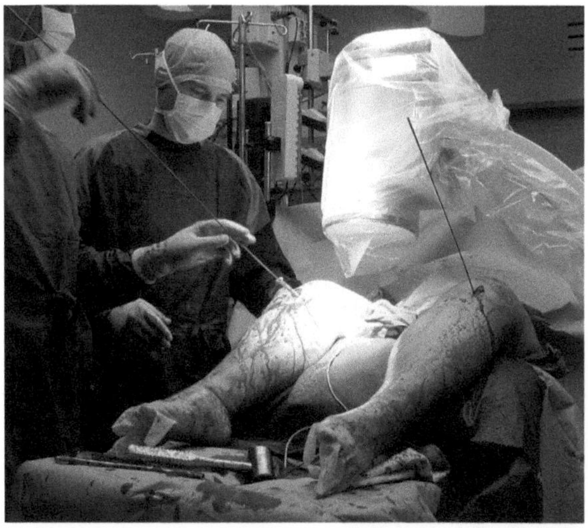

**Fig. 7.3.** Positioning a patient for retrograde nailing of the femur. In this case, a multitrauma patient underwent laparotomy, pelvic stabilization and simultaneous nailing of bilateral femur shaft fractures on the same operating table

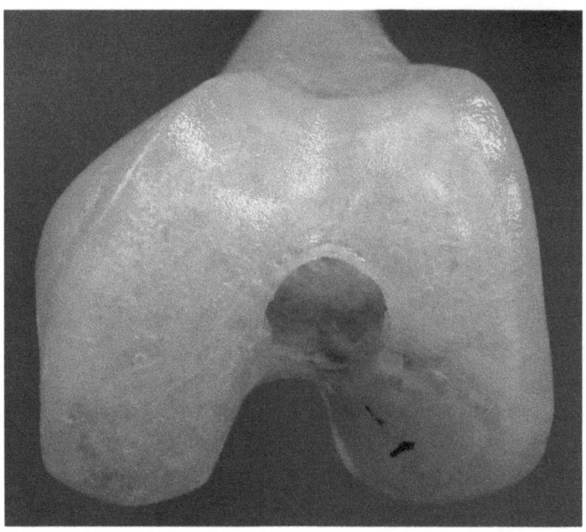

**Fig. 7.4.** Entry point of the femur for retrograde nailing

In cases with a floating knee nailing, the femur and tibia nailing procedure can be performed through the same incision. It is not necessary to visualize the entry point to the tibia if the entry point is chosen right on the edge of the tibia plateau.

We prefer to operate on tibia fractures with the aid of a temporary external fixator between the proximal tibia and the calcaneus on the medial side of the leg. When working with a floating knee, we start by attaching this fixator to the lower leg first and then proceed with the femur fracture, and lastly nail the tibia fracture. This allows easier manipulation of the leg during the entire procedure.

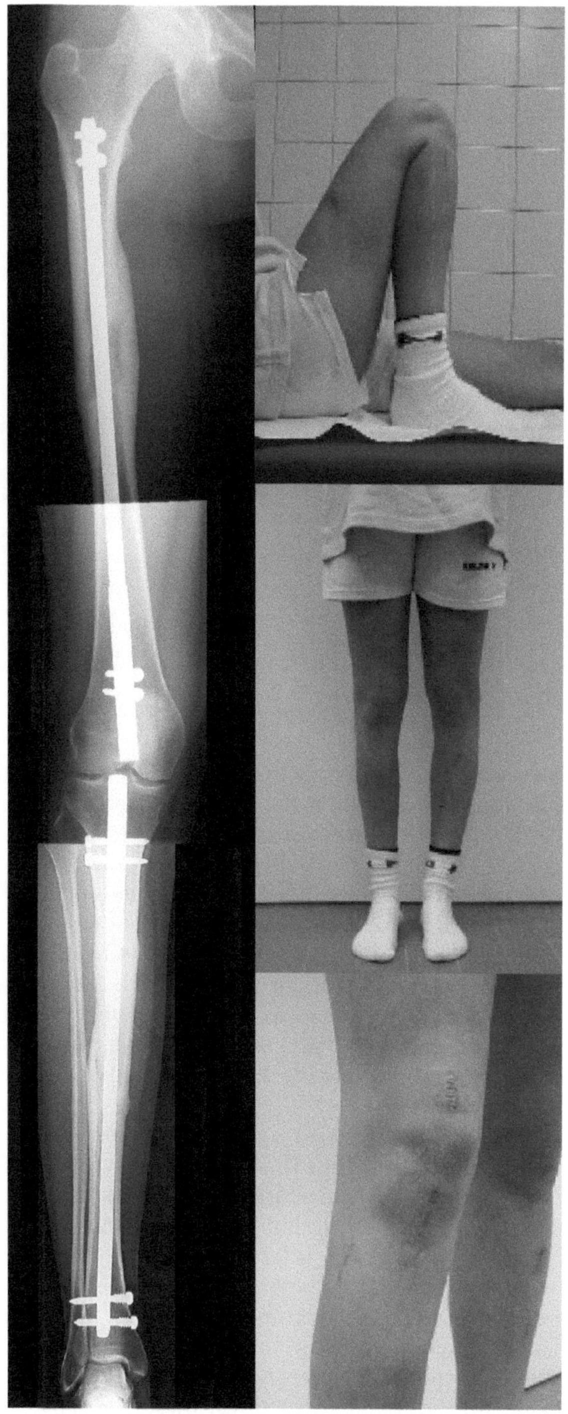

**Fig. 7.5.** Female patient, 19 years old, floating knee treated with retrograde femur and antegrade tibia nailing. Results after 1-year follow-up

## Special Nails Designed for Retrograde Nailing of Supracondylar Femur Fractures

Various types of nails have been designed for retrograde nailing of distal fractures of the femur

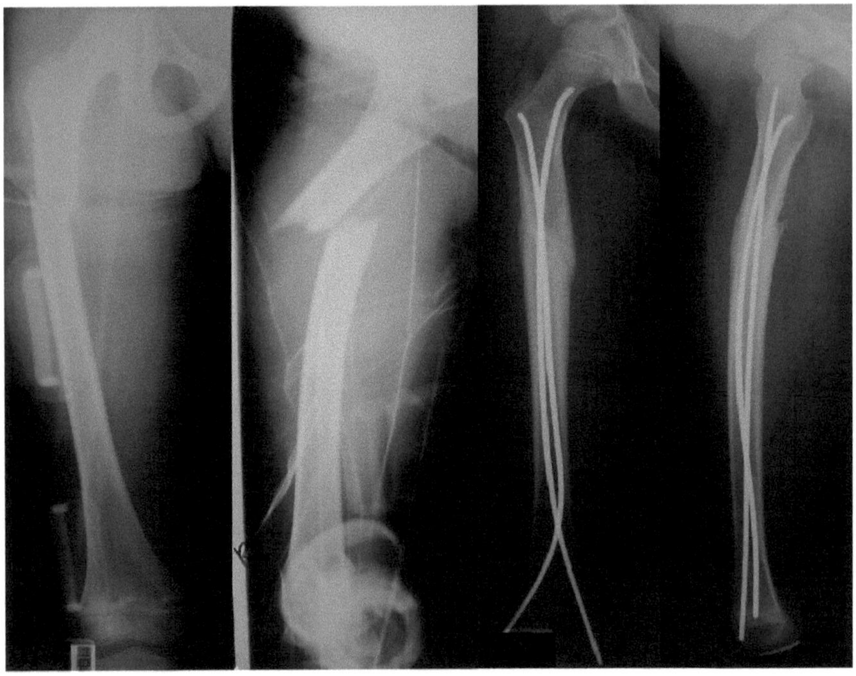

**Fig. 7.6.** Male patient, 7 years old, proximal femur shaft fracture treated with Prevot nails. Preoperative image and results after 4 months. Note that the medial nail was inserted too ventrally, causing some temporary knee complaints

since the work of Green, Seligson, and Henry [6]. These nails are especially designed for treatment of distal femur fractures, including intra-articular fractures. The nails are usually mounted on a target device, which allows distal and proximal locking. Most nails have a small curve to allow easier positioning in the distal femur. Some nails have a special type of locking screws, which have a nut-and-bolt design to allow compression over the screw. To enhance grip in osteoporotic bone, there are also web-shaped locking screws available with nut-and-bolt design.

Operative technique and tips are in general the same as for other femur fractures. However, in the case of intra-articular fractures, one should first make a reconstruction of both condyles, either provisionally with a large reposition clamp or with separate screws, before inserting the nail. Compression over the fracture in cases of intra-articular fracture can be achieved using the above-mentioned compression locking screws.

Even in type B and C fractures, these specially designed retrograde nails can result in osteosynthesis, which allows for early weight-bearing. This is of particular advantage to the elderly patient.

Special care should be taken when these nails are used in case of a fracture below a hip prosthesis. It must be realized that there is great stress force in the femur segment just distal to the stem of the hip prosthesis and proximal to the tip of the retrograde nail. The femur segment between the two should be large enough and free of bone cracks to carry this stress force successfully.

## Femoral Fractures in Children

In children femoral shaft fractures can be treated with elastic Prevot or Metaizeau nails [3, 4, 8]. Here the entry point is chosen just proximal from the distal epiphysis on the medial and lateral side of the upper leg. The entry point can be made very easily with a small awl on the posterior part of the medial or lateral aspect of the distal femur. If, as in Ender nailing, the entry point is chosen too far on the ventral side children will have many more complaints about the protruding nails near the knee joint (Fig. 7.6).

After opening the medullar canal, at least two prebend nails are inserted to stabilize the fracture.

## Tibia Fractures in Children

Proximal tibial fractures in children can be treated with retrograde nailing from entry points on the medial and lateral aspect of the distal tibia. The same operative technique is used as for the femur.

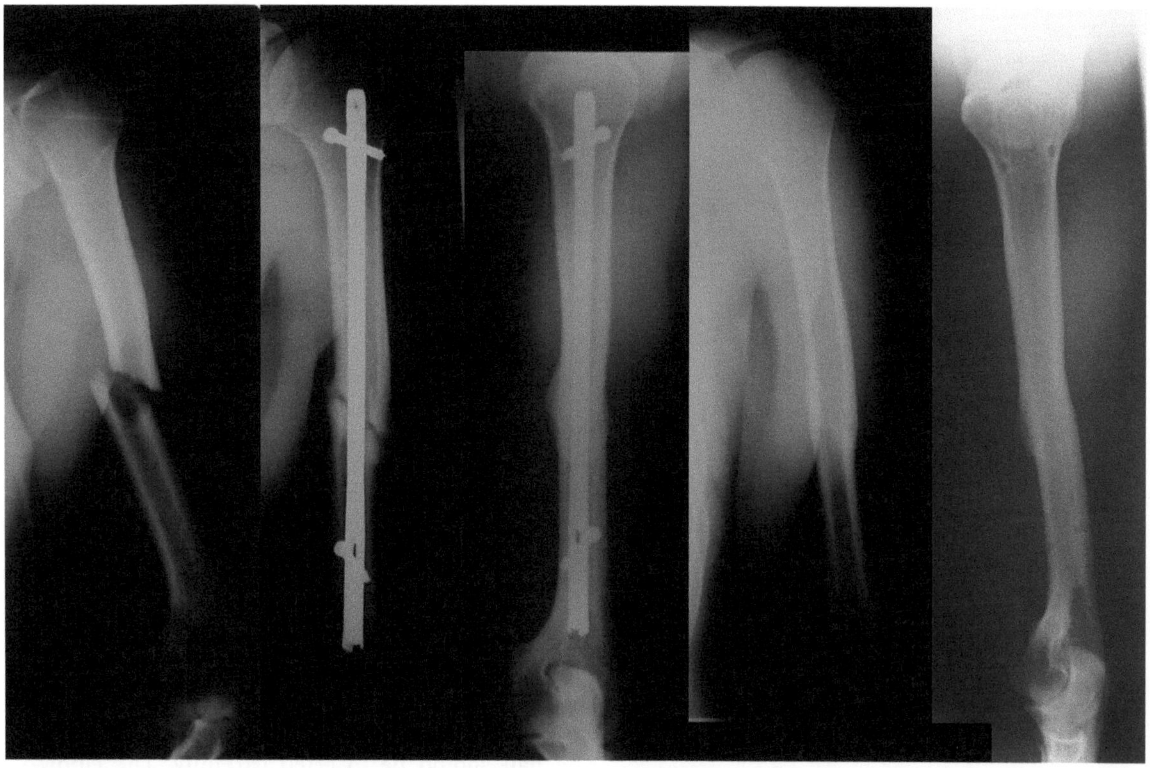

**Fig. 7.7.** Male patient, 37 years old, humerus shaft fracture with primary radial palsy. The radial nerve was found intact, riding over the fracture ends, and recovered completely. Stabilization of fracture with a retrograde telescopic locking nail. Preoperative image and results after 6 months and 22 months after nail removal

## Humerus Fractures

Humerus fractures can be treated with intramedullary nailing, both ante- and retrograde [10]. Modern nailing systems allow both approaches. The nails are usually more flexible than femur or tibia nails.

The advantage of the retrograde method over the antegrade approach is avoidance of damage to the shoulder capsule and hence there are fewer shoulder complaints. Proximal fractures are more easily treated using a retrograde approach, distal fractures with an antegrade approach. The retrograde approach is more delicate, requiring a precise entry point and smooth instrumentation to avoid fractures around the entry point.

### Indications for Retrograde Nailing

1. Proximal or midshaft humerus fractures, including open fractures, especially those fractures which seem to be less suitable for early functional treatment, e.g., spiral fractures of the proximal humerus.
2. Multiple-trauma patients with a humerus fracture, to facilitate adequate nursing care and faster mobilization. Examples are bilateral humerus fractures, floating elbow, segmental fractures in humerus fractures, and humerus fractures in combination with fractures of the lower extremity.
3. Humerus fractures combined with neurovascular injury, for example, in cases of primary or secondary radial palsy. In both cases, we visualize the radial nerve at the fracture site to allow primary repair if needed. We then proceed with nailing of the fracture (Fig. 7.7). We prefer nailing over plating in these cases in order not to have to compromise the radial nerve a second time if it becomes necessary to remove the osteosynthetic material.
4. Delayed union of humerus fractures. Care should be taken to gain solid osteosynthesis. This can be facilitated by using locking nails with a compression mechanism and encircling wire loops where needed. Also, the use of spongy-bone grafting is mandatory. The bone graft can be done locally or through the medullar canal. If solid osteosynthesis cannot be achieved

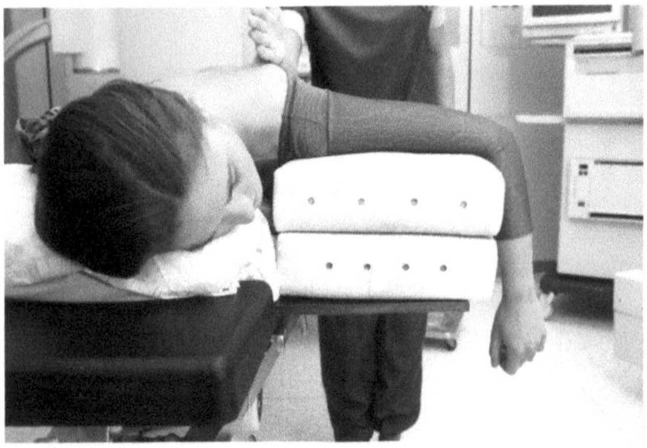

**Fig. 7.8.** Positioning the patient for retrograde nailing of the humerus

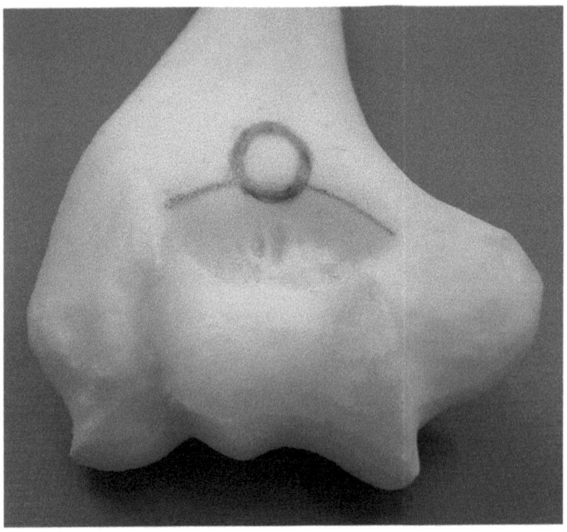

**Fig. 7.9.** Entry point of the distal humerus for the intramedullary approach

with a nailing system one should consider conventional plating as a good alternative.

5. Subcapital humerus fractures can be approached with retrograde nailing using a locking nail or multiple Prevot nails. Retrograde procedures allow early mobilization of the shoulder without further compromising the joint.
6. Pathological fractures or impending fractures of the humerus shaft.

## Operative Technique and Tips

### *Positioning the Patient*

The patient is put in a prone position with the humerus and shoulder on a small radiolucent side table. The forearm is allowed to hang free so that the elbow is flexed at 90° (Fig. 7.8).

An incision is made from the olecranon upwards, splitting the triceps tendon longitudinally.

The entry point of the humerus lies at the edge of the olecranon fossa, in line with the medullar canal of the humerus (Fig. 7.9). The canal can be opened using a small drill, drilling first at right angles with the humerus, then slowly moving the drill in line with the humeral shaft. The shaft is further opened using drills with increasing diameter in order to allow the introduction of a reamer guide and an 8-mm reamer. Repositioning the fracture is done while inserting the reamer guide. Reaming then proceeds in 0.5-mm steps until the required diameter is reached. One must never ream at the fracture site in comminute fractures, to avoid damage to the soft tissue and radial nerve. One should also avoid too much pressure opposite the entry point. Excessive reaming at this spot can make the bone thin and susceptible to an intraoperative fracture of the distal humerus.

### *Insertion of the Nail*

The nail should be inserted carefully. The elbow should be flexed maximally to keep the olecranon out of the way, thereby avoiding stress at the entry point. The humerus should not be rotated while the target device is mounted on the nail, to avoid stress fractures. AP and lateral views with a rotating image intensifier are taken to confirm the position of the nail.

Distal locking can be done with a targeting device or using the free-hand method; proximal locking is most often done using the free-hand method. Some nails have a compression mechanism which is installed after locking.

The insertion of Prevot nails follows the same procedure as IM nailing, except that reaming is not necessary. The number of nails which can be introduced depends on the size of the Prevot nails and the diameter of the shaft. Usually three to four nails can be inserted, fanning out with their tips in the humeral head.

## References

1. Gregory P, DiCicco J, Karpik K, DiPasquale T, Herscovici D, Sanders R (1999) Ipsilateral fractures of the femur and tibia: treatment with retrograde femoral nailing and unreamed tibial nailing. J Orthop Trauma 10:309–316
2. Henry SL (1995) Management of supracondylar fractures proximal to total knee arthroplasty with the GSH supracondylar nail. Contemp Orthop 31:231–238

3. Ligier JN, Metaizeau JP, Prevot J (1983) Closed flexible medullary nailing in pediatric traumatology. Chir Pediatr 24:383–385
4. Ligier JN, Metaizeau JP, Prevot J, Lascombes P (1988) Elastic stable intramedullary nailing of femoral shaft fractures in children. J Bone Joint Surg Br 70:74–77
5. Lonner BS, Lonner JH, Sadler AH (1995) Retrograde femoral nailing between an ankylosed hip and a stiff knee. J Orthop Trauma 9:266–269
6. Lucas SE, Seligson D, Henry SL (1993) Intramedullary supracondylar nailing of femoral fractures. A preliminary report of the GSH supracondylar nail. Clin Orthop 296:200–206
7. Moed BR, Watson JT (1996) Retrograde nailing of the femoral shaft. J Am Acad Orthop Surg 7:209–216
8. Oestern HJ, Rieger G, Jansen T (2000) The internal fixation of fractures in children. Unfallchirurg 103:2–11
9. Ostrum RF, Agarwal A, Lakatos R, Poka A (2000) Prospective comparison of retrograde and antegrade femoral intramedullary nailing. J Orthop Trauma 14:496–501
10. Rommens PM, Verbruggen J, Broos PL (1995) Retrograde interlocking nailing of fracture of the humeral shaft. A clinical study. Unfallchirurg 98:133–138
11. Sanders R, Koval KJ, DiPasquale T, Helfet DL, Frankle M (1993) Retrograde reamed femoral nailing. J Orthop Trauma 7:293–302
12. Tornetta P III, Tiburzi D (2000) Antegrade or retrograde reamed femoral nailing. A prospective, randomised trial. J Bone Joint Surg Br 82:652–654

# CHAPTER 8

# Osteotomies of the Femoral Diaphysis by Closed Technique

D. Grosse, D. Brinkert, I. Kempf

Locked intramedullary nailing has been shown to be effective as a fixation option for osteotomies resulting from malunions of the femur. A series of 42 cases of open osteotomies [11] revealed, interestingly, that statically locked intramedullary nailing was accompanied by a significant rate of complications when performed by open procedure. The complications occured mostly for lengthening and shortening osteomies and included nonunions, numerous infections, possibly associated with the destruction of the intramedullary blood supply as a result of reaming, and devascularization of the periosteum by virtue of the open approach to the osteotomy site.

Küntscher, however, had already suggested that correcting osteotomies of the femur should be done using closed methods because of the advantages already known. Osteotomy with an intramedullary saw using a closed technique was proposed and fine-tuned by Küntscher in 1964 [15]. Associated with locked intramedullary nailing, it combined several advantages: lower infection rates, better environment for bone consolidation and healing. We have used this technique of closed intramedullary osteotomy since 1987 for length discrepancies (lengthening or shortening osteotomies) as well as for malunions in rotation or varus/valgus.

## Materials Used

For the earlier cases in our series (until the 2nd trimester of 1993), we used Küntscher's intramedullary saw. In 1964, Küntscher [14, 15] developed a small circular saw to split long bones from the inside. The bones were reamed with an intramedullary reamer so that a circular saw blade attached on a long shaft with a protector could be inserted in the shaft.

The shaft was bowed in the area of the rotatory saw allowing the saw, after partial removal of the protector, to cut the bone with rotatory movements. This was continued until the entire bone was split. For noncylindrical bones, splitting in this way was not entirely possible and was achieved using external forces (Fig. 8.1).

Professor Küntscher developed a variety of intramedullary (IM) saws. All of them had a decisive disadvantage: inappropriate or untrained use of the saws made them dangerous and sometimes led to other injuries. Therefore we developed an easier and safer saw for all types of osteomies, bringing in the collaboration of Dr. Hempel [8, 9], who had experience with an American IM saw made by Boeing. The disadvantages mentioned in the preceding paragraph should be rectified with the new models (Figs. 8.2, 8.3).

The concept of the new saw is different from previous saws. All activities are exclusively done by hand, all the functional elements are in the upper part of the device. The shaft is flexible and therefore also adequate for use on the tibia. The graduated scale very precisely indicates the distance for the splitting level as well as the length for the shortening osteotomy.

Bone splitting is done using the progressive exit possibilities of the saw by means of a handle with a wheel. The saw blades fit to the saw-blade protector which are 14, 16, and 17 mm in diameter. The bone is cut by the blade progressively coming out through the eccentric part of the blade. The blades are equipped with a new design of cutting teeth.

So that the shaft and the protector enter more easily, intramedullary reaming should be at least 1 mm larger than the eccentric diameter to be used.

The instrument works in a cutting area of approximately 90–250 mm below the saw's point of contact.

We also use specific instruments developed by Küntscher:

- Ball-shaped reamers for thinning the cortical wall to reduce the thickness of the bone to be severed or for splitting the cylinder in cases where shortening osteotomy is required (Fig. 8.4 a)
- A retrograde, crochet-shaped chisel for splitting a severed cylinder (Fig. 8.4 b)
- A metal ruler for direct measurements (Fig. 8.4 c)

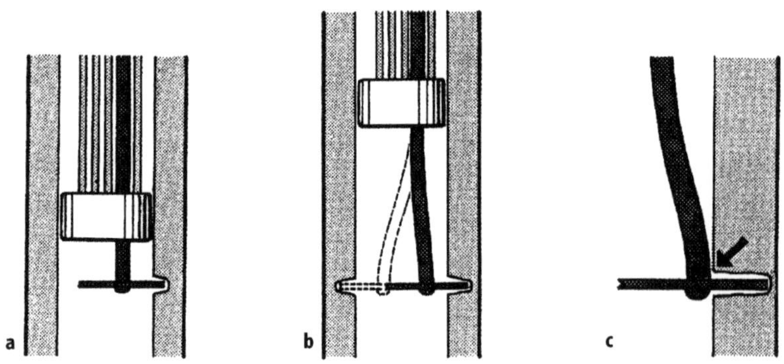


**Fig. 8.1 a–c.** Küntscher intramedullary saw with distal bend axis. **a** First introduction of the saw without bend axis. **b** With retrograde tube, the bend axis has full function. **c** The ability of the rotating saw to cut the cortical bone is limited by the axis

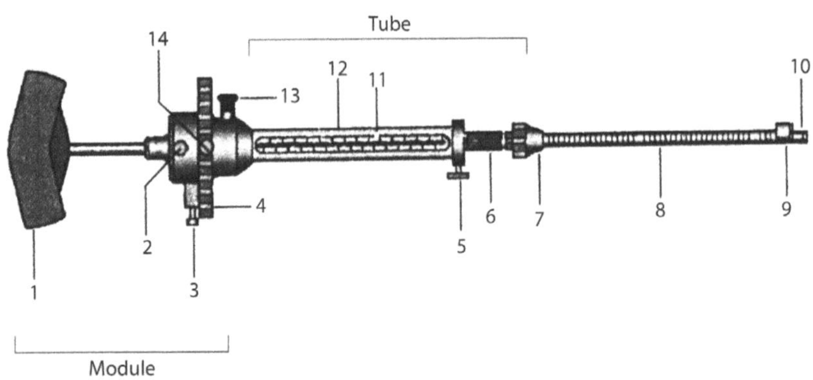


**Fig. 8.2.** The new intramedullary saw. *1*, Handle; *2*, pushbutton for locking/unlocking the saw shaft; *3*, pushbutton for setting cutting radius (measured in degrees); *4*, locking plate; *5*, screw for securing/loosening the distance rod; *6*, adjustable distance rod; *7*, taper with milled ring; *8*, flexible shaft; *9*, eccentric (saw blade protector); *10*, saw shaft with blade; *11*, position maker; *12*, tube/supporting handle with scale for displaying the distance rod setting; *13*, release button for separating module and tube components, *14*, screw for securing/loosening the flexible shaft

## Operative Technique

The patient is placed on the orthopaedic table in the supine position, with traction on the limb to be operated on, achieved by a transcondylar Steinmann pin fixed to the table by a stirrup. This is the classic positioning for IM nailing as described by Kempf and Grosse. Attention must be paid to the amount of adduction applied to the operative limb, so as to make it easy to position the IM saw the length of the patient's flank.

After fluoroscopic location of the entry point at the tip of the greater trochanter with the pointed awl, the reaming guidewire is inserted. It may be necessary at times to use a pseudoarthrosis guide for cases where there is a malunion and the canal is blocked. Preliminary reaming is completed on the full length of the femur. Then, once a reaming diameter of 16 mm has been reached, reaming is continued only to the level where the postoperatively planned osteotomy is to be undertaken. To make it easier to insert the saw into the canal, we always ream 1 mm greater than the saw used. Then the saw is inserted into the medullary canal. We recommend that the entire femur (proximally as well as distally) be reamed to at least 16 mm. This will allow the placement of a large nail, which will limit postoperative bleeding and help to avoid any secondary malposition.

The depth of the medullary cut is displayed on the graduated depth gauge. After the introduction of the saw into the canal, the adjustable stop abuts the tip of the greater trochanter. It is suggested that the cut be made at the level of the junction of the middle third and distal third of the femoral diaphysis, at the level where the femoral flare begins to open. The mechanical stresses imposed on the nail are fewer at this level than in osteotomies done in the proximal third. It is only in shortening osteotomies that certain authors have demonstrated that it is perhaps preferable to make the osteotomy higher, for better rehabilitation of the quadriceps muscle.

The instrument is inserted into the medullary cavity with the blade in a neutral position (the cursor is on 0°). Obtaining AP and lateral fluoroscopic views monitors the correct positioning of

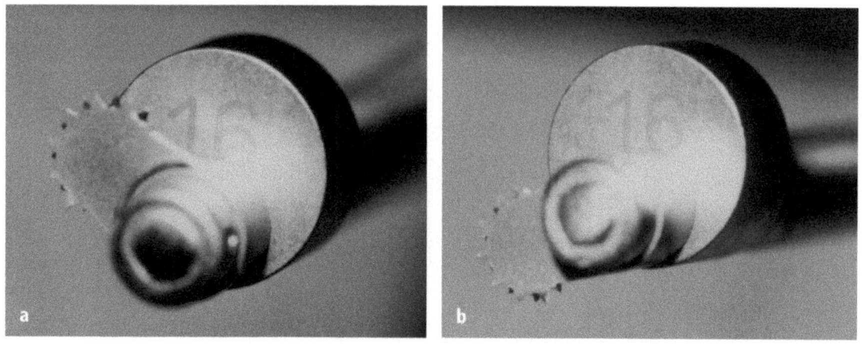

**Fig. 8.3 a, b.** Eccentric saw shaft with blade protector. **a** The saw is coming out; **b** the saw has come out completely

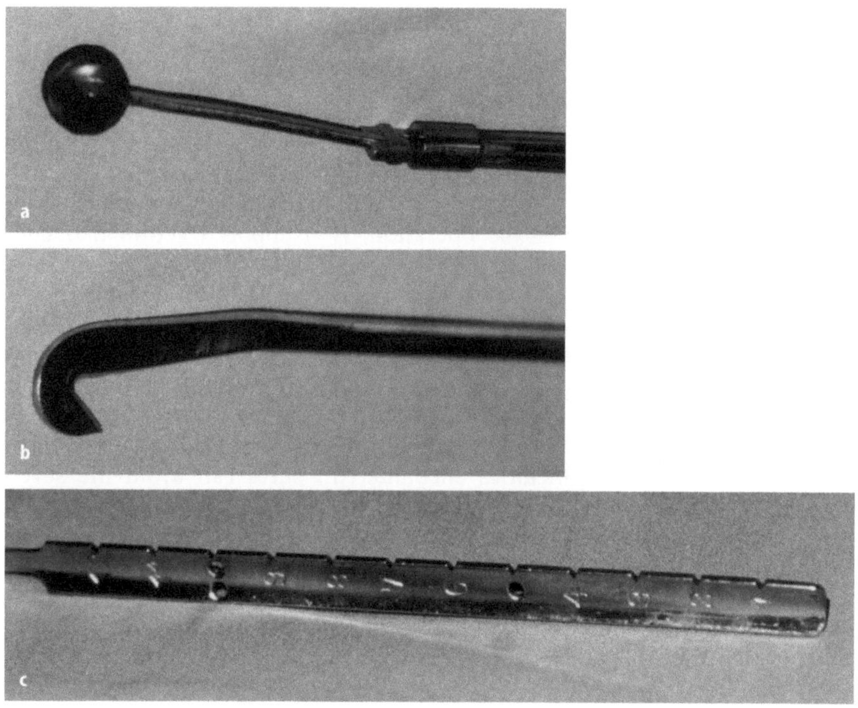

**Fig. 8.4 a–c.** Küntscher specific instrumentation. **a** Spherical reamer. **b** Special hook. **c** Graduated scale

the saw. Then the blade is progressively extended in steps of 10°, aided by the cursor on the handle.

Three complete rotations of the instrument are required for each step of the cut. If the operator feels that there is resistance, he should retract the blade by 10° and continue with cutting increments of 5°. The instrument gives the feeling of gentle grating or rasping. The amount of work that the blade is doing should be confirmed regularly, until the full 180° cut has been achieved.

Before removing the saw, it is imperative to ensure that the cursor on the handle has been returned to 0°. The saw is gently retracted, using semi-circular motions.

The severing is completed by means of an osteoclasia, usually accomplished with external manipulations by the operator himself at the operative site. The goal is to disrupt any persistent, intact cortex (most often at the linea aspera of the femur) and to stretch the periosteal connections and the osteotomy apart to achieve the desired correction. The osteoclasia procedure is made easiest when a sufficiently large medullary diameter has been reamed. A large-diameter saw blade can thus be used and the depth of the cut is therefore greater (Fig. 8.5).

Depending on the skills of the surgeon, it is sometimes preferable to reinsert the intramedullary guide to facilitate nail insertion. Once the desired correction has been achieved, static locked, intramedullary nailing is completed, as described by Kempf and Grosse. Static locking is essential in all osteotomies, in order to avoid the loss of correction described by certain authors and to avoid malposition in rotation.

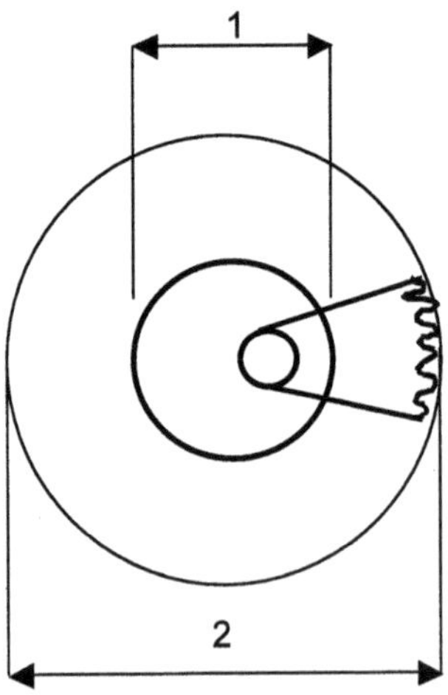


**Fig. 8.5.** Incidence of the saw diameter with the diameter from the bone section. *1*, Medullary canal diameter; *2*, maximal bone section

Blood loss, during and after the operation, is abundant, on the order of 900 ml at 100% hematocrit, on average (calculated blood loss), which corresponds to approximately 2.5 l. It is also suggested that in planning such an operation, the patient's own blood be collected for later autotransfusion so as to avoid heterologous blood transfusion.

The operative time is extremely variable, depending on the technical difficulties encountered (patent or obstructed medullary canal, etc.), the skills of the surgeon, and the type of osteotomy to be done. We have found the operative time to range from 1 h and 5 min to 4 h, the longer time caused by the Küntscher saw blade breaking.

## Special Techniques According to the Type of Osteotomy

### Intramedullary Osteotomy for One-Stage Lengthening

Based on our experience with one-stage lengthening [3, 13, 19] using open methods with in situ autologous bone grafting [13, 18], we are able to achieve a closed osteotomy with one-stage lengthening of a femoral segment and the placement of the cancellous bone graft via the medullary canal or, more recently, using a percutaneous technique. This type of grafting is sometimes insufficient and has to be completed by secondary decortication and autologous corticospongious graft.

The correction desired is measured very precisely on X-ray plates with grids for exact measurements.

Lengthening is obtained by applying traction by pulling on the Steinmann pin. This pin will support traction that generally will allow a one-stage lengthening of 2–2.5 cm. Attention should be paid to pelvic support, which must be sufficiently large and well padded. In addition, the traction should never be applied until the actual lengthening is started and the nail is inserted. When the nail has been locked distally, the traction is released as rapidly as possible. These measures can avoid the severe complication of perineum necrosis, fortunately occurring only once at the beginning of our experience.

The amount of lengthening can be determined by relating the length to the diameter of the IM saw blade. Although some authors advocate this method, due to its lack of precision, we prefer to use the graduated metal ruler designed by Küntscher. Once the lengthening has been done, material obtained from the reaming is inserted using a thoracic catheter via the medullary canal.

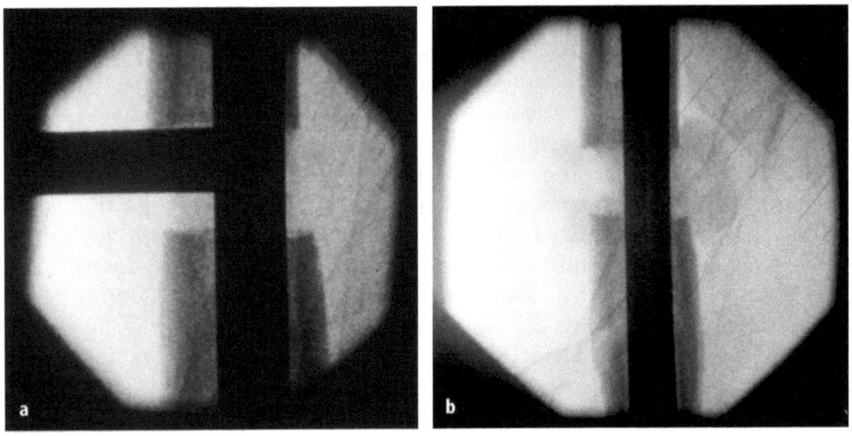


**Fig. 8.6 a, b.** Insertion of the osseous graft with a drill sleeve. **a** Positioning the sleeve; **b** the graft is in place

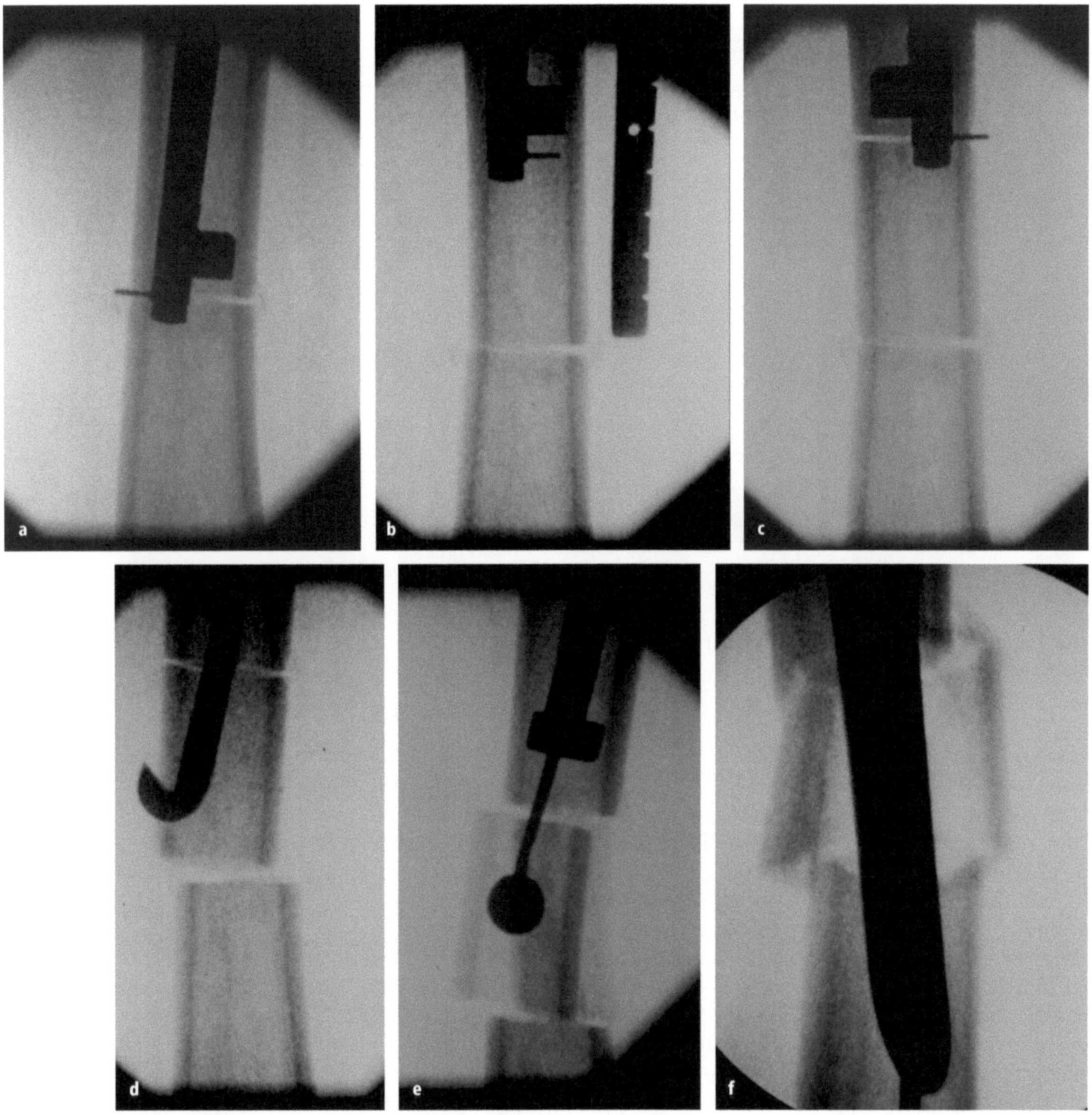


**Fig. 8.7 a–h.** Intramedullary shortening osteotomy. **a** Distal osteotomy. The saw has functioned as expected completely severing the bone. **b** Localization of the proximal osteotomy using the graduated ruler. **c** Successful proximal osteotomy. **d** Splitting of the fragment with a hook-shaped chisel. **e** The fragments are separated with a bowl-shaped reamer. **f** Insertion of the nail. **g** Impaction of the fragments by the progression of the nail and the counterpush of the transcondylar Steinmann pin. **h** Consolidation of including of the fragments of the shortening procedure

More recently, we have been placing this bone graft percutaneously using a drill sleeve from the nailing instruments under fluoroscopic monitoring (Fig. 8.6).

The time to union is long, nearly 10 months on average. When we sawed delayed unions or pseudoarthroses in our series, we felt that they were the result of too much lengthening (3 cm or greater). Union is then obtained by means of a second decortication and grafting operation. There has been no incidence of infection.

Vigilance is required so that sufficient flexion of the knee is maintained throughout the operation to avoid damaging the sciatic nerve by elongation. Moreover, in the first postoperative days, the patient's limb should be kept in flexion with a pillow while in bed. Placed under the knee, the pillow prevents undue tension on the sciatic nerve. It is only progressively that the full extension is recovered, with light physical therapy. Weight-bearing is not allowed right away. It is best to wait for the formation of a sufficient cal-

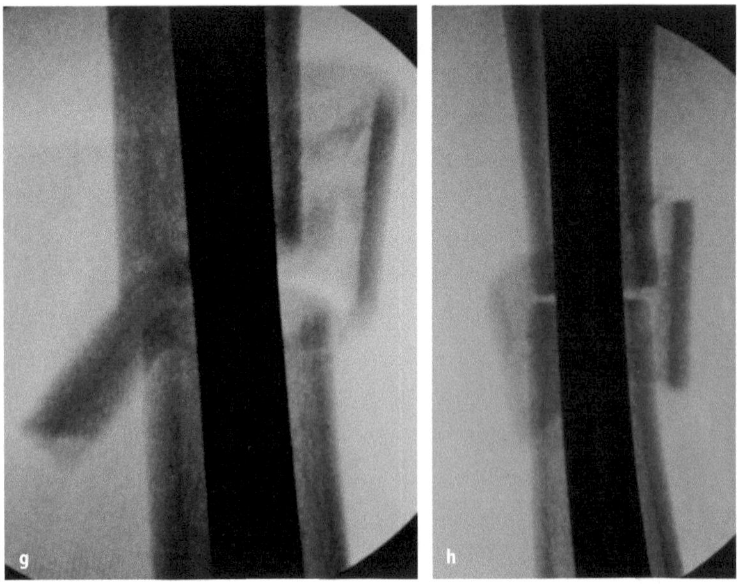

Fig. 8.7 g, h.

lous so that all of the force loads are not borne by the nail. In general, full weight-bearing is not allowed until 3 months after surgery.

## Shortening Osteotomies of the Femur

The set-up and the steps of the first osteotomy are the same as described "Operative Technique" [2, 5, 17].

A few specifics about positioning should be mentioned. It is not necessary to place a transcondylar Steinmann pin for traction. It should be noted that fluoroscopic monitoring will be needed after the shortening has been done. It may at times be necessary to position the patient eccentrically on the table, in order to have good fluoroscopic visualization of the proximal femur. Finally, it is necessary to have available a full range of nails of large and small diameters.

We recommend osteotomizing at the level of the middle and distal third of the femur where the canal begins to widen. There, the mechanical stresses are lower than at a more proximal level. Nevertheless, a more proximal resection of the bone will result in better recovery of the quadriceps muscle [10] (Fig. 8.7).

Shortening requires a second osteotomy. In order to remove the saw easily, we perform the distal osteotomy and osteoclasia and then the proximal osteotomy. Particular care must be taken with the proximal osteoclasia in order to avoid the posterior cracking described in numerous series. Here again, we insist that the canal be sufficiently reamed to maximize the efficiency of the saw.

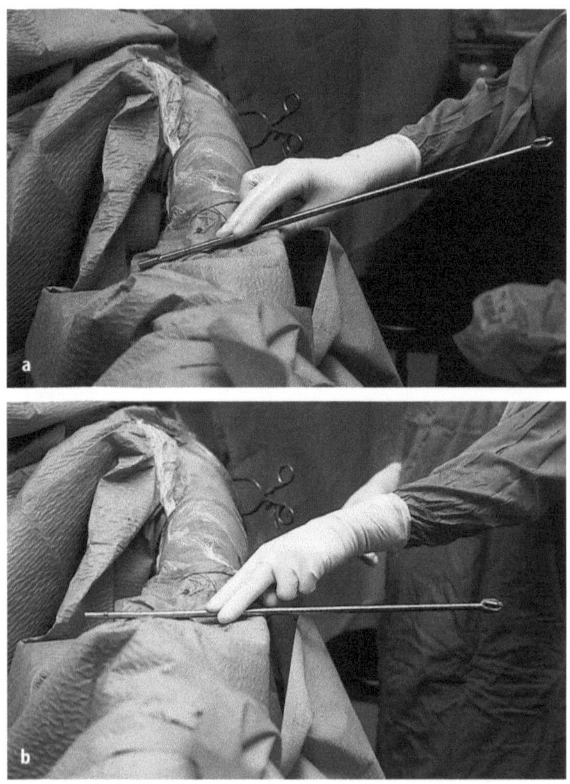

**Fig. 8.8 a, b.** Evaluation of the degrees of rotation osteotomy. **a** Preoperative angulation. **b** Postoperative angulation

The amount of shortening is determined by using the position maker on the intramedullary saw and checked by the Küntscher graduated ruler. This can be placed on the outside of the patient's thigh with a very small risk of error created by the variances caused by X-ray projection. Ideally, this ruler would be placed in the medullary canal. Some authors determine the amount of shortening to be done by comparing the actual diameter of the IM saw used (14, 16, or 17 mm) to the size projected on the screen.

Fragmentation of the intermediate osseous cylinder may be difficult. This is accomplished using a hook-shaped chisel designed by Küntscher. We use as a slightly modified model that allows us to connect the hook to a nail extraction slap-hammer. The easiest way, in our experience, is to make a false slice with the hook-shaped chisel placed tangentially to the circumference of the femoral diaphysis. Then, in orienting the chisel perpendicular to the distal cortex, it is hooked. The hooked chisel is then forcefully brought out, effectively cutting one of the cortical walls of the middle fragment. This step is carried out on the medial wall then on the lateral wall, creating hemi-cylinders anteriorly and posteriorly. The fragments are separated with the use of a bowl-shaped reamer.

Finally, inserting the nail using anteroposterior maneuvers positions both fragments well. After release of the traction, the impaction of the fragments is obtained both by the progression of the nail and the counterpush on the transcondylar Steinmann pin.

## Osteotomies in Rotational Deformities

This type of osteotomy requires a derotation angle that is as precise as possible. At the beginning of our experience, we used two pins, fixed in an angle for correction, one located in the proximal fragment and the other in the distal fragment. But problems arose when fixing the pins so that they would not be an obstacle during the intramedullary nailing procedure and in preventing deformity due to the tension of the soft tissues. We now prefer external measures.

At the beginning of the procedure, the leg is placed in rotation determined by scanning (axometry) and fixed by the stirrup. Then the osteotomy is performed and the leg is positioned vertically in order to get the patella placed on zenith during the nailing. This second method is sufficiently precise and is above all easy to carry out (Fig. 8.8). Full weight-bearing is always allowed.

## Varus or Valgus Osteotomies

In cases where correction of malunion is required, the osteotomy is ideally performed at the level of the deformity or as close as possible. For deformities such as curvature (congenital or acquired), the osteotomy must be performed at the most se-

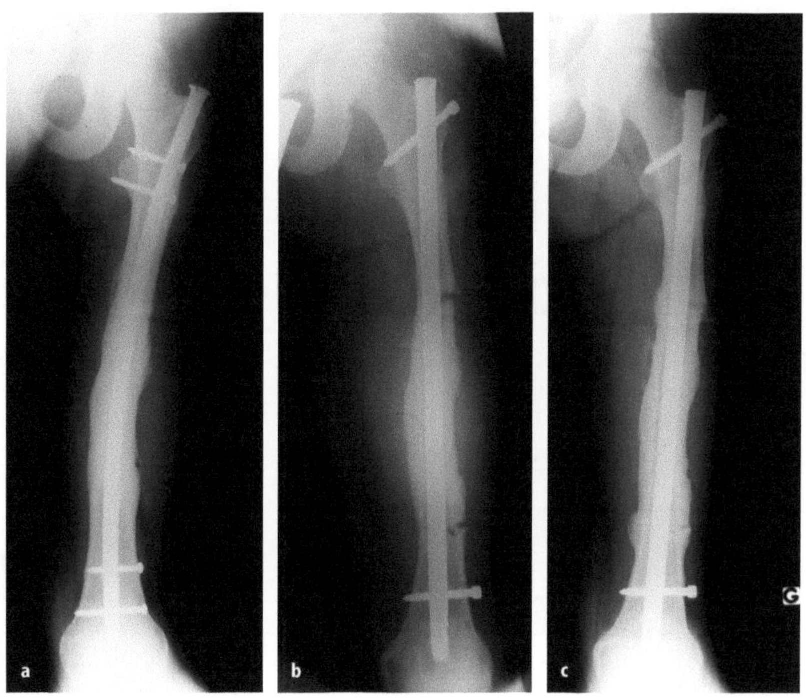


**Fig. 8.9 a–c.** Clinical case of valgus deformity. **a** Preoperative view. **b** Postoperative view. **c** Consolidation at 4 months

verely bent level. Reaming is first done until the point of the planned osteotomy. If the canal is blocked, it is often necessary to use a pseudarthrosis guidewire. Once the cut with the saw is completed, the osteoclasia could be difficult to perform. The largest saw must be used, but it is sometimes necessary to complete the osteotomy with a chisel by making a small incision. The reamer guide is inserted in the distal fragment. The operation is finished by static intramedullary nailing. Fragment alignment is easily done with a nail of a sufficient diameter. Full weight-bearing may be allowed, depending on the congruence of the osteotomy site.

## Indications

The femur, less than the tibia, is the best indication for closed osteotomy, with the intramedullary saw fixed by locked nailing.

Theoretically, this method could be used for other long bones such as the humerus, ulna, and radius, but it has not yet been developed and special instrumentation would be necessary.

For the femur, all the closed one-stage osteotomies previously described are indicated for malunions, curvatures, as well as shortening and lengthening.

For the tibia, our experience is limited to axial corrections.

Axial or rotational malunions are, indeed, indications of choice. Easy to perform, the main advantage consists in shorter consolidation time than with the open procedure [7, 12]. For derotations, our technique, based on clinical evaluation, has brought satisfaction with generally good corrections. Our method could be improved with extremely precise measurement instruments, but we think that this is not necessary.

Axial deformities of approximately 10°–15° are satisfactorily corrected using this method, which can also be used for the tibia (Fig. 8.9). Major malunions – which have become rare with the modern methods of fracture treatment – have to be treated with a minimal open approach with a wedge or a double osteotomy stabilized by nailing. In this case, a longer consolidation time is necessary.

For corrections of leg length discrepancies, shortening osteotomy is reliable, whereas lengthening osteotomy is more debatable.

For large patients, shortening osteotomy is preferred over lengthening osteotomy, although when the shortened leg has trophic, muscular, or malunion problems or predisposes to risks, lengthening is not recommended.

The technique is long and delicate, the resection of the cylinder must be done preferably in

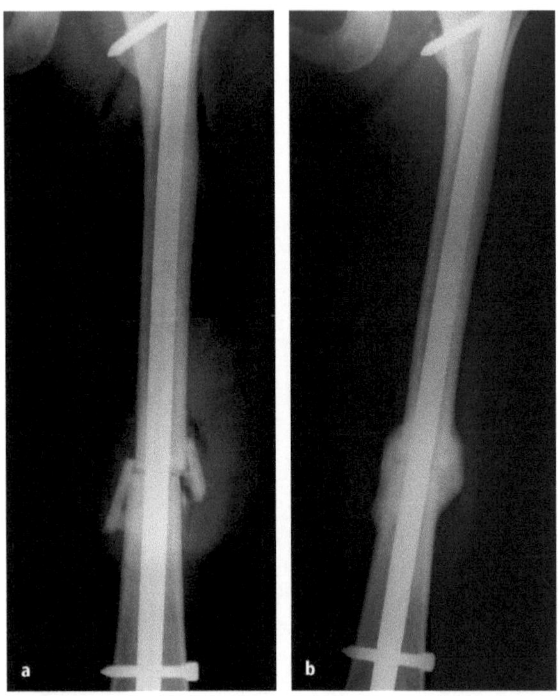

**Fig. 8.10 a, b.** Clinical case of a 4.5-cm shortening osteotomy. **a** Postoperative view. **b** Consolidation at 3 months

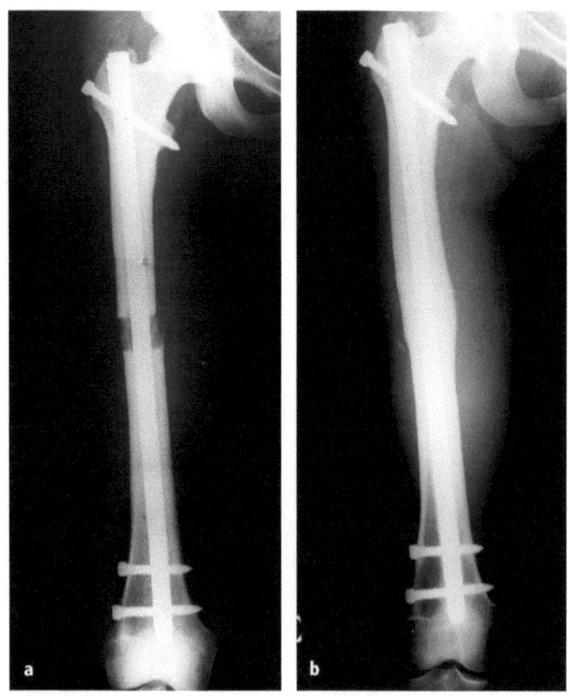

**Fig. 8.11 a, b.** Clinical case of lengthening osteotomy. **a** Postoperative view. **b** Consolidation at 6 months

the epiphyseal-metaphyseal area, where the conditions for consolidation are the best. Shortening must not exceed 5 cm because muscle recovery can otherwise be problematic (Fig. 8.10). Nevertheless, some authors have reported shortenings of more than 7 cm [20].

The main advantage that can justify the major technical difficulties remains the reduction in consolidation time. Thus, in a first series of shortening osteotomies using the open procedure, we had a mean consolidation time of 7.8 months as opposed to 3.6 months in our series operated on using the closed procedure, with a statistically significant difference ($t=2.73$ and $0.02 < a < 0.05$) [7].

However, comparing the consolidation times between lengthening and shortening shows a clear advantage for shortening osteotomies (10 months vs 3.6 months).

The lengthening osteotomy technique is complex and difficult. It is recommended for small patients with good trophic and muscular conditions; a lengthening of a maximum of 3 cm can be performed (Fig. 8.11). Otherwise, exaggerated lengthening can cause various neurological and vascular consequences. In 4 of 13 cases, consolidation problems appear and a spongy graft with decortication was necessary. Finally, distraction osteogenesis following Ilizarov's principles is much more reliable. Recently, lengthening methods with monitored nails [16] or combined with an external fixator have been developed and should dethrone the one-stage lengthening technique [1, 3, 6].

Nevertheless, the principle of closed osteotomy with the intramedullary saw remains the last and still fruitful demonstration of the genius G. Küntscher.

## References


1. Baumgart R, Betz A, Schweiberer L (1997) A fully implantable motorized intramedullary nail for limb lengthening and bone transport. Clin Orthop 343:135–143
2. Blair VP, Schoenecker PL, Sheridan JJ, Capelli AM (1989) Closed shortening of the femur. J Bone Joint Surg 71A:1440–1447
3. Caton J (1990) Allongements de membres chez l'adulte (adolescents et adultes jeunes) Cahiers d'enseignement de la SOFCOT. Conférences d'enseignement 52:79–98
4. Chapman ME, Duwelius PJ, Bray TJ, Gordon JE (1993) Closed intramedullary femoral osteotomy. Shortening and dérotation procedures. Clin Orthop 287:245–251
5. Dagrenat D (1987) L'enclouage centromédullaire avec verrouillage dans le traitement des cals vicieux des membres inférieurs. Thèse de médecine, Strasbourg
6. Guichet JM, Grammont P, Casar RS, Alexander H, Frankel VH (1994) Propriétés mécaniques du clou d'allongement progressif. In: Inégalité de longueur des membres. Masson, Paris, pp 136–138
7. Hamon P (1995) L'ostéotomie endomédullaire des diaphyses fémorales et tibiales. Etude expérimentale et clinique. Thèse de médecine, Strasbourg
8. Hempel D (1980) Korrektur von Rotationsfehlstellung an Femur und Tibia mit geschlossener Osteotomie und neuen Winkelmessgerät. Chirurg 51:480–481
9. Hempel D, Fischer S (1982) Intramedullary nailing. Thieme, Stuttgart
10. Holm I, Nordsletten L, Stehen H, Folleras G, Bjerkreim I (1994) Muscle function after mid-shaft femoral shortening. A prospective study with a two-year follow-up. J Bone Joint Surg 76B:143–146
11. Kempf I, Grosse A, Abalo C (1986) Locked intramedullary nailing. Its application to femoral and tibial axial, rotational, lengthening, and shortening osteotomies. Clin Orthop 212:165–173
12. Kempf I, Grosse A, Dagrenat D (1986) Les applications du clou verrouillé dans les ostéotomies correctrices (vol. 26). Cahier d'enseignement de la SOFCOT. Conferences d'enseignement, Expansion Scientifique Française, pp 211–227
13. Kempf I, Grosse A, Lefevre C (1982) Allongement extemporané du femur fixé par clou centromédullaire verrouillé. Rev Chir Orthop 68:575–579
14. Küntscher G (1962) Praxis der Marknagelung (vol 1). Schattauer, Stuttgart
15. Küntscher G (1964) Operationstechnik – die Innensäge. Chirurg 9:413–415
16. Paley D, Herzenberg JE, Paremain G, Bhave A (1997) Femoral lengthening over an intramedullary nail. A matched-case comparison with Ilizarov femoral lengthening. J Bone Joint Surg 10A:1464–1480
17. Peters JD, Friermood TG (1990) Closed intramedullary femoral shortening. Orthop Rev 19:709–713
18. Wagner H (1978) Operative lengthening of the femur. Clin Orthop 136:125–142
19. Winquist RA (1986) Closed intramedullary osteotomies of the femur. Clin Orthop 212:155–164
20. Winquist RA, Hansen JR, Pearson RE (1978) Closed intramedullary shortening of the femur. Clin Orthop 136:54–61

# CHAPTER 9

# Arthrodesis with Locking Nails

H. SEIDEL

## Arthrodesis of the Knee Joint

### Introduction

Fusion of the knee joint is the treatment of choice, if prosthetic reconstruction of the joint is not possible. In the past, arthrodesis with a long Küntscher nail was used to treat elderly patients with fractures (Fig. 9.1). This method is described as an exceptional operation by Arens, Beck, Lentz, Maatz and collaborators [9], and pupils of Küntscher [8]. Other methods are recommended for arthrodesis: for example, the external fixator is used by Blauth [2], Hessmann [7], Müller [10], Friedebold [5, 6], and many others. Blauth introduced compression arthrodesis with two plates. The Küntscher method was modified by Maatz [9] and Chapchal [3]. These authors performed knee arthrodesis with a short Küntscher femur nail. Cheng used a similar technique with a short locked intramedullary nail [4]. Arthrodesis with the intramedullary nail is more comfortable for the patient. It is described by Puranen [11] and Vidal [14], who prefer the intramedullary technique, as do Vander Griend [13] and Alt [1]. Küntscher nail arthrodesis is described in detail by Blauth [2]. The application of a modified long Grosse-Kempf femur nail is the further development of the Küntscher nail. The nail gives more stability and security of arthrodesis, particularly because the rotation is locked. The arthrodesis technique is less traumatic than plate arthrodesis and more comfortable than arthrodesis with an external fixator [14]. The nail is stable for bridging arthrodesis used for tumor resection [12, 15] or a failed knee prosthesis.

### Indications

The indications for arthrodesis of the knee have changed with the success of modern osteosynthesis and joint replacement. It is strictly limited to salvaging the leg after complications with other treatments, either total joint replacements or osteosynthesis. A rare indication is total instability of the knee joint in arthritis by tabes dorsalis, tuberculosis of the joint, or in combination with tumor resection. A two-step operation with the nail is preferred. If the indication for arthrodesis is infection, cleaning of the infected bone, followed by arthrodesis with the locking nail and if required bone grafts are undertaken.

### Operation Technique

Preoperative planning is important. Full-length radiographs of both legs, from the hip to the ankle, are required so that comparisons can be made between the normal leg and the damaged leg. The length of the leg, the amount of valgus-varus, and the rotation must be evaluated. A shortening of the leg usually aids in consolidation and accelerates the healing time. Any gap in the knee joint is a risk, as it subjects the nail to higher load and may result in a stress fracture of the nail.

### Patient Positioning

The patient is placed in the supine position on the traction table, traction being applied via a transcalcaneal Steinmann pin. Slight adduction is helpful for the approach to the greater trochanter of the femur. This positioning makes it easy to obtain the correct rotation of the leg.

### Approach

The nail is introduced at the tip of the greater trochanter of the femur, as in standard locking nail procedures. Where open resection of the knee joint is required, for example, if the knee joint is opened for resection of an implant, the easiest approach to both the tibia and the femur is entry from the knee joint through the resection area.

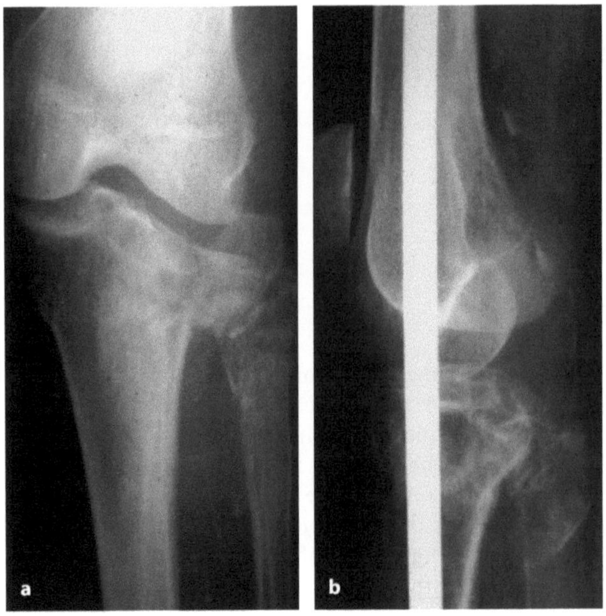

**Fig. 9.1. a** A 56-year-old male with fracture of the tibia head treated 1957 by Prof. G. Küntscher at the Hafenkrankenhaus of Hamburg. **b** Arthrodesis with long Küntscher nail

## Reaming

The reaming guidewire is pushed retrograde into the femur from the knee. It perforates the top of the greater trochanter and indicates where the skin incision should be made. The femur is then reamed, either in a retrograde or antegrade fashion.

The reaming guidewire for the tibia is placed antegrade through the knee joint. The diameter of reaming depends on the length of the nail. If the nail passes the diaphysis of the tibia, the nail diameter is determined by the diaphyseal diameter. If the nail ends in the metaphysis of the tibia, the nail diameter can have the same (larger) diameter as in the diaphysis of the femur.

## Nail Locking

In contrast to the classical Küntscher nail, the locking nail is secured with locking screws on both sides of the knee joint, to give more stability and more precision to the operation. The largest possible diameter of nail should be used to prevent nail breakage.

Nails with lengths of 400–900 mm, with diameters of 8–16 mm are available as standard. Alternatively, custom-made nails can be delivered in any length and diameter. The nail length and the nail diameter is determined at preoperative planning. Shortening, as a result of the knee resection, has to be allowed for when calculating the nail length.

## Nail Positioning

After reaming both the femur and the tibia, the reaming guidewire is exchanged for the nail guidewire, which has a length of 150 cm. This guidewire is introduced at the tip of the greater trochanter and is passed through the knee into the tibia. The nail is placed in the appropriate position by hand, over the guidewire.

Proximal locking is carried out using the locking method for the Grosse-Kempf femoral nail. Compression of the tibia against the femur is recommended to close the resection zone prior to performing distal locking. Two screws are essential to guarantee locking stability. Three distal locking screws are recommended if a large gap, packed with cancellous bone grafts, is necessary to correct the leg length.

### *Two-Step Operation*

This procedure is helpful for treating seriously infected knee joints.

1. In an initial operation, total resection of foreign material and total debridement of infected hard and soft tissue is carried out. The knee and the bone cavities are filled with antibiotic impregnated beads. The knee is then temporarily stabilized and held in extension with an external fixator or a plaster splint.
2. After draining the infection – usually after 4–6 weeks – a second operation is performed. The antibiotic impregnated beads are removed

and the locking nail is implanted with the usual technique. Antibiotic therapy from this point is routine.

## Additional Therapy

The basic indication for knee arthrodesis is infection of a prosthetic implant, with the secondary complication of implant loosing. The treatment of infection therefore must be the primary therapy.

1. Local treatment. After resection of all dead bone and foreign bodies, the joint is thoroughly cleaned with lavage and irrigation with betavidine or tauroline. Temporary implantation of antibiotic impregnated beads has a double effect:
   a. Local antibiotic treatment, with a high level of antibiotic in the infected zone
   b. Revascularization and stimulation of the bone to improve the bone.
2. General therapy. The specific antibiotic therapy must be maintained for a long time. The effect of the therapy is controlled in periods of 2, 4, and 6 weeks. It is extended later to 3 and 6 months and includes specific tests such as C-reactive protein, ASTAL (Antistaphylolysin reaction), ASL (Antistreptolysin titer) leukocytes, with X-ray control and scintigraphy of leukocytes.

## Postoperative Treatment

The construct, with the arthrodesis locking nail, is stable enough for early or immediate weight-bearing. Usually any loss of length is compensated with an orthopedic shoe. The time to consolidation depends on the bone loss. Normally, consolidation is achieved within 3–6 months. Dynamization of the nail is not required and removal of the implant is very rare.

## Complications

### *Early Complications*

In a group of 20 patients, we observed two tibial fractures. These fractures occurred at the time of operation, in one case, and within 4 days of the operation in the other patient. In both, the nail tip ended in the diaphysis and was acting as a stress concentrator. It is recommended to make sure that the tip of the long nail passes into the distal metaphysis of the tibia or that it ends in the proximal metaphysis of the tibia.

### *Late Complications*

The literature describes a 5%–20% rate of broken Küntscher nails. In our group, we had one broken nail. The reason for nail breakage is either poor osseous contact at the line of fusion or a nail that is too small. Such cases are revised by renailing with a lager diameter nail. It is essential to ream the medullary canal again, to ensure consolidation (Figs. 9.2–9.15).

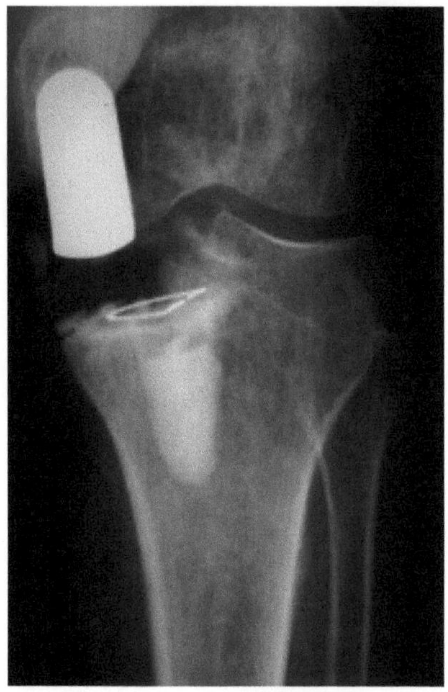

**Fig. 9.2.** Case 1: 52-year-old male patient. Failed hemiprosthesis left knee, infection

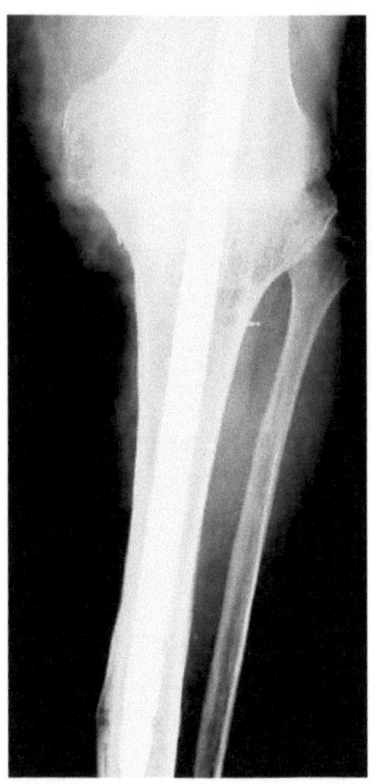

**Fig. 9.3.** Knee arthrosis with Grosse-Kempf (GK) locking nail, distal dynamization, anterior-posterior view

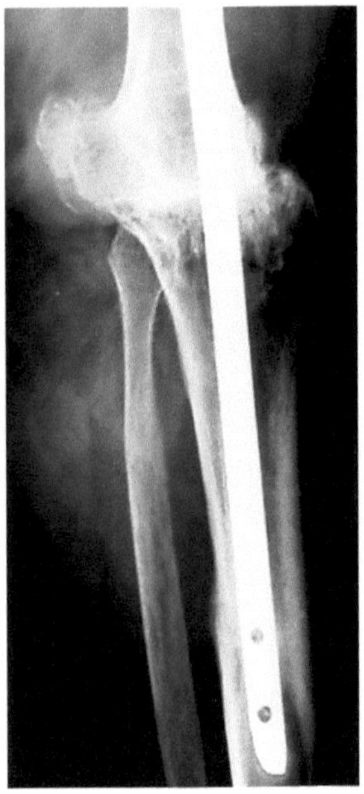

**Fig. 9.4.** Knee arthrosis with GK locking nail, distal dynamization lateral view

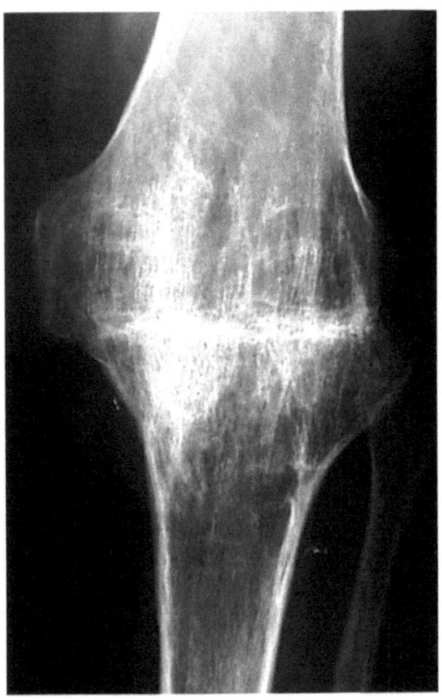

**Fig. 9.5.** Knee arthrosis with GK locking nail, nail removal, complete consolidation, anterior-posterior view

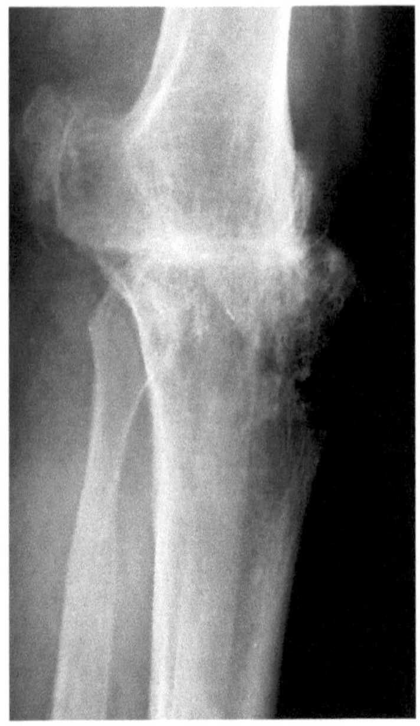

**Fig. 9.6.** Knee arthrosis with GK locking nail, nail removal, complete consolidation, lateral view

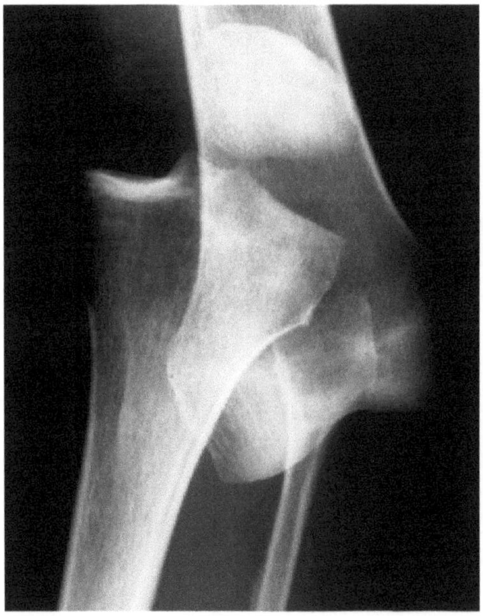

**Fig. 9.7.** Case 2: Complete dislocation of the knee joint

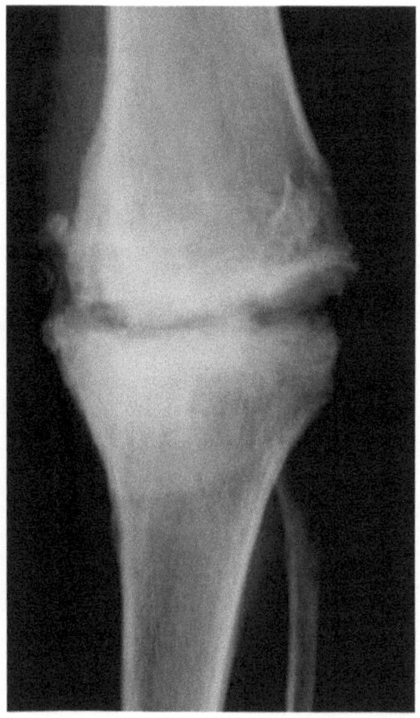

**Fig. 9.8.** Posttraumatic arthrosis after complete dislocation of the knee joint

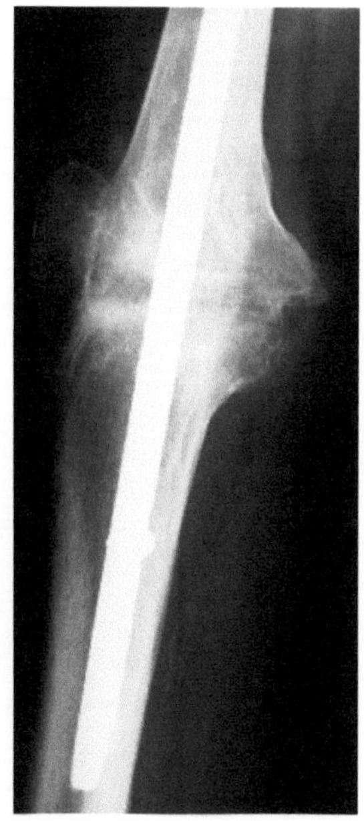

**Fig. 9.9.** Arthrodesis with a long custom-made nail lateral view

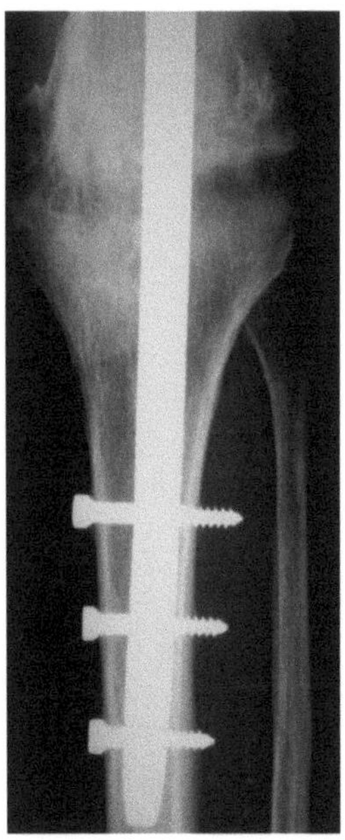

**Fig. 9.10.** Arthrodesis in consolidation anterior-posterior view

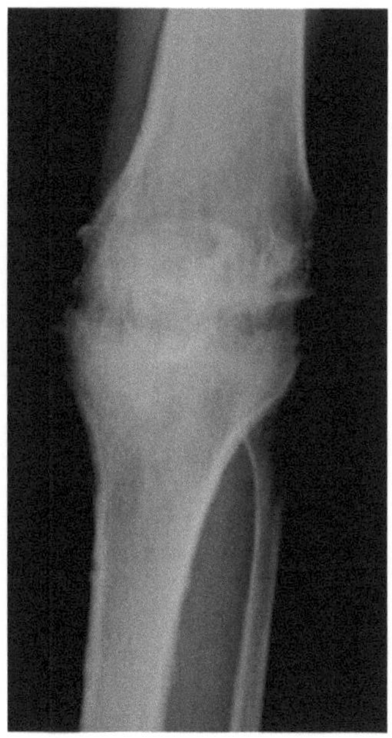

**Fig. 9.11.** Removal of the nail after consolidation of the arthrodesis

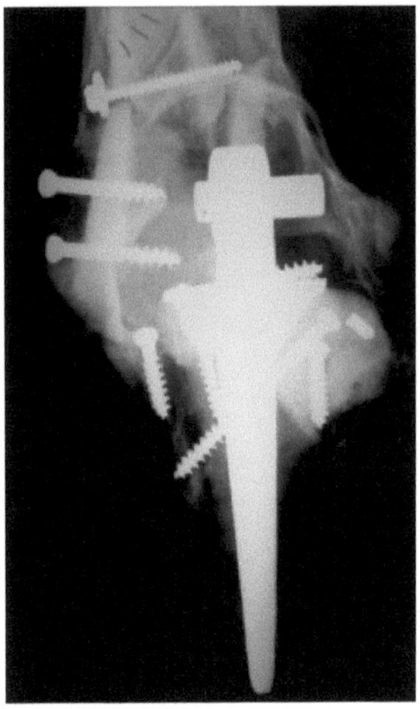

**Fig. 9.12.** Case 3: Complete loosened knee prosthesis

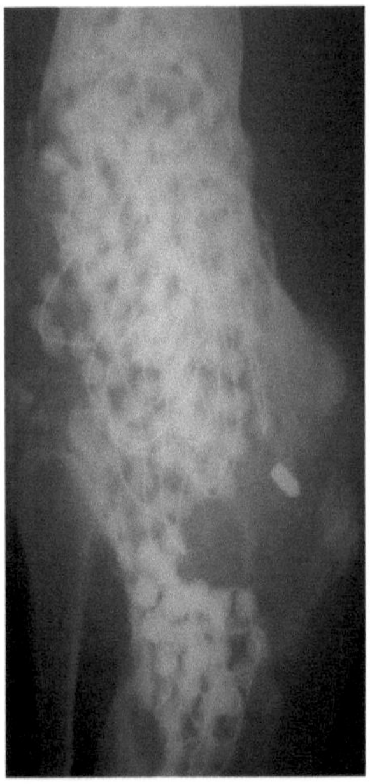

**Fig. 9.13.** Removal of the knee prosthesis, treatment of the infection with antibiotic impregnated beads

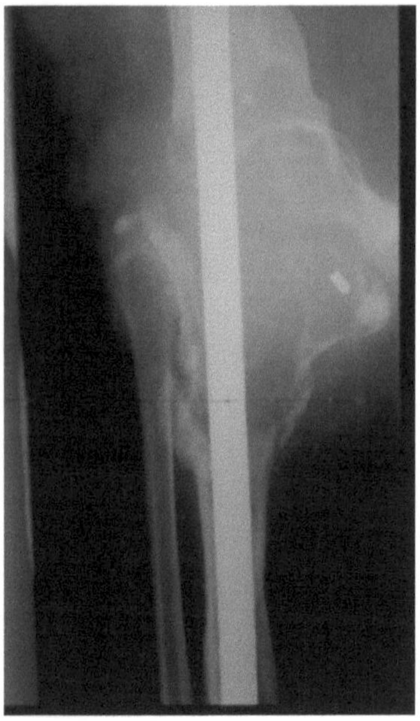

**Fig. 9.14.** Stabilization and arthrodesis with long GK nail

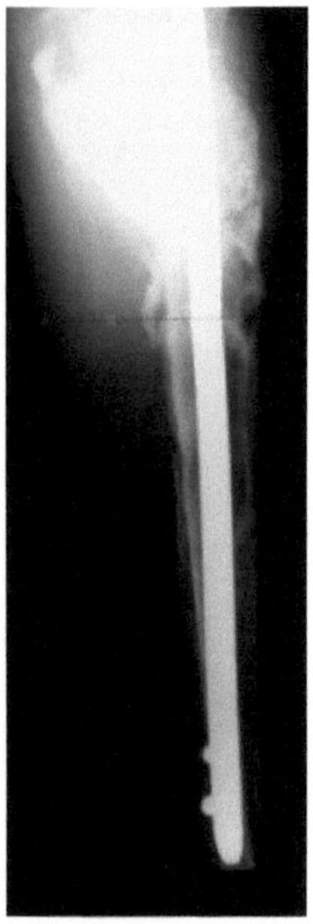

**Fig. 9.15.** Stabilization and arthrodesis with long GK nail lateral view

### Discussion

Küntscher first introduced arthrodesis of the knee joint with an extra-long intramedullary nail bridging the knee. With the advent of interlocking nailing, a higher quality of operation became possible and the complication rate was reduced. The method is more comfortable for patients and they are able to bear weight early. A less than 2-cm shortening of the leg needs no special treatment. An orthopedic shoe should be used to compensate for shortening greater than 2 cm. Since the nail is straight, the anatomical valgus of the leg is changed. Probably as a result of the shortening of the leg, patients have no pain, due to the straight axis of the leg. Hospitalization time is quite long, mainly because this is a difficult indication with infection or prosthetic loosening. However, amputation can be avoided even if the knee is extremely damaged. For such cases the two-step operation is the key to salvage.

## Arthrodesis of the Shoulder Joint

The indication for shoulder arthrodesis is rare. Painful, postoperative arthroses with infection sometimes require an arthrodesis as a last step of treatment to stabilize the shoulder and clean the infection. The nail is used as a stabilizer and as treatment of both the arthrosis and the infection. The local and general treatment of infection is required as the first step of treatment and is the precursor to treatment with the nail. If a dormant stage of the infection is achieved nail arthrodesis is performed.

The shoulder is opened frontally. Debridement is performed to remove necrotic tissue and the nail is placed in the humerus. The shoulder blade is fixed with two screws. The screws are introduced in the frontal plane through the glenoid. Antibiotic impregnated beads are used locally in addition and in accordance with the antibiotic treatment (Figs. 9.16–9.18).

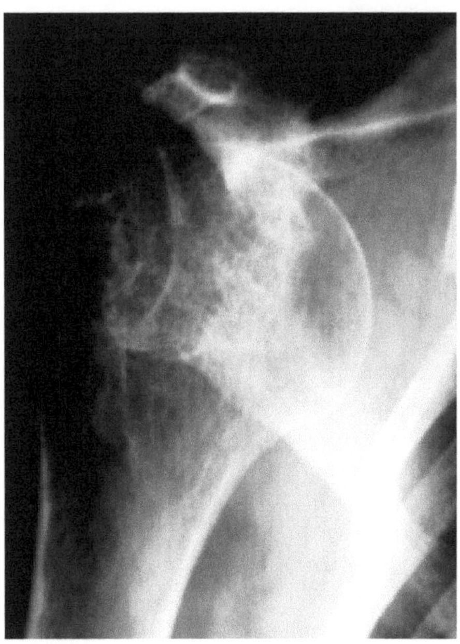

**Fig. 9.16.** Case 4: 77-year-old female patient chronic unstable dislocation of the shoulder joint

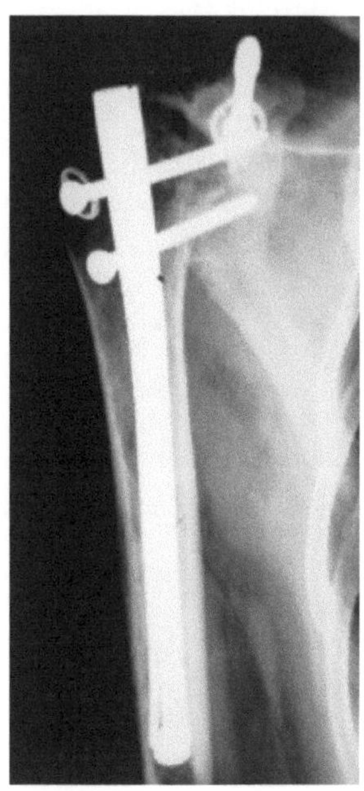

**Fig. 9.17.** Arthrodesis with humeral locking nail (HLN), anterior-posterior view

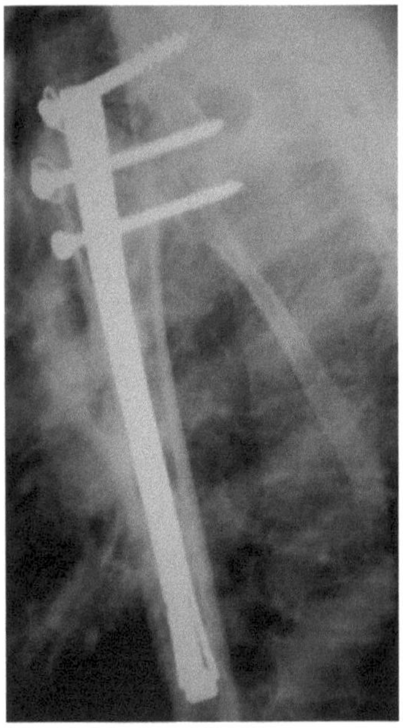

**Fig. 9.18.** Arthrodesis with humeral locking nail transthoracal view

## Arthrodesis of the Elbow Joint

The indication for the elbow joint is similar to the indication for arthrodesis of the shoulder joint. The technique for arthrodesis with the humeral locking nail is easy to perform and effective. The distal humerus is united with the ulna. The humeral locking nail is inserted through the olecranon, into the humerus. The nail is locked at first in the humerus, by expansion of the nail tip, with the spreading screw. In the second step, one locking screw is placed through the olecranon, after correct placement of the nail in the ulna.

A splint is used for 2 weeks to stabilize the montage (Figs. 9.19–9.22).

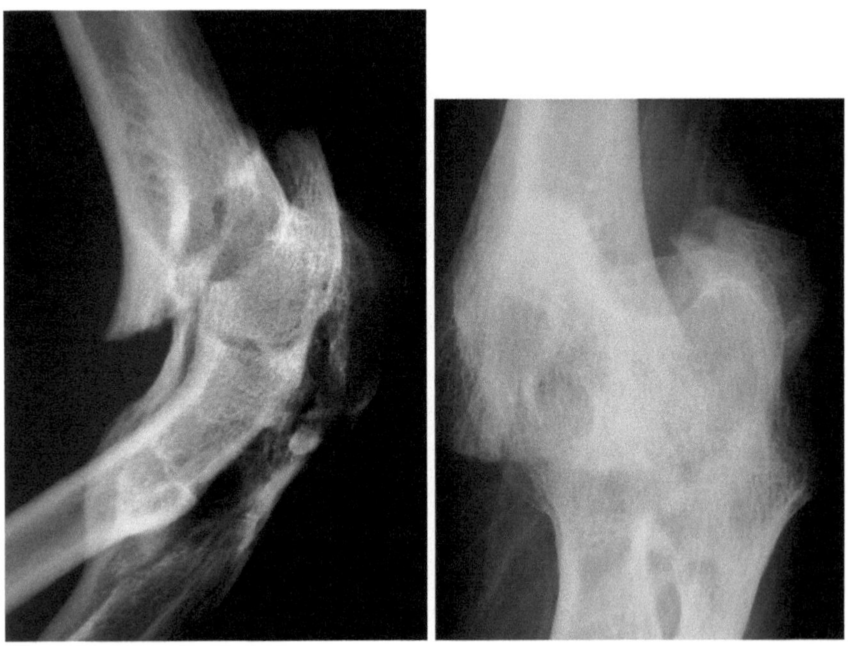

**Fig. 9.19.** Case 5: 73-year-old male patient, supracondylar humeral fracture by elbow arthrosis

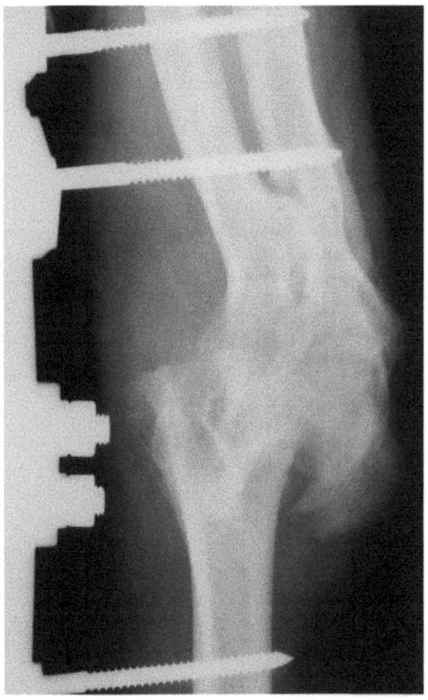

**Fig. 9.20.** Open supracondylar humeral fracture by elbow arthrosis. At first stabilization with external fixator

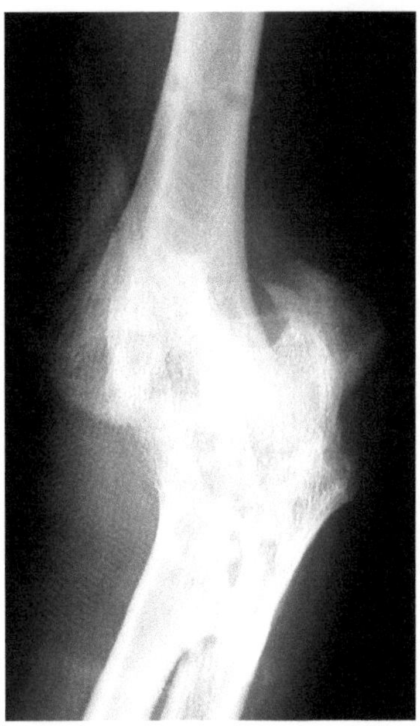

**Fig. 9.21.** Removal of external fixator

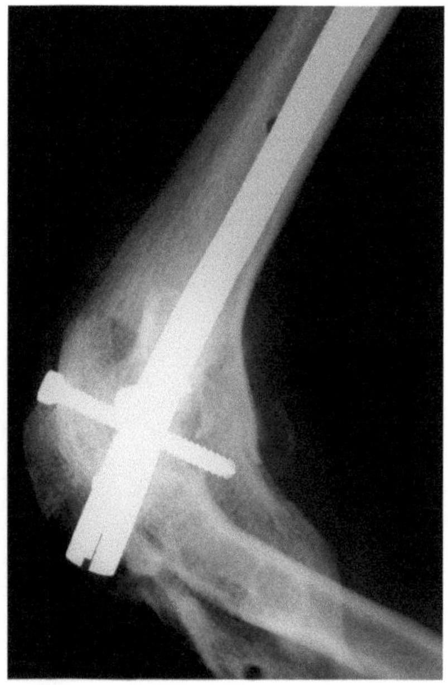

**Fig. 9.22.** Arthrosis with humeral locking nail

## Arthrodesis of the Ankle Joint

The indication for arthrodesis is the arthrotic or arthritic destruction of the ankle joint, with pain and with or without infection (Figs. 9.23–9.28). The technique is performed using an open method, in four steps:

1. Osteotomy of the fibula, in an oblique direction, in the region of the talocrural joint
2. Osteotomy of the medial ankle, at the level of the talocrural joint
3. Resection of the cartilage of the tibia and of the talus. The ankle joint is resected on both the tibia and the talus, cutting a segment of 0.5 mm off both
4. The nail is introduced via the plantar surface, through the calcaneus and talus, into the tibia. The nail tip is expanded with the internal screw. The distal locking is achieved with two crossed screws, in the lateral-medial direction and the frontal-dorsal direction.

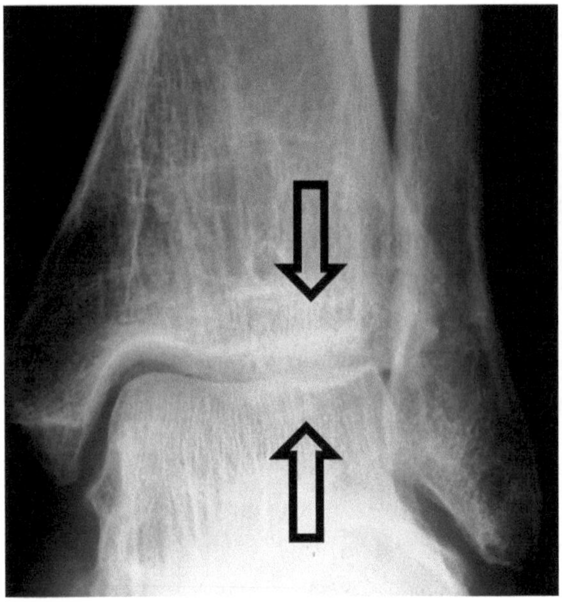

**Fig. 9.23.** Case 6: Posttraumatic arthrosis 30 years after malleolar fracture

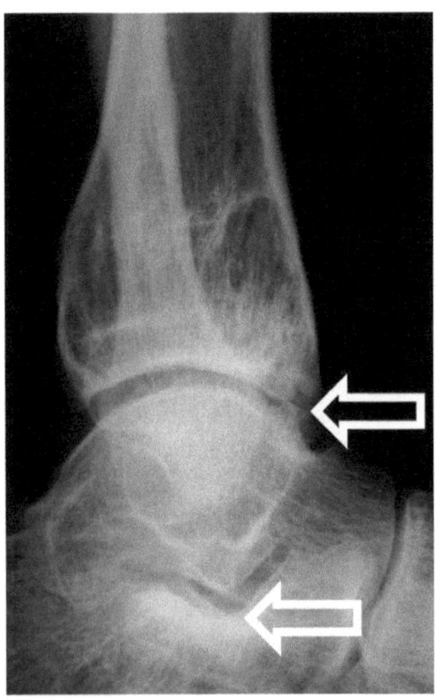

**Fig. 9.24.** Posttraumatic arthrosis 30 years after malleolar fracture

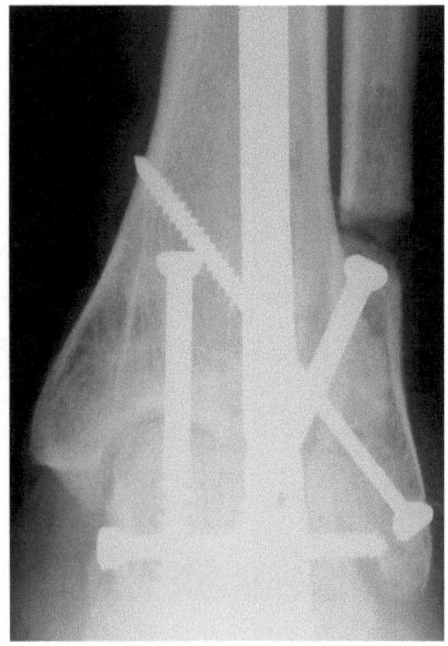

**Fig. 9.25.** Arthrodesis with humeral locking nail and screws, anterior-posterior view

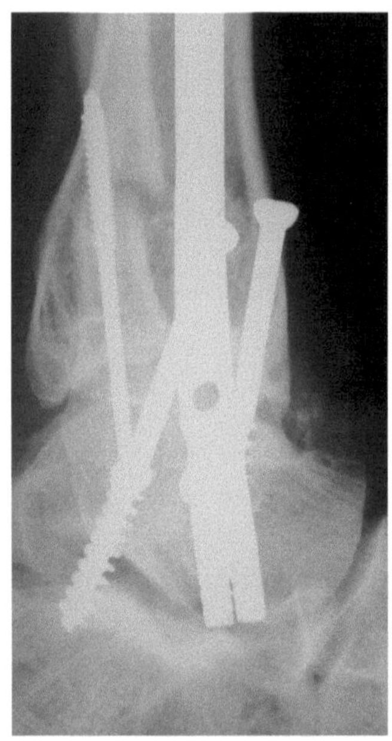

**Fig. 9.26.** Arthrodesis with humeral locking nail and screws, lateral view

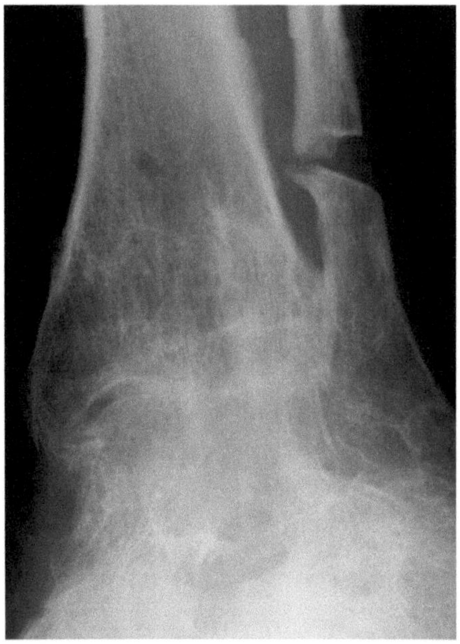

**Fig. 9.27.** Nail removal after consolidation, anterior-posterior view

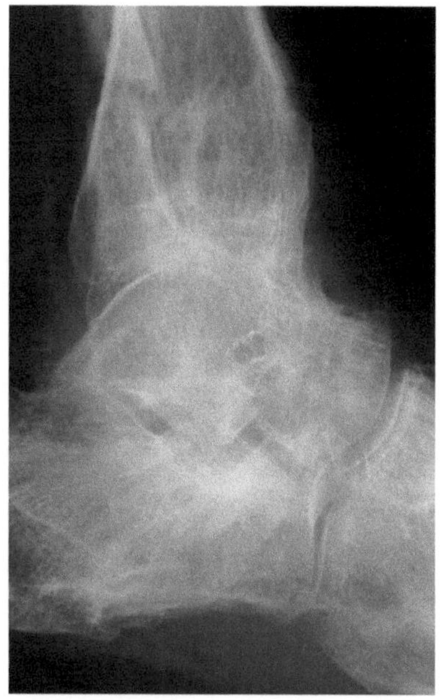

**Fig. 9.28.** Nail removal after consolidation, lateral view

## References


1. Alt V, Seligson D (2001) Knee fusion. A new technique using an old Belgian surgical approch and intramedullary nail. Acta Orthop Belg 67:49–63
2. Blauth W, Schuchardt E (1986) Orthopädisch-chirurgische Operationen am Knie. Thieme, Stuttgart
3. Chapchal G (1948) Intamedullary pinning for arthrodesis of knee joint. JBJS 30A:728–734
4. Cheng SL, Gross AE (1995) Knee arthrodesis using a short locked intramedullary nail. A new technique. Am J Knee Surg Spring 8:56–59
5. Friedebold G, Stegmann E (1966) Arthrodesis in tabetic arthropathy. Arch Orthop Unfallchir 55:272–285
6. Friedebold G, Wolff R, Steuer HG (1982) Arthritis and external fixation. Langenbecks Arch Chir 358:125–132
7. Hessmann M, Gotzen L, Baumgartel E (1996) Knee arthrodesis with an unilateral fixator. Acta Chir Belg
8. Küntscher G (1962) Praxis der Marknagelung. Schattauer, Stuttgart
9. Maatz R, Lentz W, Arens W, Beck H (1983) Die Marknagelung und andere intramedulläre Osteosynthesen. Schattauer, Stuttgart
10. Müller ME, Allgöwer M, Willenegger H (1977) Manual der Osteosynthese. Springer, Berlin Heidelberg New York
11. Puranen J, Kortelainen P, Jalovaara P (1990) Arthrodesis of the knee with intramedullary nail fixation. JBJS Am 72:433–442
12. Rodriguez Merchan EC, Sanchez Herrera S, Gonzalea Lopez M (1994) Limb salvage procedures in osteosarcomas around the knee joint. Rev Paul Med 112:661–667
13. Vander Griend R (1983) Arthrodesis of the knee with intramedullary fixation. Clin Orthop 181:146–150
14. Vidal J, Allieu Y, Goalard C, Fassio B, Connes H, Buscayrkt C (1974) Arthrodesis of the knee. External fixation device and femoro- tibial nailing therapeutic possibility in pseudarthrosis of the lower end of the femur. Rev Chir Orthop Reparatrice Appar Mot 60 [Suppl 2]:308–309
15. Yeow C, Chin CH, Ong PH (1995) Knee arthrodesis with interlocking nail after excision of gigant cell tumours of the femur. Med J Malaysia 50:414–416

# CHAPTER 10

# Tumor Surgery

S. Boriani, F. De Iure, A. Gasbarrini, S. Bandiera

## Introduction

Metastatic disease in long bones is frequent: it is assumed that about 15% of all carcinomas manifest skeletal metastases, a figure increasing to 30% if autopsic material is evaluated [3]. Bone metastases threaten the functional autonomy of patients whose life expectancy is becoming longer and longer thanks to progress in surgery, chemotherapy, and radiation therapy in the treatment of carcinomas. Fixation of pathological fractures and stabilization of impending fractures is essential in maintaining an appropriate level of function. The fixation device must allow immediate weight-bearing and create a mechanical by-pass through the pathological area for a much longer period than for the treatment of traumatic fractures.

Primary bone tumors are rare: it has been calculated that in the United States about ten cases of primary malignant bone tumors arise for each million inhabitants per year. Before the actual protocols of preoperative and intra-arterial chemotherapy were developed, the rate of amputation in the treatment of osteosarcoma of the limbs was about 90%, with a 10%–20% survival rate at 5 years. Nowadays, a limb salvage procedure through en bloc resection of the tumor can be performed after chemotherapy in more than 90% of cases, with about 70% survival at 5 years [3].

Reconstruction after limb salvage is a difficult and delicate problem: the prostheses are more frequently used for replacement of meta-epiphyseal resections; bone grafts (allografts, vascularized fibula, autogenous grafts) are used for diaphyseal replacement and meta-epiphyseal replacement (such as arthrodesis), less frequently for articular replacement (osteochondral allografts).

The fixation device required for arthrodesis or diaphyseal reconstruction must be characterized by high-performance mechanical features to allow functional recovery during the long-lasting period of graft incorporation. Plates were widely used, but their bending stiffness is poor and mechanical failures were frequent when the bone defect persisted on the opposite site. Furthermore, screw holes are weak points and may be coincident with the fracture site of the allograft. Owing to the axial position and the biomechanical features, the locked nails seemed to be an excellent reconstructive device in oncological surgery.

## Validity of the Locked Nail

It has been experimentally demonstrated [12] that the failure axial load for the Grosse-Kempf nail implanted in cadaver femora with an 8-cm mid-shaft defect was nearly four times body weight; in the same experiment, torsional stiffness of the nail was similar to the intact bone and bending stiffness was 70% of the bending stiffness of the intact femur. This data confirms the validity of this nail as a fixation device in pathological bone or as a reconstructive device after resections [1, 13, 19]. A new contribution to the treatment of tumors has been brought about by the unslotted Grosse and Kempf nail, whose bending stiffness is 20% higher than the slotted nail and torsional stiffness 20 times higher, thus reaching a 30% higher fatigue stress.

Intramedullary locked nailing in tumor surgery is indicated for:

- Fixation of pathological fractures
- Preventive stabilization of lytic lesions (impending fractures)
- Reconstruction after oncological resections

Fixation of pathological fractures and preventive stabilization of lytic lesions [11, 16, 17] require the intralesional nail, with obvious tumor spread all along the diaphysis. Preventive curettage of the lesion reduces such contamination but cannot avoid microscopic spread. This is not a major problem in cases of metastatic lesions, which will receive radiation therapy on the entire bone, in cases of pseudotumoral conditions (such as aneurysmal bone cyst), or in cases of benign, latent, and active tumors. On the other hand, nailing of a primary tumor will produce a disaster, preventing any possibility of limb salvage, due to unresectable bone and soft tissue contamination.

A few remarks about diagnosis and staging of bone tumors are therefore needed before undertaking this surgery.

## Basic Principles of Bone Tumor Surgery

In this chapter we will use the terminology proposed by Enneking [9] for bone tumor surgery.

- "Excision" means a piecemeal removal of the tumor.
- "Resection" is the en bloc removal of the tumor. This can be performed along the pseudocapsule (marginal resection) or outside the pseudocapsule, removing the tumor with a continuous shell of healthy tissues (wide resection). "Radical resection" means the en bloc removal of the tumor together with the whole compartment of origin.
- "Palliation" is a surgical procedure finalized to a functional purpose (fracture stabilization), with or without partial (piecemeal) removal of the tumor. In general, it is only intended to make a diagnosis, decrease pain, and improve function.
- "Oncological staging," proposed by Enneking, defines the biological behavior of primary tumors and has proven effective in planning the type of surgery to be performed (intralesional, marginal, wide, or radical).

This staging system divides benign tumors into three stages (S1, S2, S3) and localized malignant tumors into four stages (IA, IB, IIA, IIB). Two further stages include metastatic high-grade intra- and extracompartmental malignant tumors (IIIA and IIIB, respectively). This classification is based on clinical features, radiographic pattern, CT scan and MRI data, and histological findings [3, 9].

### Benign Tumors

The first stage of benign tumor (S1, latent, inactive) includes asymptomatic lesions bordered by a true capsule. A well-defined margin all around the circumference of the lesion is seen even on plain radiograms. These tumors do not grow or only grow very slowly. No treatment is required, unless palliative surgery is needed for fixation of pathological fracture. For example, closed locked nailing of a pathological fracture that has occurred due to angioma is a correct indication. The procedure is best preceded and followed by selective arterial embolization to reduce bleeding and treat the pathological condition.

Benign tumors stage 2 (S2, active) grow slowly, causing mild symptoms. The tumor is bordered by a thin capsule and by a layer of reactive tissue, sometimes found on plain radiograms as an enlargement of the tumor outline, sometimes pointed out by MRI. The bone scan is positive.

An intralesional excision (curettage) can be performed with a low rate of recurrence. The incidence of recurrence can be reduced further by local adjuvants (cryotherapy, embolization, radiation therapy). For example, intralesional excision of a stage 2 osteoblastoma can be followed by open locked nailing and filling of the cavity by cancellous grafting or cement.

The third stage of benign tumors (S3, aggressive) include rapidly growing benign tumors: the capsule is very thin, discontinued, or absent. The tumor invades neighboring compartments, and wide reactive hypervascularized tissue (pseudocapsule) is often found, sometimes permeated by neoplastic digitations. The bone scan is highly positive, fuzzy limits are seen on plain X-rays, the CT scan shows compartmental extension, and MRI clearly defines the contents of the tumor mass, the features of the reactive zone, its boundaries towards vessels, and nerves.

Intralesional curettage, even if augmented by radiation, can be associated with a significant rate of recurrence. A marginal resection is the appropriate treatment.

### Malignant Tumors

Low-grade malignant tumors are included in Stage I, subdivided into IA (the tumor remains inside the compartment) and IB (the tumor invades the surrounding tissues). No true capsule is associated with these lesions, but a thick pseudocapsule of reactive tissue permeated by small microscopic islands of tumor is seen.

A resection performed along the pseudocapsule often leaves residual foci of active tumor; megavoltage radiation and/or chemotherapy can be added to reduce the risk of recurrence. The treatment of choice, if feasible, is a wide resection.

High-grade malignancies are defined IIA and IIB. The neoplastic growth is so rapid that the host has no time to form continuous reactive tissue. There is continuous seeding with neoplastic nodules (satellites). Moreover, these tumors can have neoplastic nodules at some distance from the main tumor mass (skip metastases). These malignancies are generally seen on plain radiograms as radiolucent and destructive and in many cases are associated with a pathological fracture; the CT scan and MRI give details regarding the transverse and longitudinal extent of these tumors. Even a wide resection is sometimes not appropriate, due to skip metastases (small foci of the tumor at a distance from the main tumor mass). Preoperative chemotherapy allows the pseudocapsule to become a firm true capsule, making possible the en bloc resection. Different types of en bloc resection and reconstruction are indicated in stage 3 benign and in malignant long bone tumors, related to the tumor location, finalized to diaphyseal reconstruction or joint fusion, and will be discussed later on.

No staging is applied to metastases. For surgical planning, however, a complete clinical and instrumental work-up is mandatory to determine the life expectancy of the patient and the level of radiation and chemical sensitivity of the lesion. En bloc resection and prosthetic replacement (or grafting and nailing) can be decided for solitary metastatic deposit in good responder patients whose primary condition has been effectively controlled. Nailing and radiation therapy, as well as nailing and cement filling of the curetted metastasis must be considered as palliation, aiming mostly at functional recovery. The choice of closed nailing vs open nailing of a curetted and cemented cavity is based on the radioresistance of the lesion. Radiotherapy does not prevent osteogenesis and fracture healing in most myelomas and lymphomas and in about 50% of metastases; in some wide metastatic deposits (mostly lung or kidney tumors), a curettage of the lesion is advisable, filling the residual cavity with acrylic cement after nailing. This open technique is a more hemorrhagic procedure and it is therefore advisable to do it after arterial selective embolization.

## Operative Techniques

### Treatment of Primary Tumors: En Bloc Resection

En bloc resections require a careful preoperative work-up (including standard X-ray, isotope scan, contrast-enhancement CT scan, gadolinium MRI), finalized to know precisely the extension of the tumor in the canal, the involvement of muscular groups, and the relationship with nerves and vessels. Chemotherapy usually creates a firm pseudocapsule all around the tumor (Fig. 10.1 b, c), making it generally possible to dissect the tumor from the nerve and vessel sheath, and help manipulate the tumoral mass. Bone tumors never infiltrate the vessel wall, but sometimes a very huge tumor surrounds the neurovascular bundle (Fig. 10.1 c). In these cases, the surgeon must evaluate the risk–benefit ratio of sacrificing the nerve and performing a vascular anastomosis together with the en bloc resection vs amputation, vs rotation plasty in selected cases (Fig. 10.1). The skin incision does not follow the classic lines and the surgical approach is not performed through the anatomical spaces to avoid the spread of neoplastic cells. The biopsy scar as well as a continuous shell of healthy tissue must be included in the en bloc resection. Safe surgical margins in bone are achieved if 5 cm of healthy diaphyseal canal are excised.

#### *Diaphyseal Resection*

For all the long bones for which diaphyseal resection is considered – humerus, ulna, femur, tibia – the preoperative work-up determines the distance of the osteotomy lines from the articular surface. Once osteotomies have been performed and vessels and nerves have been dissected from the tumor mass by ligating the rami directed to the tumor, the resection is concluded by sectioning muscle fibers far from the tumor. The normal skin incision will be made for intramedullary (IM) osteosynthesis as well as the usual entry point on the bone. The guidewire is then inserted and the residual bone reamed. The length of the resected shaft is reported on the massive allograft; alternatively, fibula segments can be taken. Fibular segments were used as a massive graft for reconstruction after ulna resection (in this case the Lefèvre nail is inserted into the fibular graft) or around the humeral nail for humeral reconstruction.

For all considered segments, the technique is the same: the chosen nail is inserted in the proximal residual bone, then in the allograft (previously reamed at least 2 mm more than the nail diameter), then in the distal residual bone. The most difficult segment to be treated is the femur, due to the different curvatures of the allograft, the nail, the host. Consequences are fractures of the graft or imperfect contact between graft and host. To better achieve firm junction between host and graft, two different techniques are advised: cut-step junction or the use of a small plate (Fig. 10.2 b–d). The first is difficult to perform and can create stress concentration points at the angles. The second has the disadvantage of using screws around the nail and possible damage to the nail itself. Proximal and distal locking is per-

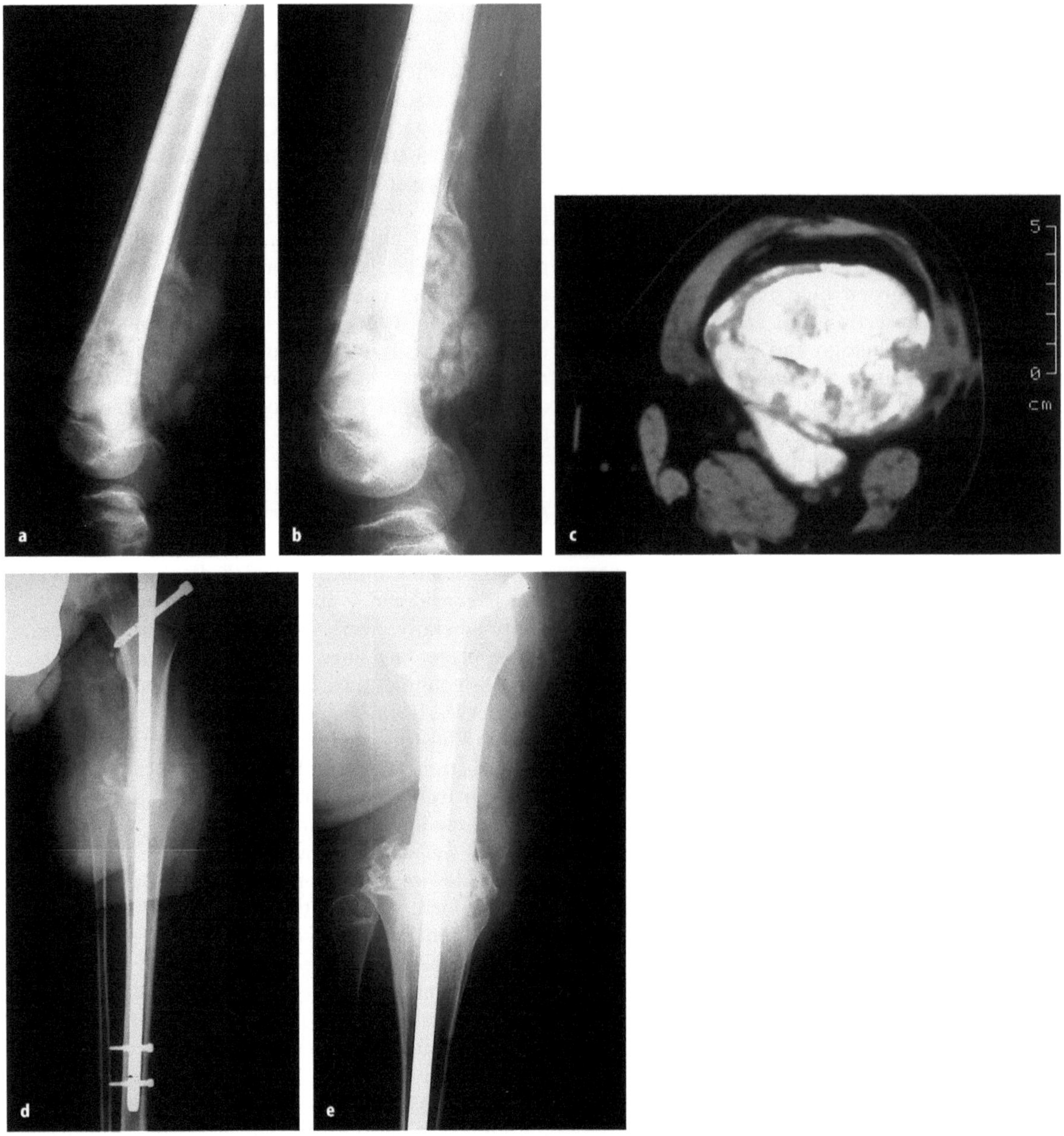

**Fig. 10.1.** **a** Osteosarcoma of the distal femur in a 10-year-old boy. **b** Radiographic picture of the same case after preoperative neoadjuvant chemotherapy: volume reduction and ossification of the tumoral mass. **c** CT scan showing the ossified tumoral mass, which includes the popliteal vascular bundle. **d** Distal femur resection including the vascular bundle and rotationplasty. The femur to tibia fixation by static locked nail can be easily performed without concern to the different shapes of the involved bones. **e** Radiograph 6 months later: bone fusion and evident callus formation

formed as usual. When the shaft reconstruction is performed by autogenous graft struts or a cement spacer, the nail is inserted leaving an empty space corresponding to the resected bone.

The autogenous graft (fibula or cortical segment of the tibia positioned opposite the frontal plane) will be positioned all around the nail and fixed by screws. Maximal care must be taken to avoid distraction because of the risk of nerve and vessel damage. The experience gained at the Rizzoli Institute has shown that using the nail in diaphyseal resection has the advantage of being a fast method of reconstruction without the risk of angle deformity; on the other hand, using allografts, particularly in femoral reconstruction and in patients with high-grade malignant tumor needing postoperative chemotherapy treatment, the complication rate is high: 11 delayed union or

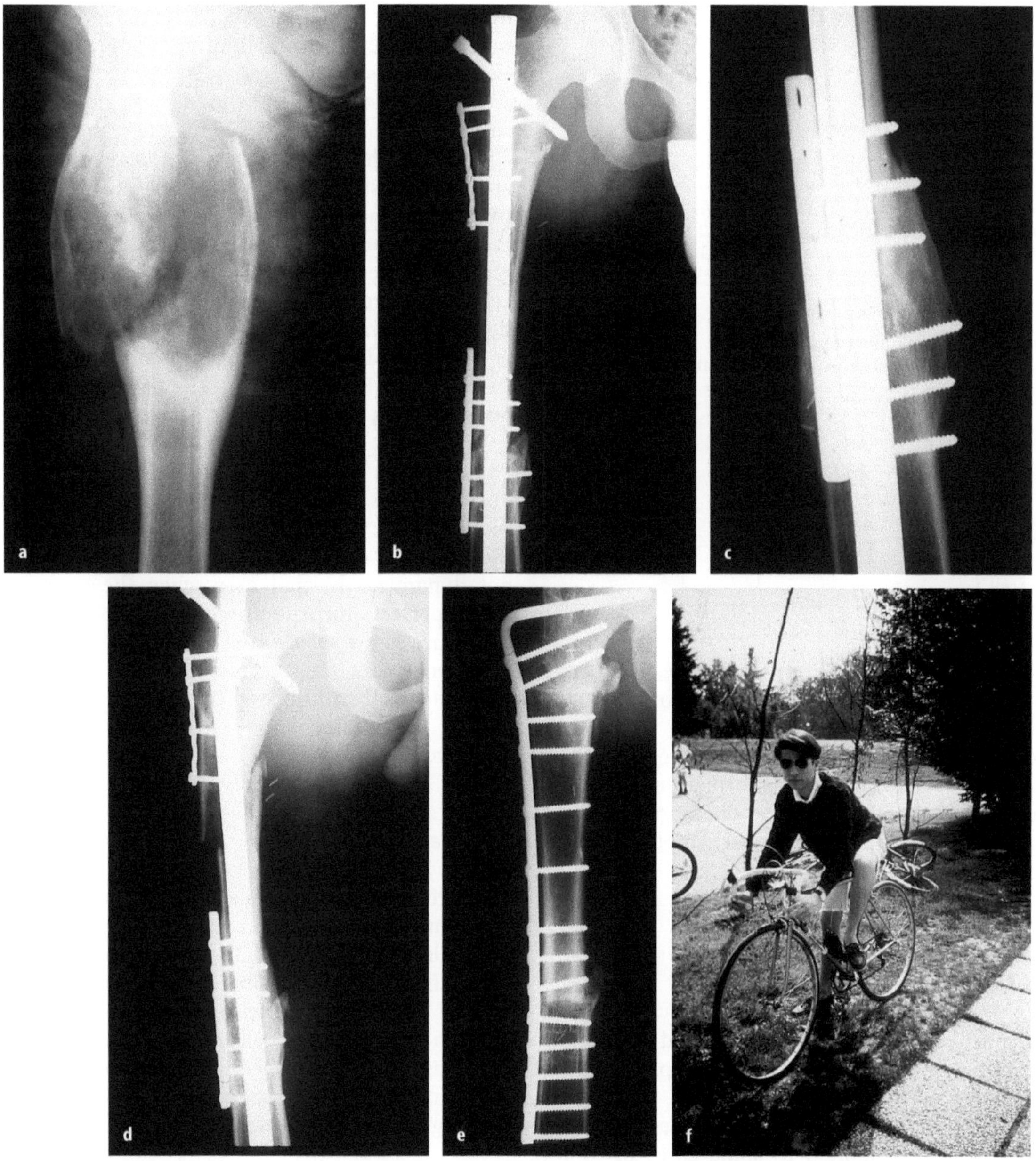

**Fig. 10.2.** **a** Pathological fracture in low-grade osteosarcoma in 12-year-old boy. **b** The patient was submitted to en bloc resection and reconstruction by allograft, GK static nailing, and plating. No chemotherapy was performed. Simple nailing of such a lesion before diagnosis would have disseminated the osteosarcoma all along the diaphysis, making necessary hindquarter amputation to achieve the same margin. **c** Favorable progression of the distal osteotomy line at 6 months of follow-up. **d** Graft fracture 8 months after resection. **e** New grafting (massive allograft), stabilization by special condylar plate. Fusion of the osteotomy lines at 10 months of follow-up. **f** Full functional recovery. No sign of disease at 3 years of follow-up

nonunion and five fractures among 13 patients treated (Tables 10.1, 10.2). At present, in these conditions, we prefer to plate the allograft (Fig. 10.2 e), preferably filled with acrylic cement, while in short bone resections (10–14 cm) that do not require substantial soft tissue excision, the locked nail associated with autografts is a good alternative (2 cases rated excellent in our series).

**Postoperative Care**

Cast immobilization is applied for 8 weeks; then the patient is allowed to proceed to joint and

**Table 10.1.** Locking nailing after shaft resection: 39 cases

| Diagnosis | |
|---|---|
| Osteosarcoma | 23 |
| Ewing sarcoma | 4 |
| Malignant fibrous histiocytoma | 2 |
| Fibrosarcoma | 1 |
| Synovial sarcoma | 1 |
| Giant cell tumor | 4 |
| Osteoblastoma | 1 |
| Aneurysmal bone cyst | 2 |
| Osteitis | 1 |

**Table 10.2.** Massive allografts and locked nail. Results of 39 cases of resection (modified from Mankin criteria)

| | Excel-lent | Good | Fair | Poor |
|---|---|---|---|---|
| Intercalary shaft reconstruction | 5 | 7 | 0 | 5 |
| Knee arthrodesis | 5 | 4 | 2 | 2 |
| Ankle arthrodesis | 4 | 1 | 0 | 0 |
| Rotationplasty | 4 | 0 | 0 | 0 |
| Overall | 17 | 12 | 2 | 7 |

muscle rehabilitation. From this time, brace and walking canes are advised with only partial weight-bearing. Full weight-bearing as a rule should be considered only when the osteotomy lines show evidence of callus formation. Usually it occurs 3–12 months after the operation, depending on the use of postoperative chemotherapy and the type of resection.

### *Distal Femur or Proximal Tibia Resection and Knee Arthrodesis*

The oncological indication is limited to tumors occurring in the epiphysis and metaphysis as an alternative to prosthetic replacement. The development of modular prostheses has reduced such indications, now limited to some cases of tumor intra-articular involvement requiring resection of the entire joint or when muscle excision is very extensive. However, it is still suggested in young and active male patients between 9 and 14 years old. From a functional point of view, a sound knee fusion allows heavy work performance but prevents normal sitting.

Special extra-long slotted nails are required: reaming must be performed separately along the tibia and femur. The entry point should be slightly more medial, to avoid excessive frontal nail impingement. Particular care is required during hammering because of the risk of neck fracture. Simple nailing has been frequently used for knee resection and fusion (the Putti-Juvara technique); the locking nail allows reducing or avoiding plaster cast time, limiting dangerous rotational stresses on the grafts.

If a massive allograft is used, it is important to select a straight graft, to reduce the risk of breakage during the introduction. If autogenous grafts are used, first the nail will be inserted, carefully respecting the length of the resected segment, then static locking will be performed; finally, the grafts will be positioned. The use of corticocancellous autogenous chips can be useful to avoid delayed union or nonunion, unless chemotherapy is not to be delivered in the postoperative period. In this case, it is better to save the bone autogenous stock in case of further delayed union [7].

**Postoperative Care**

Postoperative care is the same as in diaphyseal resection; with the use of the locking nail, cast immobilization can be reduced. It is important to not dynamize the nail even when the graft presents perfect incorporation. Rotational stresses can cause late fracture (the latest observed in our experience was after 50 months) due to the uncompleted substitution of the graft by the host, leaving a weaker bone requiring protection throughout life.

### *Ankle Resection and Fusion*

Very frequently, soft tissue involvement with vessel compression makes limb salvage procedures for malignant tumors in the distal tibia impossible. When feasible, a tibia nail longer than the normal length will be used, sized to allow distal bolts in the talus and calcaneum. Once the resection has been performed and the nail inserted, the segmented fibula (vascularized or not) or tibia grafting will be positioned all around the nail.

**Postoperative Care**

Cast immobilization is required for 4 weeks, then partial weight-bearing in a brace will be allowed for 8–12 weeks, to avoid disturbing the incorporation of autogenous grafts. When an allograft is used and/or chemotherapy delivered after surgery, no weight-bearing at all is advised for 6 months.

### *Free Vascularized Fibula Support*

Where microsurgical facilities are available, primary vascularized fibula can be considered as the procedure of choice. Usually this is not associated with an IM nail fixation. The indication recommends using minimal osteosynthesis and/or a combination with massive allograft [4]. We have used a vascularized fibula in seven cases as a salvage procedure in allografts for intercalary femoral reconstruction, always healing the graft nonunion. In this case, the free vascularized fibula is positioned on the medial site of the allograft in an effort to achieve the best possible contact, and screwed to the host proximal and distal bone. In intercalary resection, when sound osteosynthesis can be achieved, we do not advise the primary use of vascularized fibula, leaving this technique as a salvage procedure.

### *Rotationplasty*

This surgical procedure described by van Nes in 1950 [18] provides the oncological result of a thigh amputation as well as the functional result of a below-the-knee amputation in the treatment of large malignant tumors (stage IIB) of the diaphysis and distal part of the femur [5]. It requires the psychological acceptance of the patient (disturbance of his own body imaging) and his family, and the manufacture of a special prosthesis. Special physical therapy is also required to learn to use the reversed ankle as a knee.

The fixation between the proximal residual femur and the 180° reversed proximal tibia is easily performed using an intramedullary device (rather than a cortical plate, difficult to adapt to such different surfaces) and a femoral Grosse and Kempf standard nail – a proximally dynamic locked nail – is effective in obtaining rapid fusion in adults. For the more frequent pediatric indications, the smaller 10-mm unslotted nail can be too thick for the tibia shaft and is the limit of the indication for nailing in this procedure.

In the experience gained at the Rizzoli Institute, uneventful fusion (4–7 months) was achieved in four patients; one of them had previously undergone plate fixation, which resulted in pseudarthrosis.

#### Postoperative Care

Immediate active mobilization is scheduled to prevent stiffness and to achieve complete foot dorsiflexion, which allows full extension of the new knee. A special custom-made prosthesis is fit around the forefoot, giving it the shape of a leg. Weight-bearing is allowed after 40 days of spica cast immobilization, with a walking spica cast transferring the weight to the ischium. Two months later, as soon as the prosthetic limb is ready, full weight-bearing is allowed.

## Treatment of Metastases: Palliation

The surgical treatment of metastases, myeloma, and lymphomas is a priori palliation and its goal is to provide patients with maximal functional activity while performing the required local treatment (most frequently radiotherapy). Radiosensitive lesions such as metastatic lesions from breast carcinoma, myeloma, and lymphomas are generally subsequently subjected to radiation therapy. Metastases from lung or kidney tumors are less radiosensitive: intralesional curettage or even resection can be considered for longer stability. Long bone shaft metastases are considered to threaten stability when circumferential destruction is over 50% [10]: at that time a preventive osteosynthesis is already indicated.

### *Pathological Fractures*

A pathological fracture has a weak healing potential (or none at all), so a strong device is needed to obtain immediate functional recovery and weight-bearing. A standard Grosse and Kempf nail can be used in the femur and tibia, frequently the unslotted ones; the gamma nail (or better, the new long gamma nail) is indicated for the proximal femur, as well as the Seidel nail for humeral metastases and the Lefèvre nail for the ulna.

In proximal femur metastases, the alternative of a prosthetic replacement must always be considered. Factors in favor of prosthetic replacement are the radioresistent tumor, epiphyseal involvement, and femoral neck destruction in a patient with a long life expectancy.

The surgical technique is the same as for traumatic fractures. The patient is positioned as for a traumatic fracture, with the traction pin in the usual position for the femur and tibia. If the diagnosis has not been made previously, an intraoperative histological frozen section can be obtained by the direct approach. In this case, the surgical incision must be performed such that it is included in the skin incision of the possible resection if the lesion is proven to be a primary tumor. Once the diagnosis has been confirmed, there are two possibilities: suture the biopsy incision and perform the usual technique of closed IM locked nailing, or better, perform an intralesional curettage.

Other indications for closed nailing are brown tumors of hyperparathyroidism, a condition that will heal after parathyroidectomy with complete bone formation.

### *Impending Fractures*

Preventive stabilization is a valid indication when a pathological condition weakens the bone (impending fractures). This procedure is also only a palliative measure, to be limited to metastases or malignant hemopathies. In 14 cases of this series, a static Grosse and Kempf nail or a static gamma nail (standard or long) were implanted, soon followed by radiotherapy. Immediate weight-bearing was allowed.

The operative technique is the same as for traumatic fractures, the traction pin positioned in order to avoid unexpected displacement in the frequent case of intraoperative occurrence of the pathological fracture. A theoretically higher risk of fat embolism is reported when reaming on the closed medullary cavity [14]. No clinical onset of fat embolism was observed in our series; however, a particularly careful reaming technique is suggested, by increments of 5 mm, slowly and delicately, with frequent rinsing of the medullary cavity. Larger nails are to be avoided so that excessive reaming is not attempted. The maximum reaming diameter is related to bone size; however, we advise not reaming more than 14–15 mm in the femur and 12–13 mm in the tibia.

### Treatment of Fractures on Irradiated Bone

These pathological fractures occur, as a result of minimal trauma, on bone previously subjected to radiation therapy, mostly for the treatment of a neoplastic disease of the same bone segment or of a nearby tissue. The irradiated bone loses its mechanical and biological features due to extensive bone necrosis [8]. The healing process is heavily disrupted for the same reason. A high rate of pseudarthrosis must be expected as no physiological callus formation can occur in the absence of normal bone vascularity. At particularly high risk is a fracture on the irradiated tibia shaft, where the already precarious vascularity and the thin irradiated soft tissue could definitively compromise callus formation and enhance the risk of infection. The irradiated fractured bone heals by a process of creeping substitution, which will be obtained (if at all) after a very long time (months or even years). Full rigidity is required in these cases. The advantage of locked nailing is the closed procedure, which does not interfere with the blood supply and possibly brings reaming products from the healthy bone to the necrotic bone. However, the micromovements allowed by the nail (which are an advantage in traumatic fractures on normal bone –15) can negatively interfere with the healing of a fracture on irradiated bone [2, 6].

In our experience with 8 cases, Grosse and Kempf locked nailing and long gamma nails have allowed immediate functional recovery; however, autogenous bone grafting was needed in 20% of the cases and two nails broke 8 and 9 months after osteosynthesis. Particularly interesting is the case illustrated in Fig. 10.3: the fracture was demonstrated to be finally healed in the amputation specimen, despite the broken nail. The long gamma nail seems to be the best device for fractures on the irradiated femora: it provides good rotational stiffness, the proximal grip is very satisfying, and it reinforces the entire femur. The standard gamma nail is not indicated, in our opinion, as it can create further mechanical differences in a weakened bone. Before subjecting a fractured irradiated tibia to intramedullary fixation, the patient should be warned of the risk of nonunion and infection, frequently leading to amputation. Among the conservative alternatives, one should consider the resection of all the irradiated tissues (bone, skin, soft tissues) and reconstruction with a free vascularized graft, requiring, however, the possibility of good vascular anastomosis. When the skin is not heavily damaged, resection and Ilizarov reconstruction could be considered as well.

After locked nailing of a fracture on irradiated bone, cancellous bone grafting should be considered; at least as revision surgery if no callus formation is observed 8 weeks after the osteosynthesis.

## Implants

Most of the procedures described can be performed with the standard nail (humerus, ulna, standard femur and tibia, gamma and long gamma). The long gamma nail is superior to the standard femoral nail for stabilization of femoral metastases, as the lag screw introduced in the femoral neck is more effective (mostly in osteoporosis associated with metastatic bone) than the downward oblique 6.25-mm screw of the standard femoral nail. Moreover, it is an unslotted nail: its bending stiffness is 20% higher than the slotted nail and torsional stiffness 20 times higher, thus providing a 30% higher fatigue stress.

Special custom-made extra-long standard femoral nails are used for resections and fusion around the knee: these nails are slotted to avoid excessive stresses during insertion.

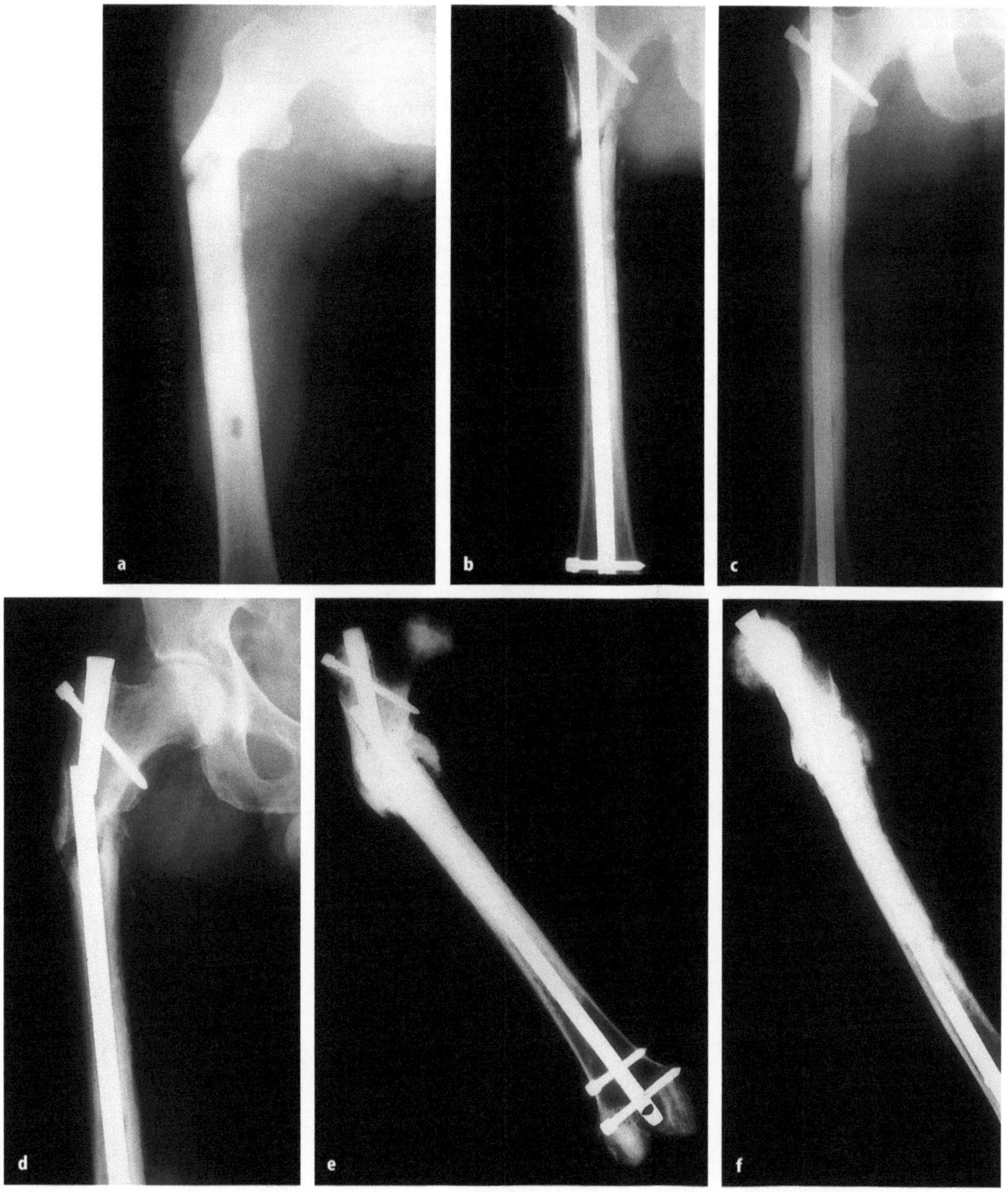

**Fig. 10.3. a** Proximal femur fracture occurring on irradiated bone (non-Hodgkin lymphoma) in a 56-year-old man. **b** Closed fixation by static locked nailing **c** Two months later, the progression of callus formation seems favorable: partial weight-bearing is allowed. **d** Refracture due to minimal trauma, associated with mechanical nail failure 8 months after the operation. No surgical revision was decided due to concomitant skin radiation-related problems. **e, f** The patient is submitted to hindquarter amputation 5 months later due to massive thrombosis and limb ischemia. The radiogram of the specimen shows fracture healing with abundant callus formation

## Errors and Potential Hazards

### Diagnosis

The most serious mistake is to nail a pathological fracture without a confirmed histological diagnosis of the disease weakening the affected bone. As previously noted, if a primary malignant tumor is nailed believing it was metastasis, no salvage procedure is possible due to the contamination of soft tissue and of the entire bone. Hindquarter amputation is the only appropriate treatment after nailing a pathological fracture because of osteosarcoma of the femoral shaft (Fig. 10.2). Conversely, closed nailing of a radiosensitive tumor, such as malignant hemopathies (Fig. 10.4) or certain metastases, can be performed, as the entire segment will be subsequently subjected to radiation therapy.

The correct attitude with a pathological fracture is to reach diagnosis by biopsy. Trocar biopsy under CT scan monitoring has proved to be safe, fast, and effective. Another solution is to perform an intraoperative frozen-section biopsy before nailing. In this case, the biopsy must be performed by a skin incision that can be included in the incision of the limb salvage procedure, in case a primary tumor is diagnosed.

## Reaming

When using an unslotted nail, 2 or 3 mm over-reaming must be performed. This way an unslotted nail cannot be used in thinner shafts or when using thin allografts.

Reaming a closed medullary cavity can increase the risk of fat embolism, as demonstrated experimentally [14]. The increase in intramedullary pressure is related to the shape of the reamer but mostly to overly forceful high-speed reaming.

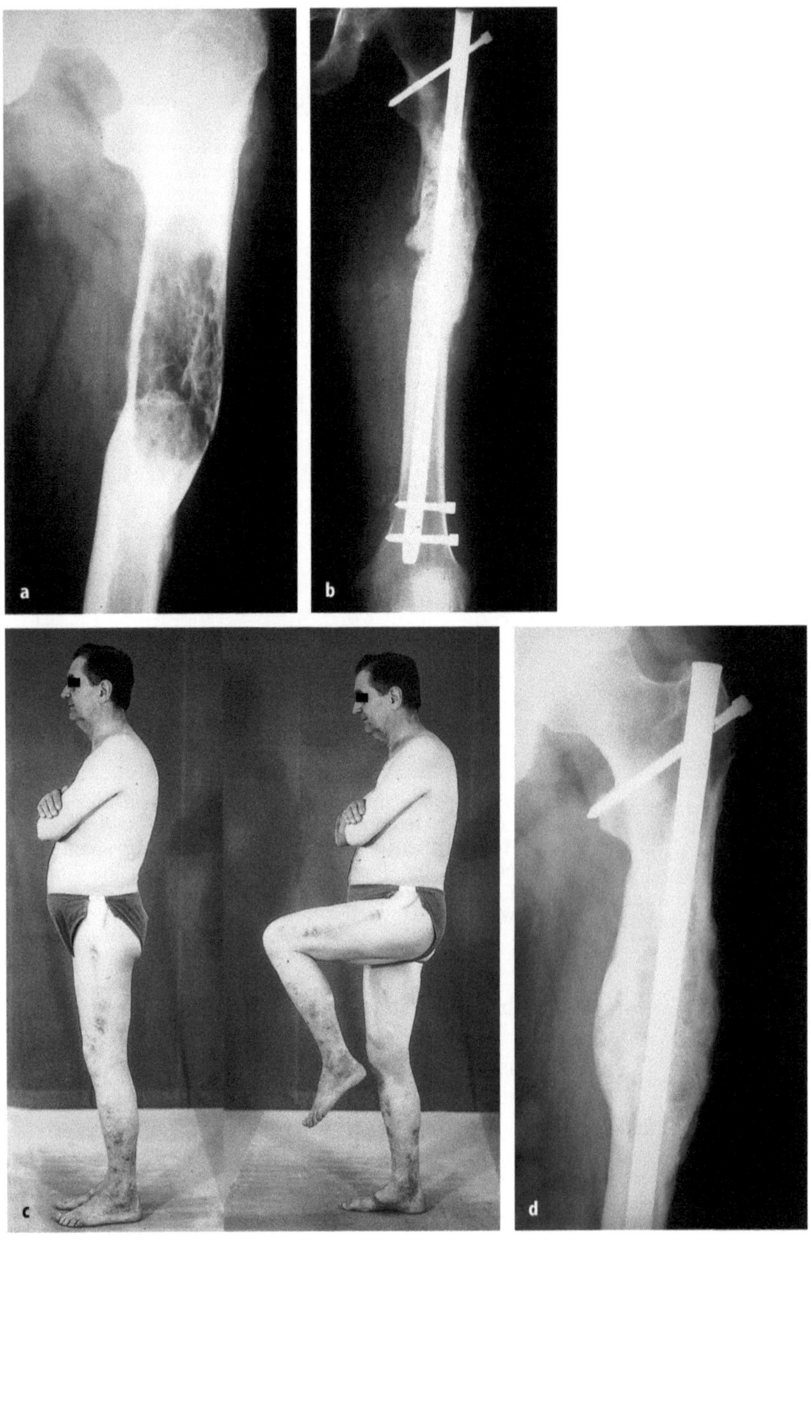

**Fig. 10.4. a** Wide osteolytic lesion in femoral shaft of a 62-year-old male patient affected by multiple myeloma. **b** Curettage of the lytic cavity, static GK preventive stabilization, filling by acrylic cement. The patient was then submitted to the protocol of chemotherapy and radiation therapy on the entire femur. **c** Immediate full functional recovery. **d** Four-year postoperative X-ray showing the persistent correct positioning of the nail and the new bone formation all around the filled cavity

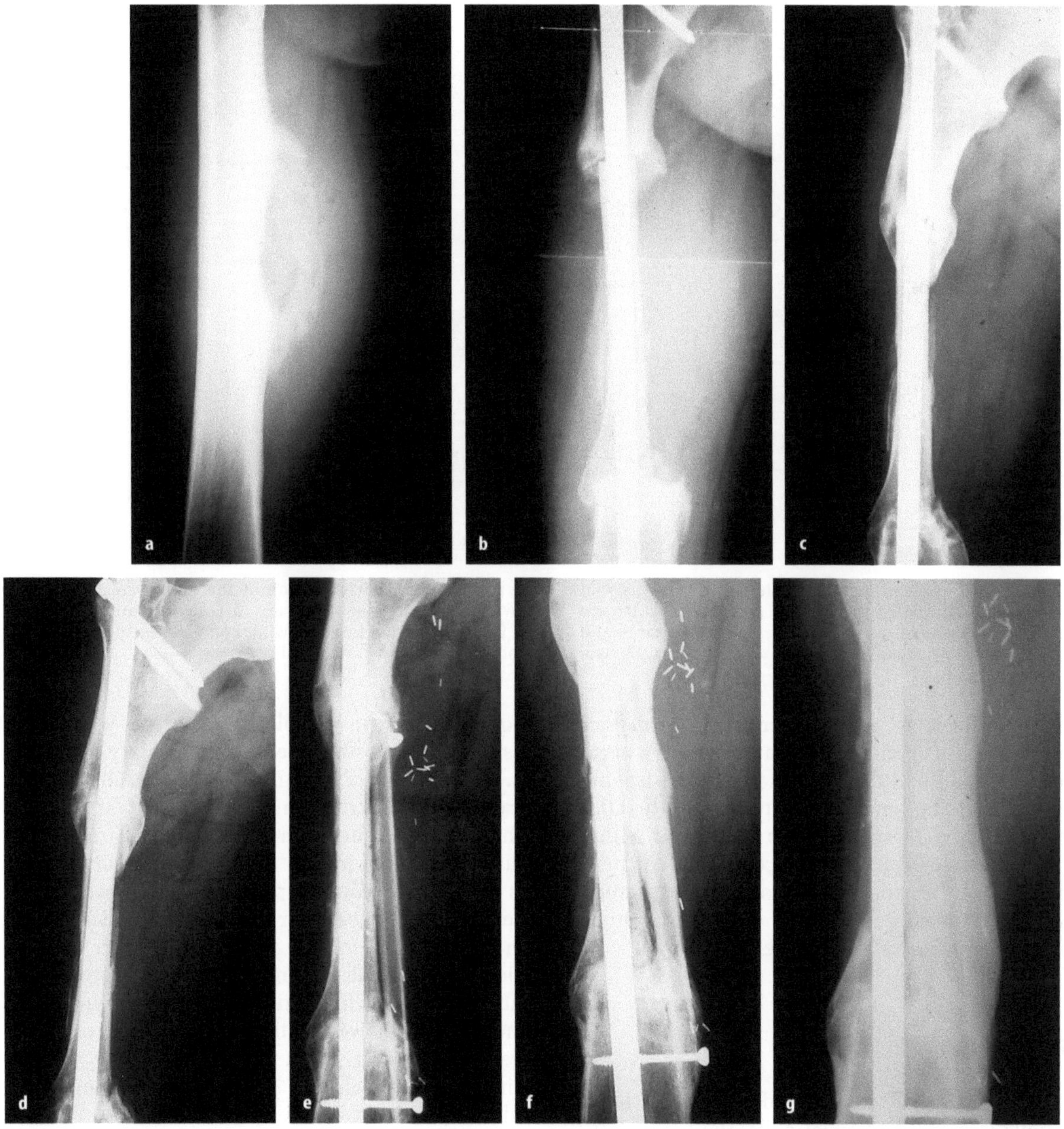

**Fig. 10.5. a** Diaphyseal osteosarcoma submitted to neoadjuvant chemotherapy, resulting in tumor necrosis and peripheral bone formation, making en bloc resection feasible. **b** The reconstruction was performed by a massive graft that was too thin (allograft tibia). Static GK nailing. **c** No weight-bearing was allowed, but 6 months later, the graft collapsed with breakage of the transverse screw. **d** An attempt to achieve fusion was unsuccessfully performed by introducing a new transverse screw, combined with autogenous cancellous grafting. **e** Vascularized fibula grafting was performed. **f** X-ray at 8 months of follow-up showing fusion of the graft. **g** Two years after fibula grafting: fusion and hypertrophy of the graft. No recurrence 5 years after the diagnosis

## Allografts

The graft must be carefully chosen because a discrepancy between host and allograft is not tolerated (Fig. 10.5). Even the longitudinal curvature must be considered, to avoid fractures during nail insertion.

## Osteotomy Lines

The process of allograft incorporation occurs by creeping substitution and therefore requires absolute rigidity and closed contact between host and graft; even a microscopic gap is very slowly filled [15] or is not filled at all. When using a nail as a reconstructive device after diaphyseal resection, it

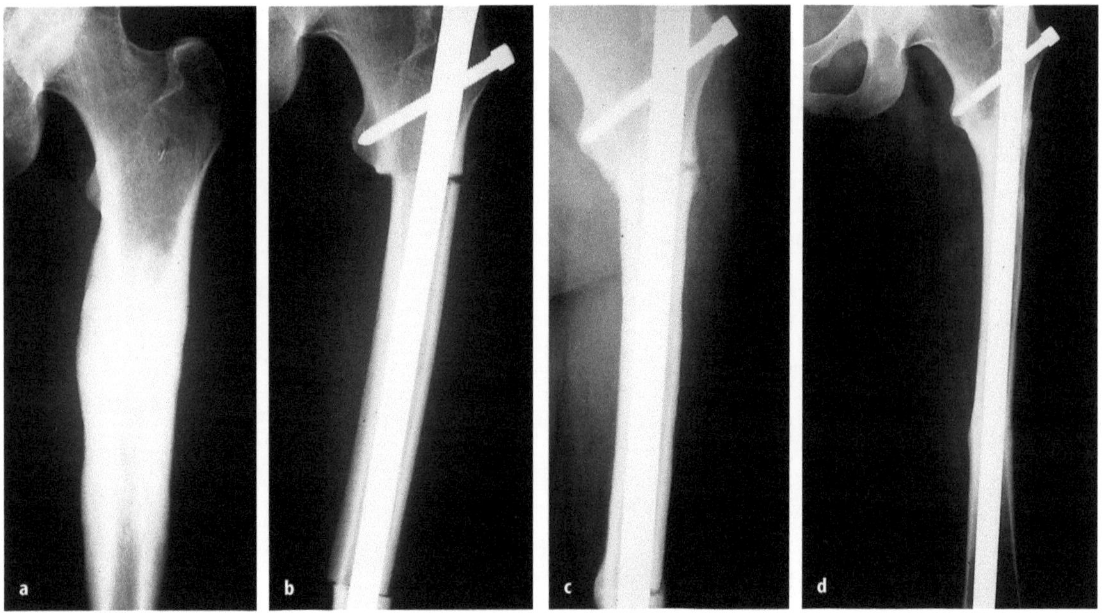

**Fig. 10.6.** **a** Chronic hematogenous osteitis in a 35-year-old female patient submitted to repeated surgical debridement procedures. **b** Extraperiosteal shaft resection (20 cm.) and reconstruction by massive allograft and static GK nail. **c** Six months later: partial fusion of the graft. Patient walking with complete weight-bearing. **d** One year after operation, follow-up radiograph showing complete fusion of both osteotomy lines. Full functional recovery

is very difficult to achieve perfect host-to-graft contact at both levels due to the different curvature of the nail and the graft. Rather than leaving a gap wider than 1 mm, it is better to fill the allograft with acrylic cement and to stabilize it with a pair of plates. It is generally incorrect to consider allograft host junction as a transverse fracture. One must consider the graft as necrotic bone with, consequently, a low chance of healing.

## Conclusions

The clinical experience acquired shows that locking nails (femoral and tibial nails, the Seidel nail, the gamma nail, the Lefèvre nail) are very effective in stabilizing pathological fractures or impending fractures given correct oncological indications. Only one mechanical failure was observed in the treatment of a fracture on irradiated bone (five cases in our series). The use of these nails is also advisable as a reconstructive device after short diaphyseal resection in benign aggressive tumor, using autogenous grafts, or in some special indications such as rotationplasty (four cases, of which one of them was treatment of plate failure with uneventful healing). For knee resection and fusion (using a special long slotted nail) and in ankle arthrodesis supplemented by an autogenous graft, the locked nail is still indicated.

Some important complications arose when a massive allograft was used in intercalary resection. In our opinion, the unsuccessful results after intercalary reconstruction with allograft are due to the differences between the biology of fracture healing and the biology of graft incorporation. This procedure requires perfect contact between bone and graft as well as rigid fixation, which has been rejected [15] for the treatment of fresh traumatic fractures. The locking nail does not provide a sufficiently rigid fixation. In cases not requiring chemotherapy, however, the results seem to be more favorable (Fig. 10.6).

Finally a few technical points must be emphasized:

- Immediate full weight-bearing can be allowed in most pathological fractures and in lytic lesions stabilized by the Grosse and Kempf or gamma nail.
- Partial weight-bearing can be allowed during radiotherapy in pathological fractures with a wide bone gap.
- Delayed weight-bearing is mandatory in the presence of grafts.
- Entry point selection and reaming must be done particularly carefully when using the unslotted Grosse and Kempf nail or the long gamma nail: at least 2 mm more than the nail must be reamed.

*Acknowledgments.* This chapter is dedicated to Prof. Mario Campanacci (†), an unparalleled teacher of tumor surgery. Further thanks are extended to Dr. Rodolfo Capanna and Dr. Mario Mercuri, who performed many of the described surgical procedures, and to Dr. Marco Manfrini for his precious support in describing the vascularized grafting.

## References

1. Babin SR, Katzner M, Vidal P, Simon P, Kempf JF, Schvingt E (1987) Résection-reconstruction diaphysaire fémorale par allogreffe massive fixée par clou médullaire verrouillé. Rev Chir Orthop 73:25-29
2. Brown KL (1991) Vascularised bone transfert for the menagement of postirradiation of pathologic fracture. Complication of limb salvage. ISOLS, Montreal, pp 585-588
3. Campanacci M (1990) Bone and soft tissue tumors, Aulo Gaggi, Bologna. Springer, Vienna New York
4. Capanna R, Donati D, del Ben M, Campanacci DA, Bufalini C, Campanacci M (1992) Innesti omoplastici in patologia neoplastica. Chir Org Mov 77:69-77
5. Capanna R, Del Ben M, Campanacci DA, Catani F, Giannini S (1992) L'intervento di giroplastica nelle resezioni segmentarie del femore. Chir Org Mov 77:135-149
6. Capanna R, Gasbarrini A, Campanacci DA, Del Ben M, Donati D, Manfrini M (1994) Le fratture patologiche in osso irradiato. Attualità in tema di osteosintesi, 5° Congresso CIOD Abstract book. Sesto di Pusteria (BZ), Gennaio, pp 23-28
7. Donati D, Capanna R, Campanacci DA, Del Ben M, Ercolani C, Masetti C, Taminiau A, Exner GU, Dubousset JF, Poitout D, Canadell J, Loty B, Langlais F (1993) Innesti ossei omoplastici massivi utilizzati per ricostruzioni intercalari ed artrodesi dopo resezione per tumore. Studio policentrico europeo. Chir Org Mov 78:81-94
8. Duparc J, Bocquet C, Frot B, Gastambide D (1977) Les radio-lésions de la hanche. Rev Rhum 44:79-89
9. Enneking WF, Spainer SS, Goodman MA (1980) A system for the surgical staging of muscoloskeletal sarcomas. Clin Orthop 153:106-120
10. Fidler M (1981) Incidence of fractures through metastases in long bones. Acta Orthop Scand 52:623-627
11. Habermann ET, Lopez RA (1989) Metastatic disease of bone and treatment of pathological fractures. Orthop Clin North Am 20:469-486
12. Johnson KD, Tencer A, Blumenthal AA, Johnston DWC (1986) Biomechanical performance of locked intramedullary nail systems in comminuted femoral shaft fracture. Clin Orthop 206:151-161
13. Mankin HJ, Dopplet SH, Sullivan TR, Tomford WW (1982) Osteoarticular and intercalary allograft transplantation in the management of malignat tumors of bone. Cancer 50:1663-1673
14. Manning JB, Back AW (1983) Fat release after femur nailing in the dog. JTrauma 23:322-325
15. McKibbin B (1978) The biology of fracture healing in long bones. J Bone Joint Surg 60B:150-162
16. René RW, van der Hulst J, Frans AJ, van den Wildenberg J, Vroemen PAM, Greve JM (1994) Intramedullary nailing of (impending) pathologic fractures. J Trauma 36:211-215
17. Sabato S, Stein H (1983) The surgical management of pathological fractures. Int Orthop SICOT 7:65-68
18. van Nes CP (1950) Rotation-plasty for congenital defects of the femur: making use of the ankle of shortened limb to control the knee joint of a prosthesis. J Bone Joint Surg 32B:12-16
19. Vincent A, Delloye C, De Nayer P (1990) Les allogreffes massives en chirurgie réparatrice. Cahiers d'enseignement de la SOFCOT. Conférence d'enseignement 1-20

# CHAPTER 11

# New Developments and Perspectives

F.C. Bakker, G.J. Eggink, M.L.M.J. Goessens, H.J.T.M. Haarman, C. Lefèvre, D. Le Nen, P. Patka, M.J.M. Segers, J.W.J.L. Stapert, J.P.A.M. Verbruggen,



## Degradable and Resorbable Nails

P. Patka, H.J.T.M. Haarman, F.C. Bakker

Throughout history man has needed to repair broken, nonfunctional bones. As knowledge and technical skills on fracture healing increased, several noninvasive and surgical techniques were designed to support the natural process of self-repair. Rational conservative treatment was developed in the nineteenth century and surgical treatment of fractures, i.e., open reduction and fixation, has been used since World War II.

Most implants currently used in surgery are manufactured from stainless steel alloys, because of their satisfactory mechanical properties and ready availability. However, significant problems are associated with stainless steel implants for fracture fixation, including the stress-shielding phenomenon, the risk of late infection or toxic reactions, and the necessity for removal of some implants [37, 41].

For many years, degradable implants have been thought to offer many potential advantages over nonabsorbable analogs.

A material that would be absorbed slowly by means of hydrolysis or enzymatic degradation would be advantageous, especially as bone implant. A second operation would not be necessary and stress-shielding would not occur, resulting in a better product from bone remodeling.

In 1971, Kulkarni et al. first described implants for fracture fixation made from biodegradable polymers [22]. Since then, a large variety of biodegradable materials have been tested in vitro and in vivo [2, 3, 32, 35]. From these reports, it seems that the mechanical properties of the polymers show considerable variation. The distribution of molecular weights plays an important role. Crystallinity, the amount of free monomers, and the stereotactic configuration are other factors that influence the mechanical properties of the biodegradable material.

A biodegradable material used for fracture fixation must supply the injured bone with sufficient support for a sufficient length of time. In several animal studies, poly-L-lactic acid (PLLA) pins or screws haven used as fracture fixation devices. The ultimate strength of PLLA rods resembles the ultimate strength of cortical bone, i.e., 10–150 Mpa. Polylactic acid with a high mean molecular weight (260,000), a large degree of crystallinity, and a small number of free monomers may contribute to a development of a long-term biodegradable interlocking nail for fracture fixation [5, 44].

### Biocompatibility

The development and application of surgical and orthopedic implants made it necessary to give increasing attention to the materials used for the manufacture of such implants. These materials, which are also referred to as biomaterials, have to meet certain chemical, physical, and biological requirements in order to ensure optimum and long-lasting function of the implant and success of the implantation procedure. The chemical and physical requirements include such properties as strength, wearing friction behavior, and corrosion resistance, as well as workability and sterilizability. Acceptance by living tissue and stability within the body also constitute important biological requirements.

Biocompatibility is determined by the extent of chemical and biological interaction between host and implant and the stability (mechanical integrity) of the implant. Rapid and inexpensive in vitro techniques can be used to predict the quantity and cytotoxicity of moieties released by an implant. These techniques can also be used to predict changes in mechanical properties of a material during implantation. This can be important in selecting materials as candidates for definitive preclinical animal experimental and clinical studies.

A compatible implant would have no effect on the adjacent tissue, the nearby cells would show no abnormalities, no variant cell types would appear, there would be no inflammatory reactions, and there would be no cell necrosis. The histology of the tissue surrounding the implant would be altogether normal.

The implant recognized by the recipient as a foreign body will be isolated by encapsulation.

Commonly, the thickness of the encapsulating fibrous tissue membrane is often taken as a measure of the compatibility of the implant in relation to the surrounding tissue. The thinner the membrane, the better the compatibility of the implant.

Animal studies of biocompatibility are necessary because of the complexity of chemical, biological, and physical (mechanical) implant–host interactions. Strong dependence of the tissue response on the biomechanical conditions along the interfaces has been demonstrated in experimental studies. The amount of motion between the implant and the adjacent tissues contributes greatly to the biological response. Any histological evaluation of biomaterial for bone replacement must be accompanied by a careful description of the load and changes that have been applied to the bone–implant interface. The portion of the interface from which the histological sample was taken has to be noted.

Unfortunately, methods to determine compatibility are not standardized. This complicates any comparison of different studies of a specific implant material. Sometimes it makes such comparison impossible. Therefore, a rigid system to determine material biocompatibility by standardized test controls has been proposed. Implant materials should be subjected to biological tests in a stepwise standarized procedure. As is well known, no general agreement on this has yet been reached. In general, either a material has slowly evolved to fulfill a long-established clinical need or a new material has been tried on a somewhat arbitrary basis to explore clinical and commercial possibilities. It is likely that most biomaterials have become known to us in this fashion. This situation is less satisfactory than a thoroughly scientific approach to the development of biocompatible materials.

## Biodegradability, Bioactive and Bioinert Material

The terms "biodegradable," "bioactive," and "bioinert" are related to the biomechanical response the implanted material provokes in the surrounding tissue and relates to the notion of biocompatibility. The tissue reactions caused by relative movement between the implant and the adjacent tissue are not covered by these terms. The term "biodegradable" (bioresorbable) has been used for material that, after insertion into host tissue, is dissolved without provoking any adverse tissue reaction. Some of the calcium phosphate ceramics possess such a property.

The terms "bioactive" and "bioinert" are related to the biochemical response induced by the material at the site of implantation. The bioactive materials induce the same reaction as natural bone mineral would at the same implant area while the bioinert materials cause no reaction at all. Bioactive ceramics can form a tight junction with the osseous tissue, analogous to the natural bone mineral. This seems to be a biochemical phenomenon, but there is still no explanation for this behavior of bioactive materials.

## Current Bone Repair Technology

Most implants currently used in traumatology for bone repair are made of stainless steel, due to its satisfactory mechanical properties and availability. However, significant problems are associated with stainless steel implants for fracture fixation, such as stress shielding, the risk of infection, corrosion problems, even sensitivity, and mostly, the necessity to remove implants [34, 37, 41].

Bioresorbable fracture fixation materials without these disadvantages and without the need for a removal operation could be very useful in fracture treatment. Bioresorbable fracture fixation materials, derived from the resorbable suture materials developed in de 1960s, can be completely metabolized in a biological system. There is no need for an operation to remove these implants, providing a medical, financial, and psychological advantage to the patient.

At present, the most important degradable implant materials are:

- Poly-L-lactic acid (PLLA)
- Poly-DL-lactic acid (PDLLA)
- Polyglycolic acid (PGA)
- Polydioxanone (PDS)
- Polyorthoester (POE)
- Poly-C-capralactone (PCL)

Different biodegradable materials for fracture fixation haven been tested in the research laboratory and in a clinical setting [8, 16, 30, 39, 42, 46]. In a prospective randomized study on fractures of the ankle joint, PLLA/PGA (Biofix) biodegradable implants (Fig. 11.1) were tested in patients [7]. Forty-three patients with fracture dislocation of the ankle joint were treated by open reduction and fixation with either steel or biodegradable implants. Results in both groups were favorable and the biodegradable material appears to be useful for some fracture fixations to obviate the need for a second operation.

The use of biodegradable implants is not, however, without problems. The most commonly occurring postoperative complication of these implants is the delayed inflammatory reaction resulting in a sterile sinus or delayed wound swelling. The patient has no local or systemic signs of a problem within the wound in the immediate postoperative period. The main interval between fixation of the fracture and the clinical manifestation of the reaction is 12 weeks. The overall complication rate due to delayed inflammatory reaction with PGA implant is approximately 8%. The rate of inflammation-related complications is estimated to be around 1.5% in PLLA implants [46].

The histological characteristics of specimens obtained during debridement of the sinus tracts demonstrate a nonspecific foreign-body reaction with abundant giant cells phagocytosing the debris from the polymer. This polymer debris possesses a high crystallinity.

In experimental studies, several investigators have demonstrated that implants of polyglycolic acid, polylactic acid, or polyparadioxanone are completely absorbable within bone tissue. New bone is deposited on and within the implant as degradation proceeds [32].

In animal experiments, large biodegradable implants for the fixation of femur fractures were also recently tested (Fig. 11.2). Polylactic acid, with a high mean molecular weight (260,000), a large degree of crystallinity and a small amount of free monomers was used in pigs. The tissue response to PLLA vs stainless steel intramedullary nails was studied after 1 and 3 months of implantation. Fracture healing characteristics as well as chemical and mechanical properties deteriorated during implantation; chemical properties changed significantly within 1 and 3 months of implantation. PLLA and stainless steel implants induced similar tissue reactions. Both implants were completely surrounded by a fibrous tissue layer.

However, in another study, semi-crystalline poly-L-lactic acid (PLLA) wire was implanted in the medullary canal in rat tibiae to evaluate the fracture healing processes and the tissue reaction on the PLLA in a fractured bone [32]. The fracture healing after PLLA implantation was compared to that in the sham-operated animals. In all animals with intramedullary PLLA wire implantation, newly formed intramedullary bone formation was seen

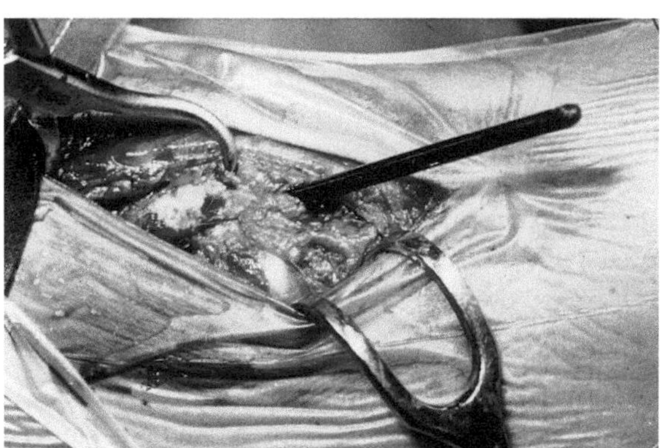

**Fig. 11.1.** Biofix rod in use for fixation of an ankle fracture

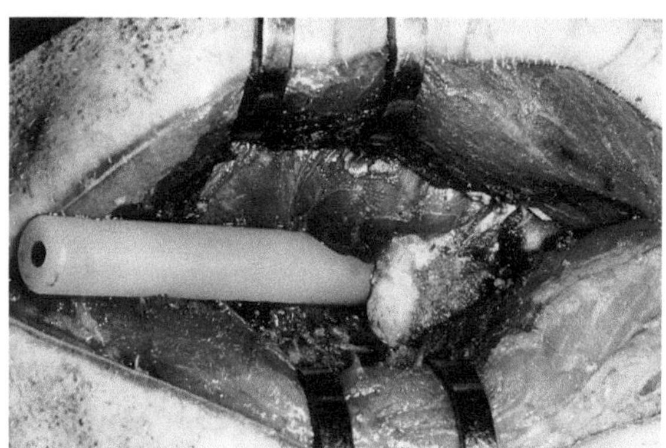

**Fig. 11.2.** Implantation of a polylactic acid rod (diameter 10 mm, length 100 mm) for a stabilization of a femoral shaft fracture in pig

immediately against the implant 2 and 6 months after implantation (Fig. 11.3) None of the sham-operated animals showed newly formed intramedullary bone formation other than fracture healing callus and normal trabecular bone.

A burst phenomenon was simulated in vivo by implantation of a large amount of a PLLA monomer. The tissue reaction on the release of a large amount of depolymerized monomer showed no adverse reaction on bone tissue [45]. This is important because it was shown that degradation of a solid implant proceeds faster in the center than at the surface due to the increasing amount of degradation by-products. Thus, after a certain interval, there is an intact outer layer filled with a jelly-like mass of monomers of high crystallinity.

When breakage of the outer layer occurs, the contents of this reservoir can be released in a short period of time: the burst phenomenon. To study this phenomenon, PLLA interlocking nails were implanted in the femur of pigs after a midshaft osteotomy. After 4 weeks, the pigs were reoperaterd. The PLLA rods were removed and a low molecular weight PLLA powder was inserted. After 4 weeks the animals were killed and the femora were studied histologically and mechanically. Active bone remodeling was seen without an inflammatory response.

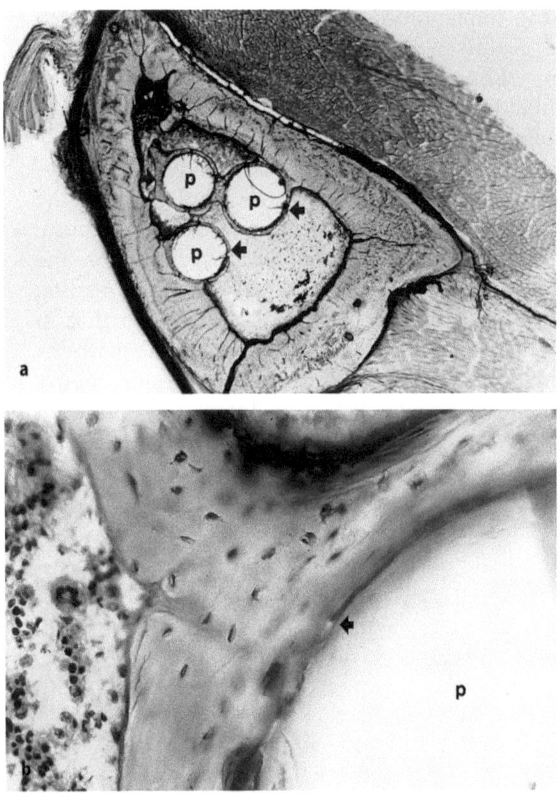


**Fig. 11.3 a, b.** Histological cross-section of tibia of rat 6 months after implantation of PLLA wires (*P*). (**a**) Overview of newly formed bony sheet (*arrow*) around PLLA wires (×20). (**b**) Enlarged part of the interface between PLLA and newly formed bony sheet around PLLA wire. The newly formed bone seems to have direct contact with the PLLA wire (×80)

Resorbable implants are promising options for fixation of fractured bone in trauma surgery. However, some problems remain to be solved before general use of these implants in surgery.

Examples of these problems are:

1. The progress of the resorption process
2. The control of mechanical properties
3. The effect of the decreased pH
4. The burst phenomenon
5. The possibility of mutagenicity

It is obvious that the optimal degradation characteristics of an implant for tissue protection and for improving tissue strength during the healing process of bone fractures remains to be found.

The clinical potential for the use of biodegradable osteosyntheses is enormous. The first successful steps using degradable implants in clinical practice have just been undertaken.

## The Telescopic Locking Nail: A Third-Generation Locking Nail for the Femur, Tibia, and Humerus

M.L.M.J. Goessens, J.P.A.M. Verbruggen, G.J. Eggink, J.W.J.L. Stapert

### Introduction

Küntscher was the first to develop a practical system for intramedullary nailing [24]. The first design of the Küntscher nail was an unreamed model. Later the design was changed to a reamed nail to enlarge the field of indications [29]. During the last 20 years, with the development of the interlocking nail, the scope for intramedullary osteosynthesis has broadened to a point where it has virtually replaced all other forms of internal fixation in the treatment of fractures [18, 20, 29, 49]. Opinions about the necessity for absolute rigid fixation in osteosynthesis, as advocated by the Swiss AO, have changed. While good results were obtained with functional bracing and early weight-bearing in conservative fracture treatment [36], in the use of external fixation there was also a trend toward more elasticity and dynamization [6]. Experimental studies seem to confirm that micromovements and cyclic loading at the fracture site and a less traumatic fixation technique are important factors in fracture healing [12, 13, 33].

Because of the excellent results in the treatment of closed fractures, the interlocking nail is also increasingly used in open fractures with soft tissue injury, obviously with better results than the external fixator, given its problems of pintrack infections and delayed union [4, 28].

Especially for use in open fractures with severe soft tissue damage and as a first strep in treatment, unreamed nails were developed as a refinement of the atraumatic technique in intramedullary nailing. When applied to this indication, these small-diameter nails have important advantages: a simple and safe operation technique and less damage to intramedullary circulation [23, 48]. The small diameter, however, causes a decrease in mechanical stability in comparison to the older generation of reamed locking nails. While these nails are increasingly used in patients with less severe bone and soft tissue injury, these patients will be confined to a treatment that does not allow full weight-bearing, because of the mechanical limitations of the implant. Moreover, the solid types of locking nail offer a great change to the surgeon who is confronted with an implant failure. As intramedullary nailing became more popular as a method of fracture treatment, many different nailing systems were developed for the femur, tibia, and humerus. This has made fracture treatment more complicated for operating room staff, as they have to become familiar with many different instrumentation sets, each with its own user's manual.

All of the developments outlined above have led us to try to develop a simple practical method of dynamic intramedullary fixation.

## Design and Development

Our criterion was a load-bearing device capable of maintaining the axis and rotation of the limb while permitting dynamic axial compression at the fracture site when walking. As the device functioned as an internal fixator, most of the features of existing intramedullary (IM) implants, such as the clover-leaf cross section, the slot, and the Herzog bend for the tibia, would be superfluous [17]. Instead we proposed a 9-mm nail of circular cross section, whose telescopic form would permit a degree of movement along the axis of the bone. Because of the telescopic form, the nail was necessarily straight. With some simple modifications, it could also be used as a static locking nail and as a device for lengthening or compression of the fracture (Fig. 11.4). Apart from interesting biomechanical properties, the system also simplifies the work of the operating room staff, since the same design of nail and instruments are used for treating femur and tibia fractures. For the humerus, the nail's design is modified; it is inserted, however, with the same set of instruments as for the femur and tibia.

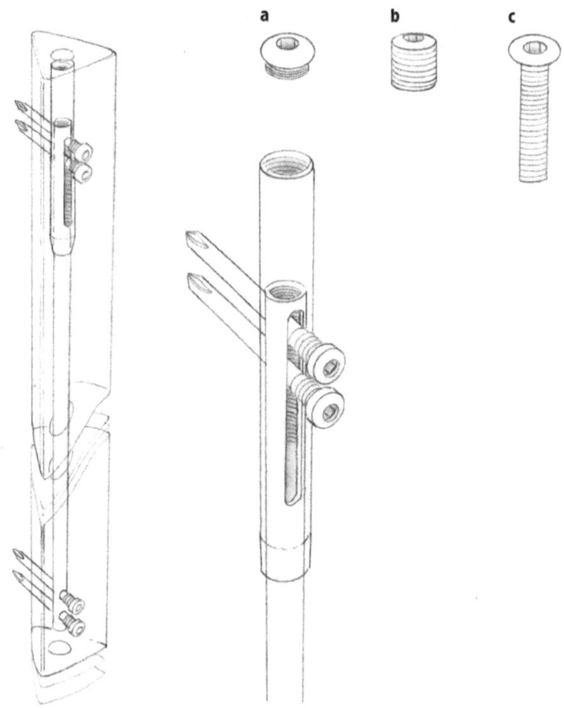


**Fig. 11.4.** The telescopic locking nail consists of a 9-mm inner nail which can move in axial direction in a 12-mm outer cylinder. The nail can be used in a dynamic configuration (*a*), as a static interlocking nail when the distraction screw (*b*) is applied and with compression when the compression screw (*c*) is inserted on top

### *Diameter of the Telescopic Locking Nail: To Ream or Not to Ream?*

Unreamed insertion of an IM nail is restricted by the diameter and the elastic properties of the implant. In young individuals, the diameter of the medullary canal of the femur is 9–10 mm. In the tibia it is smaller, 7–8 mm. Even with nails of 8 and 9 mm, limited reaming is inevitable in young patients with femoral or tibial fractures. In the classification of fractures, the morphology of the fracture matches the severity of the injury. High-energy traumatic lesions will present with comminuted or segmental shaft fractures. Low-energy lesions will present with simple two-fragment fractures. In fact, reaming is only necessary in simple fractures, where the anatomy of the medullary canal is intact. In those fractures, a reamed locking nail with a sufficient diameter to allow early full weight-bearing is an excellent treatment. In patients with a limited injury of the bone and soft tissue, the negative effect of reaming has no consequences for the duration of union and the restoration of function [19]. In the more serious type of injury with comminuted fractures, the anatomy of the medullary canal is disturbed and nails can often be inserted without reaming. As a consequence of the above-mentioned observations, in general, a nail diameter should be chosen that allows full weight-bearing in simple cases. In severe comminuted fractures, a nail of a moderate diameter can be inserted without reaming because of the disturbed anatomy of the medullary canal. For the telescopic locking nail (TLN), a thick-wall hollow 9-mm nail was chosen. A 9-mm nail will make reaming necessary in young individuals, but can be used without reaming in older patients and patients with comminuted fractures.

### *A Straight Nail?*

Because of its telescopic form, the TLN is necessarily straight. To see whether fractures of the femur, tibia, and humerus can be treated with a straight nail, a pilot study was conducted. In this study, a total of 43 nailing procedures were performed in 14 femora, 19 tibiae, and 10 humeri with a 9-mm straight nail without a telescope mechanism. The results of treatment with this nail were comparable to those of other interlocking nail systems (unpublished data). At the end of this pilot study, we concluded that it was possible to treat femoral, tibia, and humeral fractures with the same 9-mm straight nail. This was an important requirement for the further development of the TLN.

### *Biochemical Performance*

The first prototypes of the TLN were tested in the laboratories of the Mechanical Engineering Faculty of the University of Twente. The results enabled us to finalize the design, which was then extensively tested in the design support laboratories of Howmedica in Kiel, Germany. The final concept of the TLN proved to be 50% more elastic under bending stress and 143 times more stable under torsion than the widely used Grosse and Kempf 12-mm slotted nail. It withstood 970,000 dynamic cycles under an axial, torsional, shearing, and bending load increasing to 1600 N without any sign of plastic deformation [43].

The diameter of the nail stipulates the diameter of the locking bolts. In a 9-mm nail, the diameter of the hole for locking bolts can be 4.6 mm. The most important parameter for the stability of a locking bolt is the core diameter. In the current designs for locking bolts, the core diameter is significantly reduced by the thread of the bolt. In the TLN locking bolt, the thread was therefore not removed from the core but added to the core of the locking screw. Consequently, the thread was located directly under the head of the bolt, to secure the bolt into the bone. In this way a very stable bolt was developed with a core diameter of 4.5 mm. In a comparative biomedical study, Gäbler et al. showed that the TLN locking bolt was significantly more stable than other locking bolts that are fully threaded [9].

## Operative Technique

### *Femur*

For surgery, patients are positioned supine on a fracture table. The fracture is reduced under image intensification prior to draping. Via a small incision, the medullary canal is opened on the medial aspect of the tip of the greater trochanter. After insertion of a guidewire, the medullary canal of the femur is reamed to beyond the isthmus of the medullary canal, up to a diameter of 11 mm. The distal metaphysis of the femur is never reamed. The proximal 12 cm of the femur are further reamed up to 13 mm to accommodate the wider telescopic part of the nail. After measuring the length of the medullary canal, a nail that is up to 25 mm shorter than the measured length is chosen. The TLN is than inserted in its shortest fashion, with its telescope mechanism blocked. Proximal locks are inserted first. After unblocking the telescope mechanism, the inner nail is driven forward, using a small hammer, using fluoroscopic monitoring, until its tip is at the desired position in the distal fragment. Thus the implant is always the exact length of the medullary canal, which makes this nail very suitable for distal fractures. After this step, the distal locking bolts are inserted, using the freehand technique. Finally a top lock, a distraction screw, or a compression screw is inserted on top of the telescopic part to produce a dynamic or a static osteosynthesis or to exert compression at the fracture site, respectively (also see Fig. 11.4). If there is enough cortical contact between the two main fracture elements to allow weight-bearing, the TLN is inserted in the dynamic mode. In case of fractures with a comminution zone between the two main fracture elements, the distraction screw is used for static interlocking. When the indication for operation is nonunion, the compression screw can be used to exert compression between the fracture elements (Fig. 11.5 a, b).

### *Tibia*

For tibial osteosynthesis, patients are positioned supine on a standard radiolucent operating table. Tibial fractures are reduced and then temporarily fixed with a radiolucent distractor-type external fixator. The proximal Steinmann pin used for this external fixator is positioned from the anteromedial to the posterolateral aspect of the proximal tibia, the other one through the calcaneus. The advantage of this method is that the extension table is not needed and that the knee can be flexed maximally without loss of reduction.

Because the TLN is a straight implant and does not have the proximal Herzog bend like other tibial implants, the insertion point is not at the tibial tuberosity but higher, at the ventral edge of the tibial plateau ventrally to the tibial tubercle. This point is closer to the axis of the medullary canal than the conventional insertion point, which makes insertion of a straight nail easier. The knee has to be bent maximally for optimal access to this insertion point. This point is reached via a transverse incision through the skin between the tuberositas and the patellar apex, cleaving the patella tendon longitudinally. The remainder of the procedure is the same as described for femoral fractures.

### *Humerus*

As the principle of cyclic dynamic loading is not applicable to the humerus, the TLN for the humerus is somewhat modified from the original TLN [10]. The TLN humerus does not have the telescope mechanism; instead a compression screw can be inserted in the end of the nail. This makes it possible to exert a large amount of compression between the fracture elements, for instance in case of nonunion.

Our policy is to insert the nail retrograde in cases of proximal and midshaft fractures and anterograde in case of distal humeral shaft fractures.

In cases of retrograde nailing, the medullary canal of the humerus is opened with a small drill 2 cm proximal to the fossa olecrani. In the case of anterograde nailing, an awl is used for opening the medullary canal medial to the tuberculum majus.

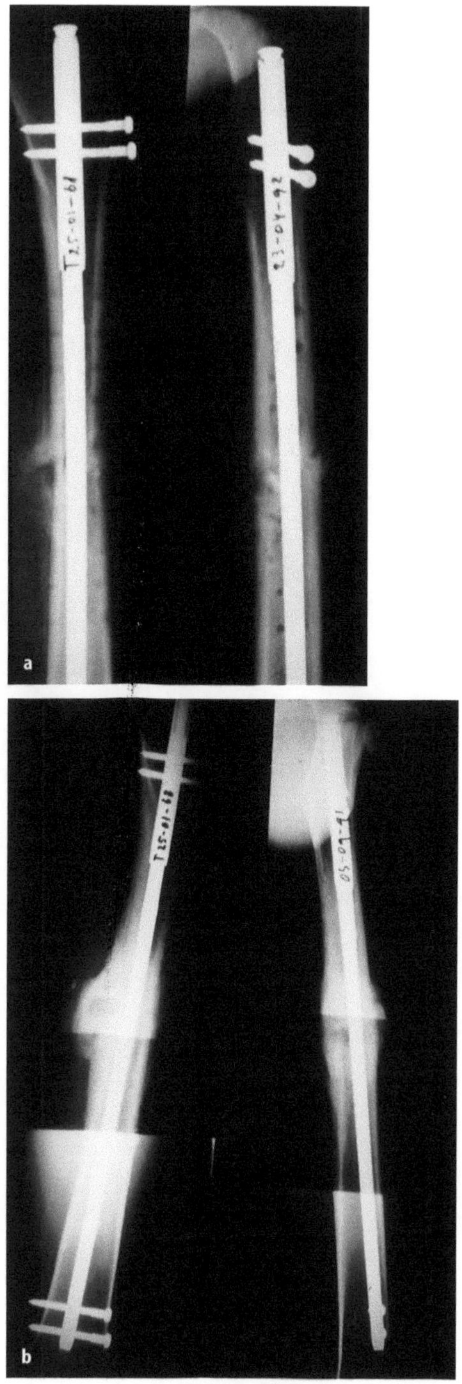


**Fig. 11.5 a, b.** Male patient, 24 years old. Three months after osteosynthesis with a plate there was a delayed union and a remarkable degree of antecurvation. The plate was removed, the antecurvation corrected, and fixation with a TLN was performed (**a**). Full weight-bearing was possible 7 days after osteosynthesis, radiological consolidation 6 months later (**b**)

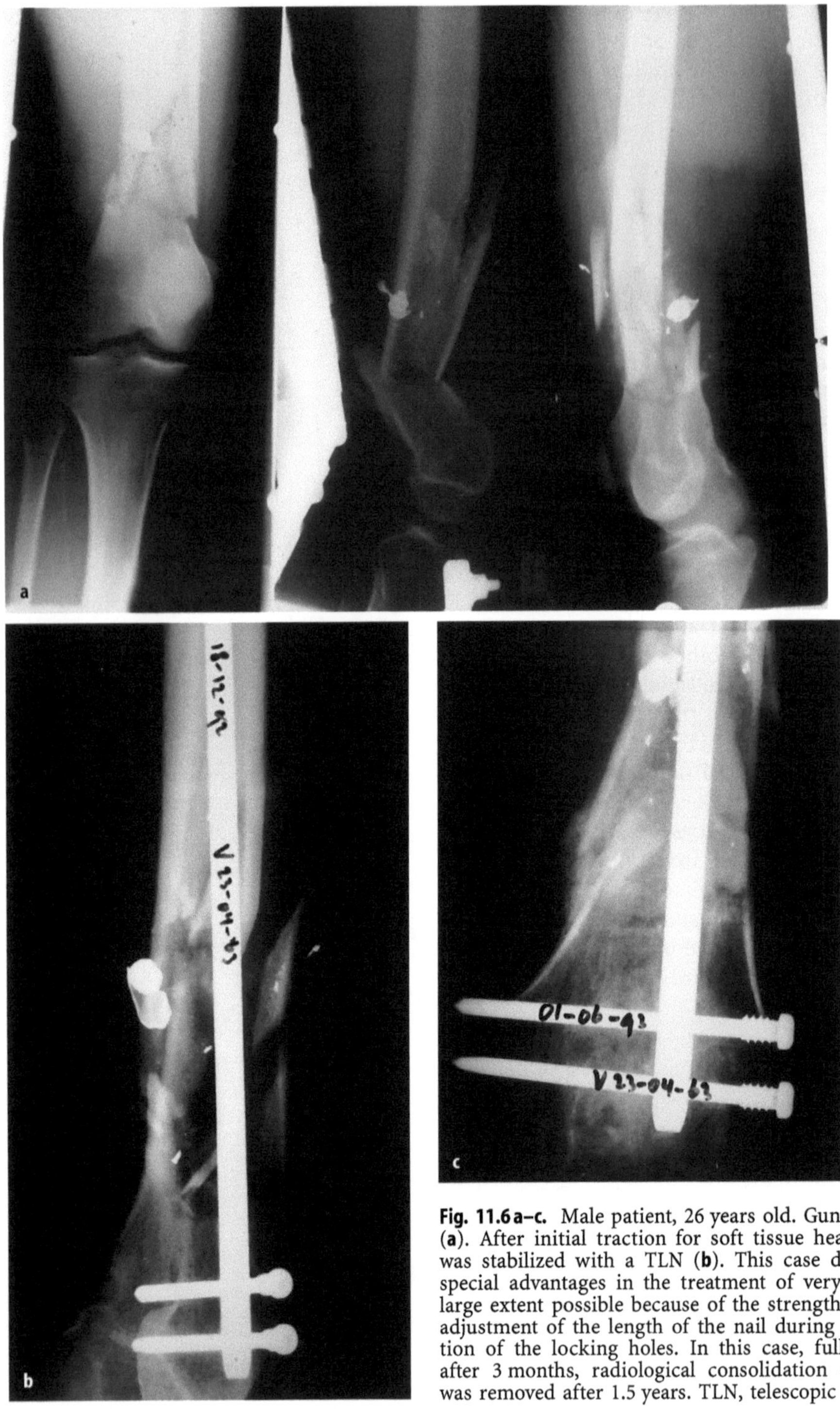


**Fig. 11.6 a–c.** Male patient, 26 years old. Gunshot injury of the distal femur (**a**). After initial traction for soft tissue healing for 3 weeks, the fracture was stabilized with a TLN (**b**). This case demonstrates that the nail has special advantages in the treatment of very distal fractures. This is to a large extent possible because of the strength of the TLN locking bolts, the adjustment of the length of the nail during operation and the distal location of the locking holes. In this case, full weight-bearing was possible after 3 months, radiological consolidation after 6 months (**c**). Hardware was removed after 1.5 years. TLN, telescopic locking nail

The medullary canal is then reamed over a guid wire up to 9 mm, the distal humerus to 11 mm, to reduce the risk of a distal fracture on nail insertion. Proximal locking is performed using the same radiolucent targeting device as is used for femoral and tibial nailing, for distal locking the freehand technique is used. After proximal and distal locking, the compression screw can be inserted in the end of the nail, which produces compression between the fracture elements.

#### *Postoperative Management*

After recovery, patients immediately start with exercises for joint mobilization and muscle strengthening under the supervision of a physical therapist. In cases of dynamic osteosynthesis and when the general condition enables mobilization, partial weight-bearing is started the first day after operation to a level at which the patient does not perceive any pain at the fracture site. Patients are then allowed to increase their weight-bearing as tolerated. Some patients with acute fractures are thus fully weight-bearing within 1 week after operation. In the case of static osteosynthesis, full weight-bearing is postponed until there is callus formation at the fracture site on X-ray examination.

### Clinical Experience with the Telescopic Locking Nail

After the pilot study with a straight nontelescopic nail and after extensive biomechanical testing of the final design of the Telescopic Locking Nail, a clinical trial was conducted in a single center setting [11]. Seventy-one consecutive patients were treated with the TLN, 24 patients with femoral, and 47 patients with tibial fracture or nonunion. In 8 of these 71 cases, the nail was statically locked, the others were treated dynamically.

#### *Femur*

For acute femoral fractures treated with the TLN, the union rate was 100% and the mean time to radiological union was 31 weeks. For these patients, the mean time lapse till full weight-bearing was 7 weeks. The malunion rate was 6.3%. There were no deep infections.

Eight cases of femoral nonunion treated with a TLN united after a mean period of 52 weeks. Two of these cases needed a secondary operative procedure before union was achieved.

#### *Tibia*

In the treatment of 29 acute tibial fractures, a primary union rate of 96% was achieved, the mean time lapse till radiological union being 23 weeks. The malunion rate was 6.9%, the infection rate 3.5%. These patients were fully weight-bearing after a mean period of 6 weeks. In 21 cases of tibial nonunion available for follow-up, union was achieved after an average period of 25 weeks. In two of these cases a secondary operative procedure was necessary to achieve bony union.

During the nailing of femur and tibia with the TLN we did not encounter specific design complications. Although in the majority of cases the nailing was performed in a dynamic fashion, this did not lead to significant limb shortening. Because of the lack of an anteversion bend in femoral nailing, we saw a slight recurvation of the femur in a few cases of less than 3°; this did not have any consequences on functional outcome. In most cases, the TLN will bend a little to follow the antecurvation of the femur.

Using a more proximal and dorsal insertion point for tibial nailing with the TLN did not lead to more postoperative knee complaints. In our study, 13% of the patients had knee complaints after tibial nailing, a significantly lower figure than reported in other studies [11]. Possible reasons for this finding are that with this more proximal and dorsal entry point, there is less irritation of the patellar tendon and that the nail is not protruding through the anterior cortex.

Although the patients in this series were fully weight-bearing after a relatively short period, we did not encounter a nail or locking bolt breakage. The combination of a 9-mm nail with a circular cross section and locking bolts with a core diameter of 4.5 mm seems to make early weight-bearing possible. Patients treated with unreamed nails are often confined to postponed weight-bearing to prevent nail or locking bolt breakage. We consider this as a step back in the practice of intramedullary nailing.

With the telescope mechanism of the TLN, the length of the nail can be adapted to every length of femur and tibia. This is very advantageous in distal fractures, as the tip of the nail with the distal locking holes can be precisely maneuvered beyond the fracture (also see Figs. 11.7, 11.8).

#### *The Telescopic Locking Nail for the Humerus*

Open fractures, neurovascular lesions, floating elbow, bilateral fractures, polytrauma, pathological fractures, pseudarthrosis, and inability to maintain reduction are absolute indications for operative treatment of humeral fractures. In order to treat these problem fractures, a stable implant with strong locking bolts is needed. In this view, the telescopic locking nail for the humerus was developed.

In developing the humeral nail we started from the experience gathered with the tibial and femoral nail. The strong locking bolts of 4.6 mm needed a minimal nail thickness of 9 mm. Locking bolts with full threads of this caliber give good purchase in the bone. A 9-mm straight nail, however, is to rigid and causes iatrogenic fractures and breaking out of the nail. Therefore, the central part of the nail was thinned to 7.6 mm, giving the necessary elasticity

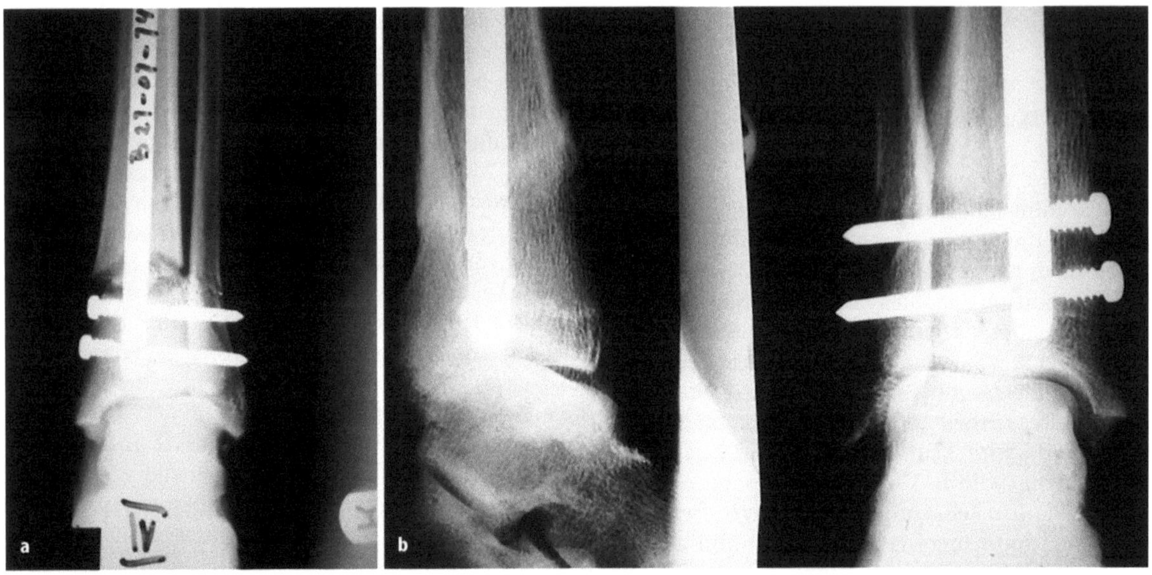

**Fig. 11.7 a, b.** Male patient, 16 years old. Failure of nonoperative treatment on a very distal tibial fracture (**a**, **b**). After 4 weeks, osteosynthesis was performed with a TLN (**a**). Patient was able to walk with full weight-bearing after 10 days. Good dynamization of the nail was observed. Full consolidation seen after 7 months (**b**)

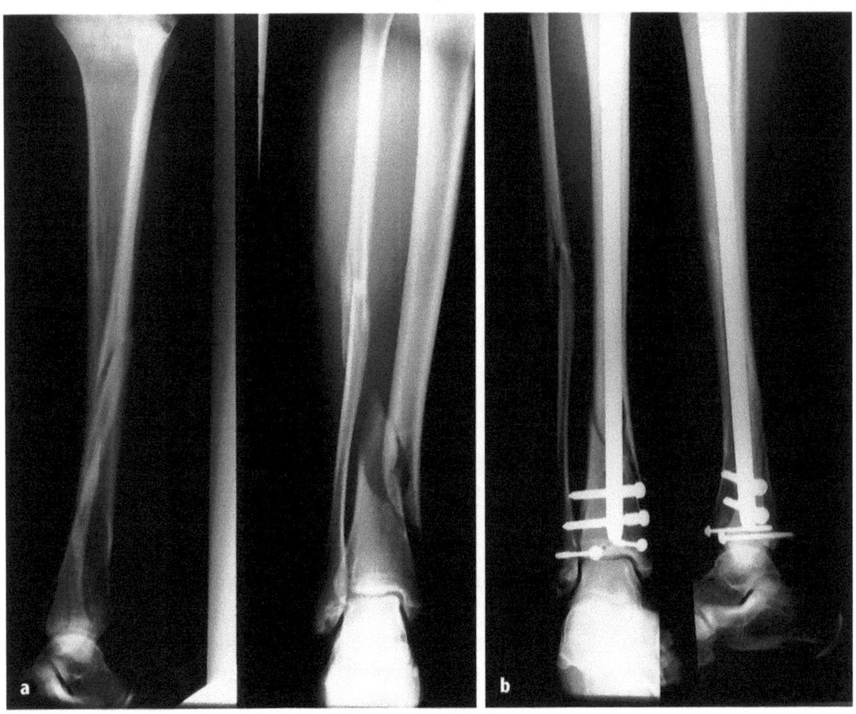

**Fig. 11.8 a, b.** Female patient, 42 years old. Distal spiral fracture of the tibia and a fissure in the third malleolus (**a**). The third malleolus was stabilized with two percutaneous cannulated screws. The shaft fracture was treated with a TLN that was adjusted during the operation. It was possible to position the tip of the nail just above the subchondral bone of the tibia-talar joint. Patient left the hospital with partial weight-bearing 7 days after the accident (**b**)

needed for insertion and fracture healing. Proximal interlocking is possible through two locking holes oriented in the same plane as the distal oblong hole and one at right angles with it. Distally an oblong locking hole makes dynamic and static interlocking possible. To give compression over the fracture site, a special screw is inserted at the proximal end after dynamic interlocking of the nail. This screw is tightened and takes support on the locking bolt, through which the nail is backed out again until the fracture gap is completely closed. This technique is used with pseudarthrosis and transverse fractures.

The nail can be inserted antegrade and retrograde. The antegrade introduction site is the same as described with other nails, just medial to the tuberculum majus. We use small incisions to avoid damaging the rotator-cuff. For the retrograde entry there are two possibilities. The supracondylar portal as described by Rommens et al. and the fossa olecrani portal is described by Linn et al. and Ingman et al. We use the fossa olecrani portal because it lies more in the axis of the intramedullary canal. This makes it easier to introduce a straight nail.

Because of the 9-mm diameter at proximal and distal ends, reaming is necessary to 10.5 mm, the entry hole to 11 mm.

The first clinical experience led to good healing results. Primary healing of acute fractures in our own patients was as high as 98%.

The secondary interventions had a healing rate of less than 50%. This was an unexpected result. In the treatment of humeral nonunion, the classic technique described is decortication with rigid plate fixation and bone grafting. These principles apply for the technique used with the TLN. The reaming provides for the necessary cancellous bone graft and the straight 9-mm nail gives stability due to its contact with the cortices. The compression is gained through the compression screw. Nevertheless, an intramedullary nail alone seems inadequate for the treatment of pseudarthroses of the humerus, as was also described by other authors.

In the treatment of (impending) pathological humeral fractures, the stability of the TLN led to good functional results with adequate pain relief and good quality of life.

The telescopic locking nail for the humerus is a suitable and stable implant for the treatment of humeral fractures, shown in the healing rate of the acute fractures.

The treatment of nonunions and pseudarthroses, however, remains a problem despite the stability of the implant and the use of compres-

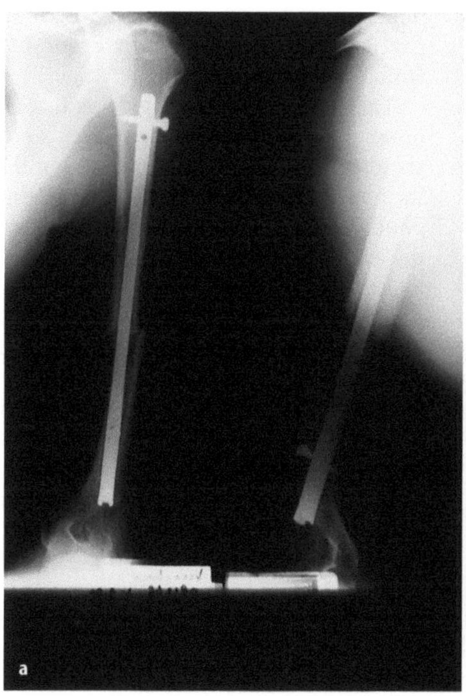


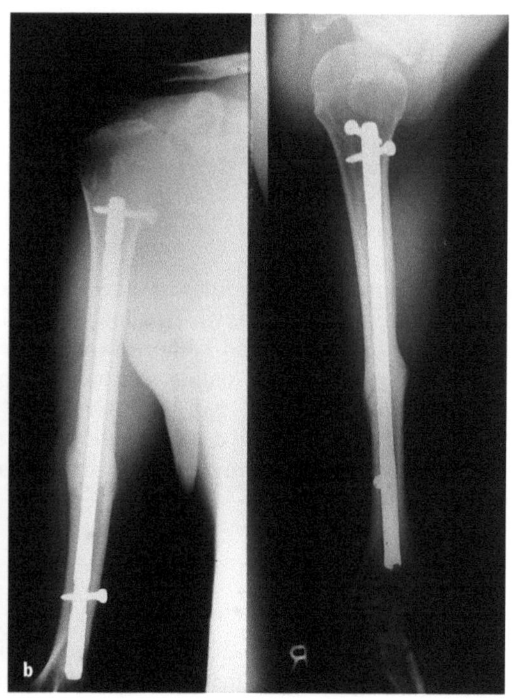


**Fig. 11.9 a, b.** Male patient, 26 years old. Injury of the right arm with an antebrachial fracture and a humeral fracture (**a**). On the day of the account, the humerus was stabilized with a TLN and the antebrachial fracture with plating. A very fast recovery was seen in the right arm and fracture healing after 3 months (**b**)

sion. For this specific problem, we recommend the use of the TLN in combination with an open cancellous bone graft. Using the TLN in elderly patients, one should consider the effect of antegrade entry on the already damaged rotator cuff. Depending on the fracture location, a retrograde entry should be used.

### Conclusion

After these first clinical experiences with the telescopic locking nail, we concluded that this nail is suitable for the treatment of fractures of the femur, the tibia, and, in a modified form, the humerus. It is a universal system, because for all these fractures the same instrumentation is used, making its application easier for surgeons and surgical staff. Dynamization of the nail under weight-bearing was observed under both laboratory and clinical conditions. One of the interesting properties of the nail is that it can be lengthened after proximal locking, which makes it especially useful in cases with very distal fractures.

The telescopic locking nail has the mechanical quality of a normal locking nail, making early weight-bearing possible. Often the nail can be inserted without reaming. Besides a dynamic configuration, the nail also has the possibility for static interlocking and compression. Thus the telescopic locking nail can be applied in a wide range indications.

## The Radial Locking Nail

C. Lefèvre and D. Le Nen

There is no intramedullary osteosynthesis, as described to the present time, which allows simultaneously rotation control and compression loading of bone fragments of the radius. Encouraged by the results with the ulna nail, we developed a locking radial nail an ideal system for both bones of the forearm, i.e., an entire nailing process by closed procedure.

### Principles

To succeed in designing a radial locking nail, many technical problems, mainly due to the morphology of the radius and to its anatomical environment had to be solved: the articular joints of the epiphysis require an epiphyseal approach, near the wrist, and not at the elbow, because of the radial nerve next to the radial head which does not allow a proximal locking from the outside towards the inside.

The medullary canal of the radius is unique. It is narrow at the neck, then enlarges at the level of the tuberosity, before becoming narrow again, to enlarge progressively towards the distal epiphysis. A centromedullary implant cannot, therefore, have broad cortical contact. This led to the idea of proposing a prebent nail, placed via a posteromedial approach in the axis with the bending of the radius.

The appropriate entry point of the nail is, therefore, at the lower or epiphyseal distal radius. The styloid approach is problematic, because of the risk of injury to the tendons, the branches of the radial nerve, and the intolerance to the tip of the implant. Furthermore, a straight nail placed by styloid approach would straighten the curvature of the diaphysis. A prebent nail should have a double bend, which would require complex manufacturing and involve high costs.

The easier posteromedial, extra-articular approach was finally chosen: it allows easy insertion of a prebent nail, which is designed according to the radiopronator curvature. The only disadvantage of this approach is the presence of extensor tendons near the entry point of the nail. This requires total sinking of the implant into the bone, in order to avoid risks of tendon rupture, particularly of the long extensor of the thumb, which is directly vulnerable.

The nail is prebent, rigid, and hollow, with one outer diameter measuring 5 mm, and it comes in six different lengths ranging from 17 to 22 mm. Its upper portion ends with three fins, which expand by a screw inserted using a screwdriver in the cannula of the nail. This will ensure proximal locking. The oblong hole can allow translation of the nail, depending on the locking screw placement for achieving compression (Fig. 11.10).

The instrumentation has been reduced to a minimum. It consists of a nail driver with a guide-sleeve, a bolt fixing the implant on the nail driver, a driving sleeve, and a flexible, long screwdriver. The remaining tools (reamers, drills, screwdriver, etc.) are the same as those used for the ulnar nail.

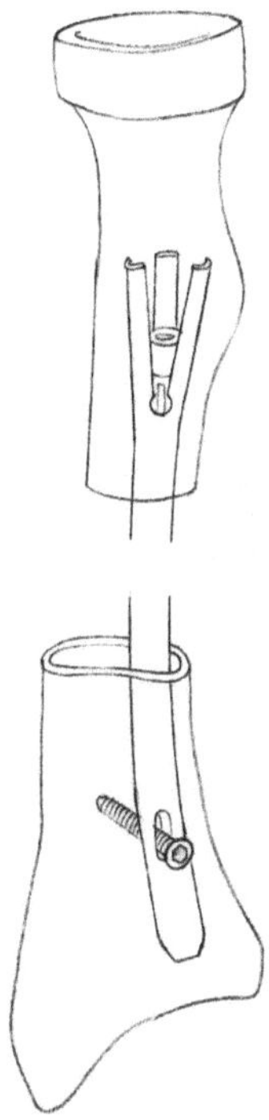

**Fig. 11.10.** Locking principles

## Operative Technique

### *Positioning*

The patient is positioned in the supine position, the upper limb on an arm support.

### *Approach*

The wrist is positioned in pronation on a rolled drape. A 20- to 30-mm incision at the level of Lister's process is made with careful protection of extensor tendons. The bone of the tubercle is removed. The extra-articular entry point is achieved with a pointed awl directed from distal to proximal.

### *Reduction of the Fracture*

This often is less problematic with the ulna because the diameter of the medullary canal simplifies the driving of the reaming guide (use simultaneous traction and supination). This could be done more easily with a repositioning frame for fractures of both bones of the forearm. Presently in the project stage, this frame will reposition and the stabilize the fragments during the different operating stages. The tip of the reaming guidewire is then pushed to the radius head.

### *Reaming*

The passage of the reamers is easy. The medullary canal becomes narrower only in the proximal third of the diaphysis. Reaming up to 5.5 mm is sufficient.

### *Guidewire Exchange*

The medullary calipering done by reaming is usually sufficient to manage the changing of the guidewire. After having removed the reaming guide, the nailing guide, precurved if necessary, must be placed until it stops in the radial head. There is no problem for placing the guide in the center of the head, as in the femur of the tibia.

### *Measurement of the Nail Length*

Inserting the nail, on the nail-holder, is done easily, if the curve of the implant is turned upward to reach the middle third of the diaphysis. The curvature of the nail must then be taken into account and must be in the same frontal plane as the diaphyseal, anatomical curvature. The tip of the nail has to be totally sunk into the bone, in order to avoid any tendinous complication.

### *Distal Locking*

Locking is obtained with the screwdriver going through the cannula of the nail holder and the nail. The principle is the same as for the distal locking of the humeral Seidel nail. Check with the image intensifier to assure that expansion of the fins is sufficient.

### *Proximal Locking*

Check the position of the extensor tendons and retract them before using the guide sleeve, which must be directly in contact with the bone, with no other tissue interposition. Drill the hole, then measure the length of the screw. The appropriate screw is placed without any pretapping.

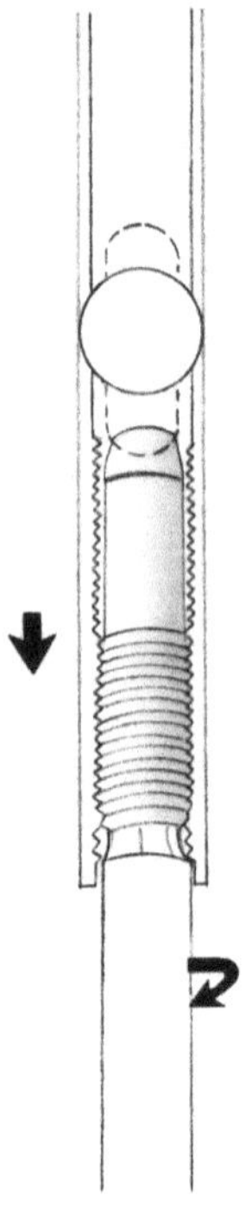

Fig. 11.11. Details of the distal end

### *Compression of the Fracture or Pseudarthrosis Site*

After removal of the nail holder, put the compression screw into the nail. Its upper tip rests against the locking screw and so directs the nail towards the wrist. This gives a compression effect at the fracture or pseudarthrosis site (see Fig. 11.11). This compression effect must be checked by the image intensifier, especially if the fracture is a fresh one.

## Preliminary Results

Seven radius nails have been used for the following indications: simple bifocal fractures or comminuted fractures of the radius, closed or open, isolated or associated with both bones of the forearm, and pathological fractures. Aseptic pseudarthrosis also seems to be a good indication, combining reaming and compression, advantages which had already been seen clinically with the ulna nail.

With each intervention, we find the technique to be easier than the ulna technique. All cases have consolidated. We noted one complication: the injury to the long extensor of the thumb, which required a secondary suture. This short experience which has, of course, no statistical prevalence, has given rise to ideas for improvements on the initial prototype. Making the nail wall thicker than 1 mm at its lower segment will avoid the deformation of the edges of the oblong hole during rotation movements of the nail at insertion (no implant breakage was observed during removal of the implant). Furthermore, the initial lower portion has two chamfers, for use of the device on either the right side or on the left side. We observed that if the curvature of the nail was not strictly in the frontal plane, the edges of the chamfers became very aggressive knives, which explains the tendinous complication. To avoid this problem, the tip of the next prototype will be rounded off around its entire circumference (Fig. 11.12). Furthermore, the initial instruments' material proved to be too delicate: the nail holder and the guide sleeve have, therefore, been re-enforced.

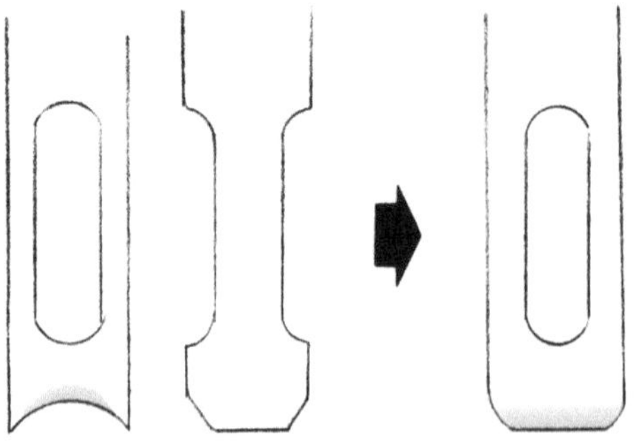

Fig. 11.12. Modifications of the distal end of the radial nail

## Conclusion

This short experience with radius nailing is encouraging. With the help of new improved prototypes, the next step will be a clinical multicenter study with the support of test sites motivated by intramedullary osteosynthesis of the forearm. Only the results of such a study will provide conclusions which are statistically valid from a clinical point of view.

## The Principles of Computer-Assisted Navigation in Intramedullary Fracture Treatment

M. J. M. Segers and H. J. T. M. Haarman

### Introduction

Fluoroscopy has enhanced the development of different intramedullary techniques for fracture treatment, especially intramedullary locked nailing of diaphyseal fractures of the femur, tibia, and humerus. In fact, the intraoperative use of a mobile C-arm can be considered as one of the oldest methods of image-guided surgery. Fluoroscopic images are familiar for all surgeons in operative trauma care. These images facilitate closed or semi-closed fracture reduction and facilitate reduced surgical access in different procedures. One of the shortcomings of conventional fluoroscopy is that a surgical action at any given time can only be directly combined with a single planar view. Obtaining multiplanar visualization requires constant repositioning of the C-arm, which can be ergonomically challenging for both the surgeon and the radiologist. In addition, every fluoroscopic planar view means an increase in radiation exposure for the medical personnel as well as the patient. These shortcomings of conventional fluoroscopy can be resolved by linking a computer to the C-arm, which creates virtual multiplanar fluoroscopic images: computer-assisted navigation.

Computer-assisted navigation is an enabling technique that combines a real-time surgical action with any desired combination of planar views. The basic principle is a fusion of preoperative (CT, MRI) or intraoperative (fluoroscopy) acquired image data with the patient's anatomy and subsequent graphic visualization of superimposed calibrated surgical instruments.

### CT-Based Computer-Assisted Navigation

In spinal surgery, CT-based computer-assisted navigation is becoming increasingly popular as the misplacement rate for transpedicular screws is significantly decreased [1, 25, 26, 38]. This kind of navigation requires registration of the spatial relationship between the patient's anatomy and the preoperative CT image data. The registration is based on both a matching of anatomical landmarks (paired point registration) and a matching of random surface points (surface registration) between the anatomical object and a 3D reconstructed CT model [27, 47]. During this registration and the actual surgery, optical electronic positioning sensors are rigidly attached to the spinous process of the instrumented vertebra by means of a dynamic reference frame. Because the configuration of the active (infra-red emitting diodes, IREDs) or passive (reflective) positioning sensors on this frame is very precisely defined, any movement of the anatomical object can be described as a rotation (rX, rY, rZ) and translation (tX, tY, tZ) in three dimensions. The spatial position of the vertebra can be localized by optical electronic cameras with a very fast refreshment rate and the dynamic reference frame compensates for any change in patient or camera position. Simultaneously, the orientation of calibrated surgical instruments with attached positioning sensors can be tracked by the same localizing cameras. The computer then mathematically defines the relative spatial orientation of the anatomical object and the surgical instruments in multiple desirable planar views. Real-time graphic visualization of superimposed surgical instruments will appear on these "virtual" planar CT-scan views. The surgeon has intelligent sagittal, look-ahead or probe's-eye views at his disposal and is able to anticipate before a decisive surgical action.

### Fluoroscopy-Based Computer-Assisted Navigation

In long bone surgery, CT-based computer-assisted navigation has some obvious disadvantages: high-volume CT scanning to obtain a 3D model means a significant radiation exposure for the patient, sharply defined anatomical landmarks are difficult to identify during operation, and surface registration of long bones will require a large surgical exposure of the anatomical object. Furthermore, trauma surgeons are much more familiar with fluoroscopic images in intramedullary fracture treatment. Considering the above, the combination of standard C-arm fluoroscopy and computer-assisted navigation technology seems a natural development. Fluoroscopy-based computer-assisted navigation offers the best of both worlds: fluoroscopic radiation exposure is strongly reduced, multiple planar views can be visualized simultaneously, and after obtaining the separate planar views and fusion of these images with the anatomical object, the C-arm can be completely withdrawn from the operating room, leaving the surgeon an unprecedented amount of space for freehand locking of intramedullary nails.

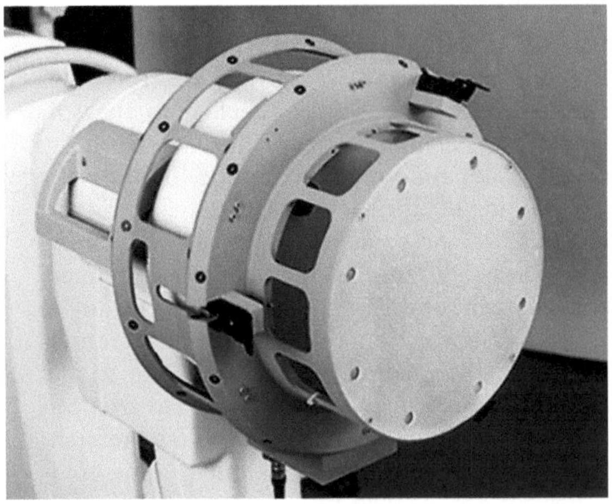

**Fig. 11.13.** C-arm with attached navigation ring containing a pin-cushion calibration target and multiple infrared emitting diodes. (Courtesy of Medtronic SNT)

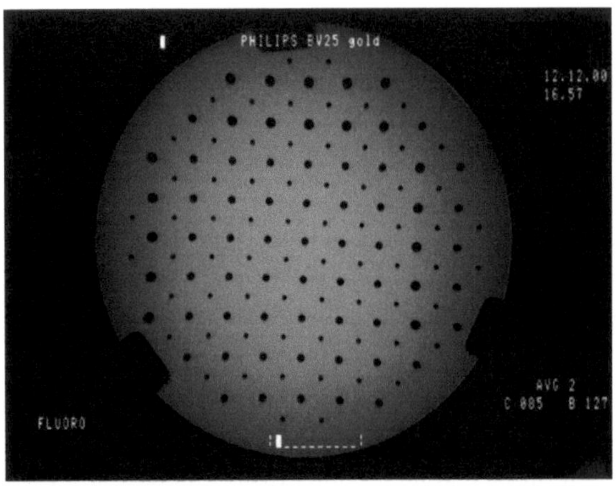


**Fig. 11.14.** Fluoroscopic view of the pin-cushion calibration target; this calibration view can be deactivated during actual navigation. (Courtesy of Medtronic SNT)

Like CT-based navigation, fluoroscopy-based computer-assisted navigation implies some basic requirements [14, 31]:

- Import of the desired fluoroscopic images in a computer for subsequent mathematical processing using a video-out signal of the C-arm or a digital connection (DICOM network protocol).
- Exact definition of the spatial relationship between these images and the patient's anatomy by employing optical electronic localizing cameras and positioning sensors rigidly attached to both the anatomical object (dynamic reference frame) and the C-arm. In contrast with a dynamic reference frame used in spinal surgery, in long bone surgery this frame is attached with a self-tapping monocortical screw, facilitating a percutaneous procedure (it is obligatory to employ two separate frames for navigation of the main proximal and distal fragments). The C-arm is mounted by a ring-shaped device containing a calibration target circumferentially fitted with positioning sensors (Fig. 11.13). The positioning sensors can be either passive reflective markers or active IREDs.
- Distortion correction of every single fluoroscopic image by calibrating these images with a pin-cushion calibration target attached to the C-arm (Fig. 11.14). This calibration target has a highly defined geometrical appearance and after calibration, the computer mathematically translates any spatial position relative to the patient as a projection onto the fluoroscopic image. Renewed calibration and mathematical computation of the geometric projection on every acquired planar image is necessary to compensate for mechanical nonrigidity of the C-arm and interference by other electromagnetic sources in the operating room. During actual navigation, the pin-cushion calibration grid can be deactivated.
- Graphical visualization and tracking of calibrated surgical instruments with attached positioning sensors, superimposed on multiple, previously acquired fluoroscopic images. The monitor settings allow personal preferences in single or multiplanar views for different procedures (Fig. 11.15). The mathematical power of the computer can also provide the surgeon with real-time quantitative information about the spatial position of his surgical instrument, i.e., the distance in millimeters from the tip of the instrument to a predefined anatomical point or the angle in degrees of the instrument in a nonvisualized plane relative to one or more processed fluoroscopic planar views (Fig. 11.16).

### Use of Fluoroscopy-Based Computer-Assisted Navigation in Intramedullary Fracture Treatment

Several investigators have confirmed the accuracy and efficacy of fluoroscopy-based computer-assisted navigation in ex vivo studies and compared these results with the performance of CT-based navigation [14, 31]. In clinical experiments, the main fields of interest comprise posterior spinal instrumentation, sacroiliac stabilization, and long bone fracture treatment using intramedullary locked nails.

A variety of operative steps in intramedullary nailing can be facilitated with computer-assisted navigation:

- Reduced surgical exposure in antegrade femoral nailing can be achieved by virtual lengthening of the tip of a surgical probe. Especially in morbid obese patients, the correct entry point in the proximal femur can more easily be identified using this technique.
- Percutaneous access in retrograde femoral nailing is facilitated with graphic visualization of a

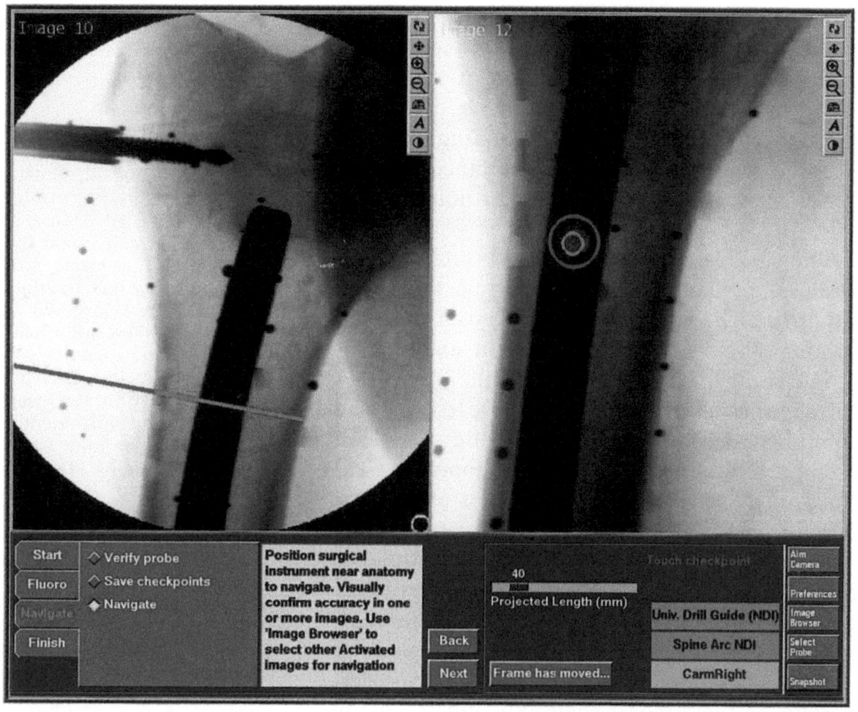


**Fig. 11.15.** Biplanar view (postero-anterior and lateral planes) of the distal femur; real-time graphic visualization of a superimposed calibrated surgical instrument (trackable drill guide), facilitating screw length measurement and correct screw insertion. (Courtesy of Medtronic SNT)

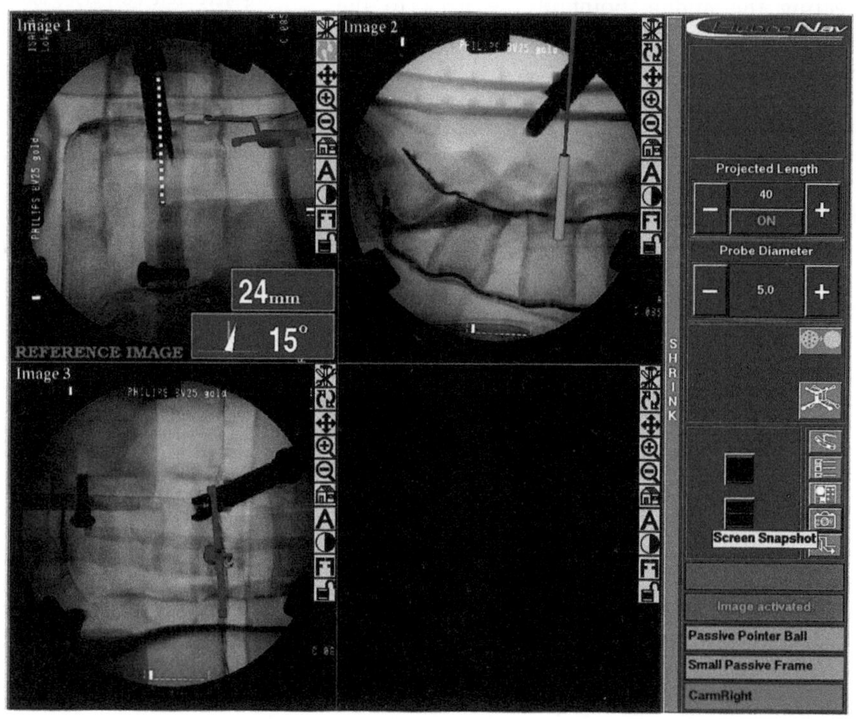


**Fig. 11.16.** Triplanar view (postero-anterior, lateral and 150° transpedicular planes) of a lumbar spine model. In the left upper quadrant, quantitative information describes the distance in millimeters from the midline joining the spinous processes of L4 and L5 and the angle of the superimposed surgical instrument (trackable ball pointer) towards the sagittal plane. (Courtesy of Medtronic SNT)

surgical instrument, e.g., calibrated drill guide or awl, on simultaneous posteroanterior and lateral fluoroscopic views of the distal femur.

- Drastic reduction in radiation exposure is accomplished during freehand locking [40]. Freedom of movement is enabled by the absence of the C-arm. Drilling can be performed with a normal, nonradiolucent, nonangled drill. As the smaller-diameter drill bits show some flexibility at the tip of the instrument, the rigid drill guide rather than the air-drive drill itself should be equipped with positioning sensors. Graphic visualization can be obtained in perpendicular planar views simultaneously (Fig. 11.15).
- By virtual lengthening of the tracked drill guide and quantitative computation, the screw length can be accurately predicted. Time-consuming screw length measurement and fluoroscopic controls are made redundant.
- In femoral shaft fractures, fluoroscopy-based computer-assisted navigation can be used as a method for the exact pre- or intraoperative estimation of the femoral antetorsion angle. Dynamic reference frames have to be attached to both main fragments of the femur. Biplanar fluoroscopic images of the distal and proximal parts of the femur are transferred to the computer. Then the spatial positions of the plane of the posterior regions of the femoral condyles, parallel to the femoral shaft axis and the plane of the mid-section of the femoral neck, connecting the middle point of the neck to the center of the femoral head are computed. The angle between these planes shows the femoral antetorsion angle in a way comparable to a CT scan method using multiplanar reconstructions. Preoperatively, the same measurements can be done for the nonfractured, contralateral femur, using a percutaneous access for the dynamic reference frames. This technique for determination of the femoral antetorsion angle provides reliable results (±1.10°) without intra- or interobserver dependencies in ex vivo experiments [15, 21]. The usability of this method in clinical practice is currently being investigated.

Computer-aided surgery will surely develop into an integral part of daily practice in operative trauma care in the next 2 decades. In contrast to medical robotics, fluoroscopy-based computer-aided navigation requires only minor adjustments in the operating room environment. Trauma surgeons are fully familiar with fluoroscopic views in intramedullary fracture treatment. Therefore, the learning curve for this kind of image-guided surgery will be short and trauma surgeons will experience the benefits of multiple real-time planar views with superimposed surgical instruments. Those benefits include smaller surgical access, improved control of fracture reduction, less radiation exposure, and more precise screw insertion in freehand locking.

## References


1. Amiot LP, Lang K, Putzier M, Zippel H, Labelle H (2000) Comparative results between conventional and computer-assisted pedicle screw installation in the thoracic, lumbar and sacral spine. Spine 25:606–614
2. Bostman O, Hirvensalo E, Vanionpaa S et al (1987) Biodegradabe internal fixation for malleolar fractures. Br Edit Soc Bone J Surg 69B
3. Christel PS, Vert M, Chabot F et al (1984) Polylactic acid for intra-medullary plugging. Biomaterials and Biomechanics 1983. Elseviers Science, Amsterdam
4. Court-Brown CM, McQueen MM, Quaba AA, Christie J (1991) Locked intramedullary nailing of open tibial fractures. J Bone Joint Surg 73B:959–964
5. Daniels AU, Chang MKO, Andriano KP (1990) Mechanical properties of biodegradable polymers and composites proposed for internal fixation of bone. J Appl Biomat 1:57–58
6. de Bastiani G, Aldegheri R, Renzi Brivio L (1984) The treatment of fractures with a dynamic axial fixator. J Bone Joint Surg 66B:538–545
7. Dijkema ARA, van der Elst M, Breederveld RS, Verspui G, Patka P, Haarman HJThM (1993) The surgical treatment of fracture dislocaltions of joint with biodegradable implants. J Trauma 34:82–85
8. Eitenmuller J, Gerlach KL, Schmickal T, Muhr G (1987) Semirigide Plattenosteosynthesen unter Verwendung absorbierbaren Polymere als temporare Implantate. Chirurg 58:831–39
9. Gäbler C, Tschegg EK, Greitbauer M, Stanzl-Tschegg S, Wozasek GE, Laube W, Vécsel V (1999) Ermüdungsfestigkeit von Verriegelungsbolzen für die unaufgebohrte Tibianagelung. Unfallchirurg 102:29–34
10. Goessens MLMJ, Van den Wildenberg FJAM, Eggink GJ, Stapert JWJL (1996) The telescopic locking nail for humerus. Implant design preliminary clinical results. Osteo Int 4:270 –274
11. Goessens MLMJ, Van den Wildenberg FAJM, Eggink GJ, Stapert JWJL (1999) Treatment of fractures of femur and tibia with the telescopic locking nail: design of a new implant and the first clinical results. J Trauma Injury Infect Clin Care 46:853–862
12. Grundnes O, Reikeras O (1991) Mechanical effects of function on bone healing – nonweight bearing and exercise in osteotomized rats. Acta Orthop Scand 62:163–165
13. Heitemeyer U, Claes L, Hierholzer G (1990) Die Bedeutung der postoperative Stabilität für die ossäre Reparation einer Mehrfragmentfraktur. Tierexperimentele untersuchungen. Unfallchirurg 3:49–55
14. Hofstetter R, Slomczykowski M, Sati M, Nolte LP (1999) Fluoroscopy as an imaging means for computer-assisted surgical navigation. Comput Aided Surg 4:65–76
15. Hofstetter R, Slomczykowski MA, Krettek C, Koeppen G, Sati M, Nolte LP (2000) Computer-assisted fluoroscopy-based reduction of femoral fractures and antetorsion correction. Comput Aided Surg 5:311–325
16. Hollinger JO, Schmitz JP (1987) Restoration of bone discontinuities in dogs using a biodegradable implant. J Oral Maxillofacial Surg 45:594–600

17. Inhofe DP (1992) Biomechnical considerations in intramedullary fixation of lower-extremity fracture. Orthop Rev 21:945–952
18. Kempf I, Grosse A, Taglang G, Bernhard L, Moui Y (1991) L'encoulage centromédullaire avec verrouillage des fractures récentes du femur et du tibia. Chirurgie 117:478–487
19. Kessler SB, Hallfeldt KKJ, Perren SM, Schweiberer L (1986) The effects of reaming and intramedullary nailing on fracture healing. Clin Orthop 212:18–25
20. Klemm KW, Börner M (1986) Interlocking nailing of complex fractures of the femur and tibia. Clin Orthop 212:89–100
21. Krettek C, Hofstetter R, Koeppen G (2000) Computer assistance for antetorsion angle correction during femoral fracture reduction. Abstract of the 5th international symposium on computer assisted orthopaedic surgery (CAOS), Davos, p 38
22. Kulkarni RK, Moore EG, Hegyeli AF, Lenonard F (1971) Biodegradable Poly (lactic acid) polymers. J Biomed Mater Res 5:169–181
23. Kuner EH, Seif El-Nasr M, Münst P, Staiger M (1993) Die Tibiamarknagelung ohne Aufbohrung. Unfallchirurgie 19:278–283
24. Küntscher G (1940) Die Marknagelung von Knochenbrüchen. Langenbecks Arch Klin Chir 200:443
25. Laine T, Schlenzka D, Mäkitalo K, Tallroth K, Nolte LP, Visarius H (1997) Improved accuracy of pedicle screw insertion with computer-assisted surgery. Spine 22:1254–1258
26. Laine T, Lund T, Ylikoski M, Lohikoski J, Schlenzka D (2000) Accuracy of pedicle screw insertion with and without computer assistance: a randomized controlled clinical study in 100 consecutive patients. Eur Spine J 9 [Suppl 1]:35–40
27. Lavallee S, Sautot P, Troccaz J et al (1994) Computer assisted spine surgery: A technique for accurate transpedicular screw fixation using CT data and a 3-D optical localizer. Proc 1st Int Symp Med Robot Comput Assist Surg (MRCAS) 323–328
28. Lhowe DW, Hanen ST (1988) Immediate nailing of open fractures of the femoral shaft. J Bone Joint Surg 70A:812–820
29. Maatz R et al (1986) Intramedullary nailing and other intramedullary osteosyntheses. Saunders, Philadelphia
30. Matsusue Y, Yamamuro T, Yoschii S, Oka M et al (1991) Biodegradable Screw Fixation of Rabbit Tibia Proximal Osteostomies. J Appl Biomat 2:1–12
31. Nolte LP, Slomczykowski MA, Berlemann U, Strauss MJ, Hofstetter R, Schlenzka D, Laine T, Lund T (2000) A new approach to spine surgery: fluoroscopy-based surgical navigation. Eur Spine J 9 [Suppl 1]:78–88
32. Otto TE, Patka P, Haarman HJThM, Klein CPAT, de Vries R (1994) Intramedullary bone formation after polylactic acid wire implantation. J Mater Sci Mater Med 5:407–411
33. Pennig D (1990) Zur Biologie des Knochens und der Knochenbruchhheilung. Unfallchirurg 93:488–491
34. Perren SM (1979) Physical and biological aspects of fracture healing with special reference to interal fixation. Clin Orthop Relat Res 138
35. Rokkanen P, Bostman O, Vanionpaa S et al (1985) Biodegradable implants in fracture fixation: early results of treatment of fractures of the ankle. Lancet 1422–1424
36. Sarmiento A (1972) Functional bracing of tibial and femoral shaft fractures. Clin Orthopaedics 82:2–13
37. Schuster J (1972) Die Meetallose. Chirurg 43:114–116
38. Schwarzenbach O, Berlemann U, Jost B et al (1997) Accuracy of computer-assisted pedicle screw placement. An in vivo computed tomography analysis. Spine 22: 452–458
39. Springer MA, Binsbergen EA van, Patka P, Bakker FC, Haarman HJThM (1998) Resorbierbare Stäbe und Schrauben zur Fixierung von Knöchenfracturen; eine randomisierte klinische Prospectivstudie. Unfallchirurg 5:377–381
40. Suhm N, Sati M, Jacob LA, Nolte LP, Regazzoni P, Messmer P (2000) Computer assisted nailing osteosynthesis of long bone fractures. Abstract of the 5th international symposium on computer assisted orthopaedic surgery (CAOS) Davos, p 38
41. Tonino AJ, Davidson CL, Klopper PJ, Linclau LA (1976) Protection from stress in bone and its effects. J Bone Joint Surg 58B
42. Tormala P, Vasenius J, Vaniopaa S et al (1991) Ultra-high-strength absorbable self reinforced polyglycolide (SR-PGA) composite rods for internal fixation of bone fractures. J Biomed Mater Res 25:1–21
43. Stapert J, Wolters JW (1992) Howmedica GmbH design support. Telescopic locking nail tests. Prüfbericht 91-030:1–15
44. van der Elst M, Dijkema ARA, Klein CPAT, Patka P, Haarman HJThM (1995) Tissue reaction on PLLA versus stainless steel interlocking nails for fracture fixation. An animal study. Biomaterials 16:103–106
45. van der Elst M, Kuiper I, Klein CPAT, Patka P, Haarman HJThM (1996) The burstphenomenon, an animal model simulating the long-term tissue response on PLLA interlocking nails. J Biomed Mater Res 30:139–143
46. van der Elst M, Patka P, van der Werken C (2000) Resorbierbare Implantate für Frakturfixierungen. Aktueller Stand. Unfallchirurg 103:178–82
47. Visarius H, Berlemann U, Schwarzenbach O (1999) Concept and clinical aspects of computer assisted spine surgery. In: Nolte LP, Ganz R (eds) CAOS – Computer Assisted Orthopaedic Surgery. Hogrefe and Huber, Bern, pp 81–88
48. Whittle AP, Russel TA, Taylor JC, Lavelle DG (1992) Treatment of open fractures of the tibial shaft with the use of interlocking nailing without reaming. J Bone Joint Surg 74A:1162–1171
49. Winquist RA, Hansen TT, Clawson DK (1984) Closed intramedullary nailing of femoral fractures. J Bone Joint Surg 66A:529–539

CHAPTER 12

# Atlas of Clinical Cases

S. Boriani, R. Pascarella, G. Taglang, C. Lefèvre, D. Le Nen, H. Seidel

## Femur

S. Boriani and R. Pascarella

### Case 1: 25-Year-Old Male Patient, Car Accident

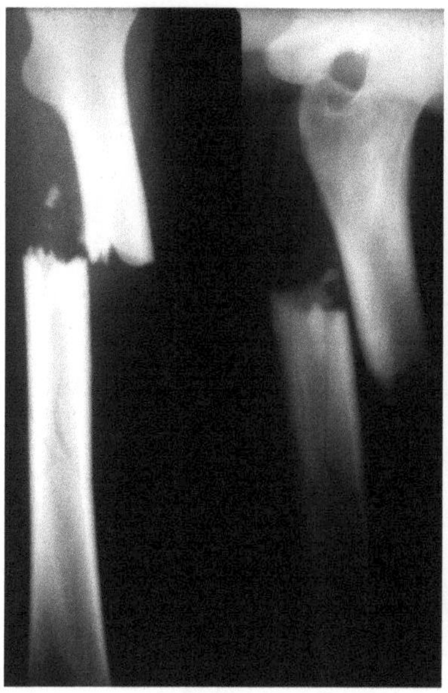

**Fig. 12.1.** AO classification 32A3

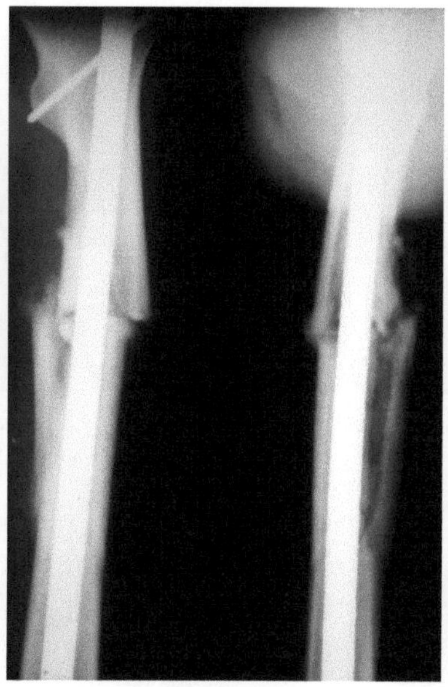

**Fig. 12.2.** Three-month follow-up

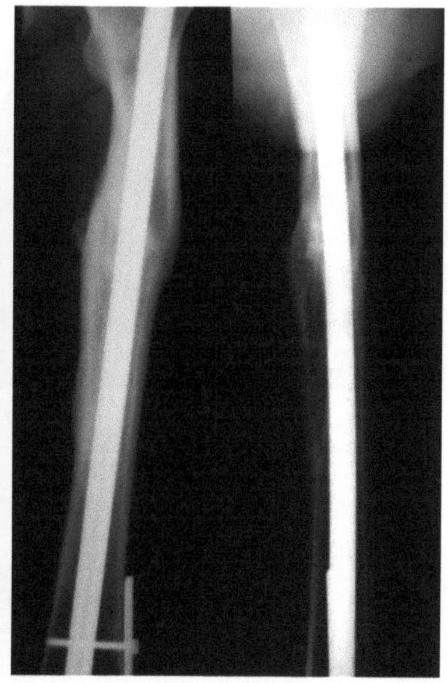

**Fig. 12.3.** Ten-month follow-up

### Case 2: 42-Year-Old Male Patient, Car Accident

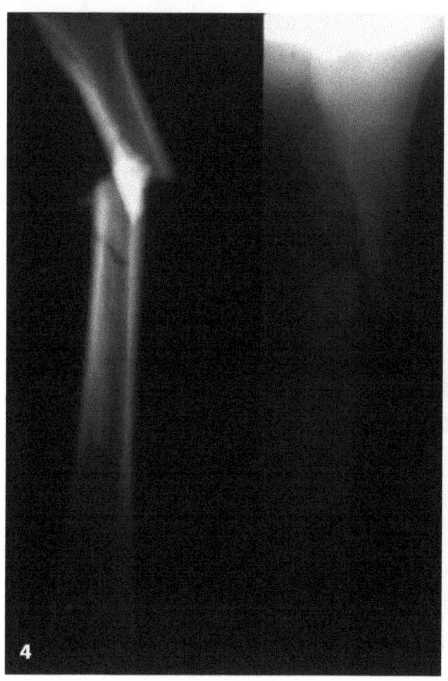

**Fig. 12.4.** AO classification 32A3

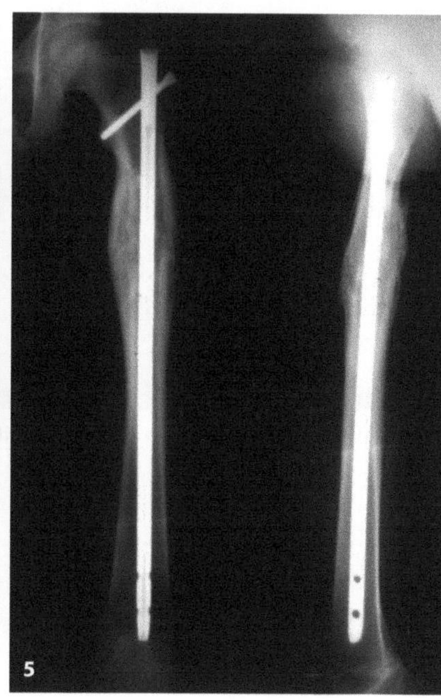

**Fig. 12.5.** Dynamic nail, 1-year follow-up

## Case 3: 42-Year-Old Male Patient, Motorcycle Accident

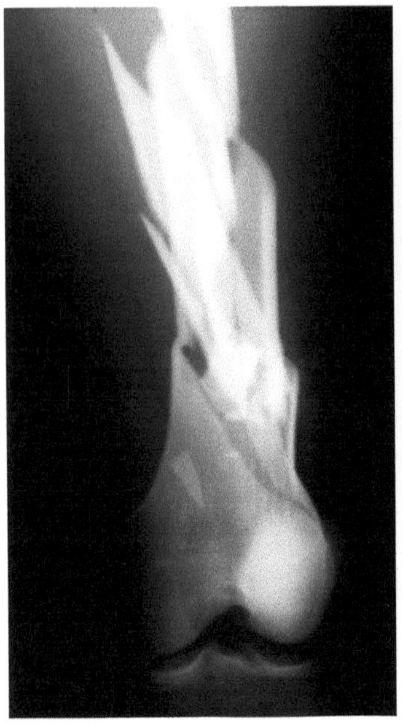

**Fig. 12.6.** AO classification 32C3

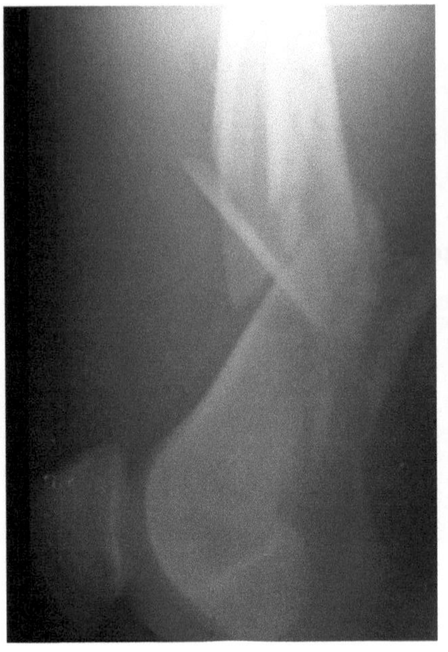

**Fig. 12.7.** AO classification 32C3

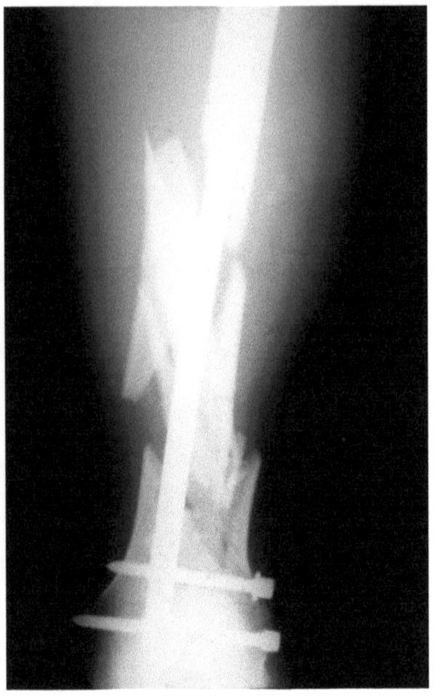

**Fig. 12.8.** Static nail postoperative picture

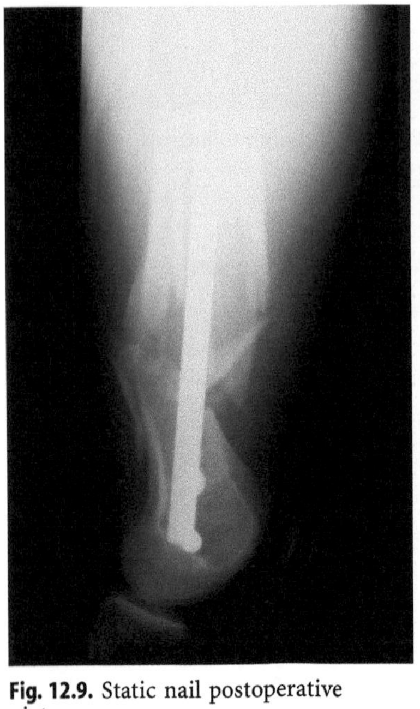

**Fig. 12.9.** Static nail postoperative picture

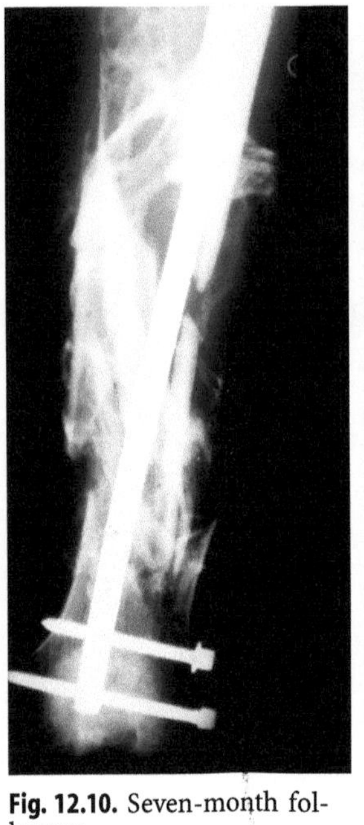

**Fig. 12.10.** Seven-month follow-up

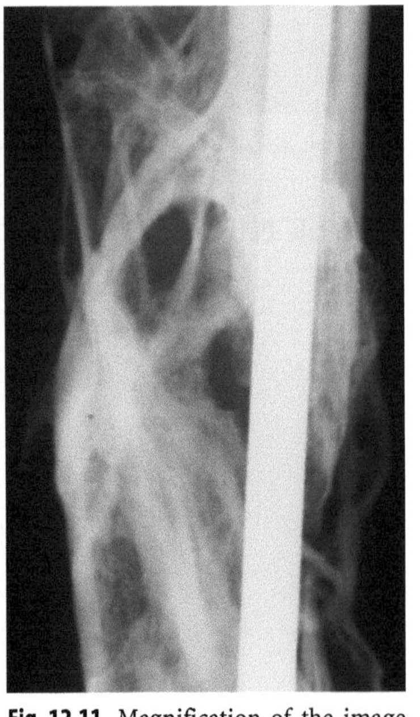

**Fig. 12.11.** Magnification of the image of callus formation

**Fig. 12.12.** Magnification of the image of callus formation

**Fig. 12.13.** Lateral view, 12-months follow-up

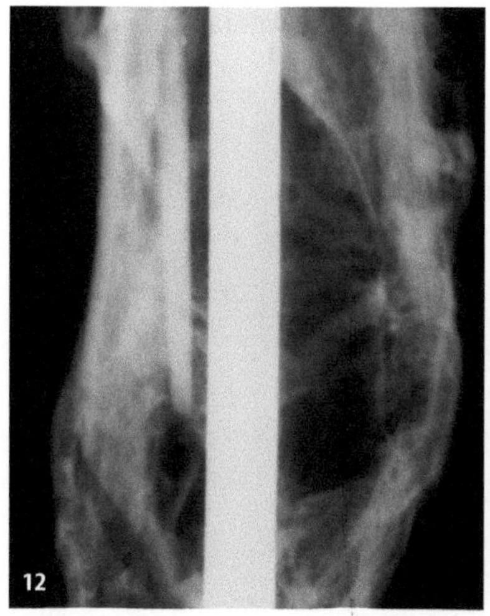

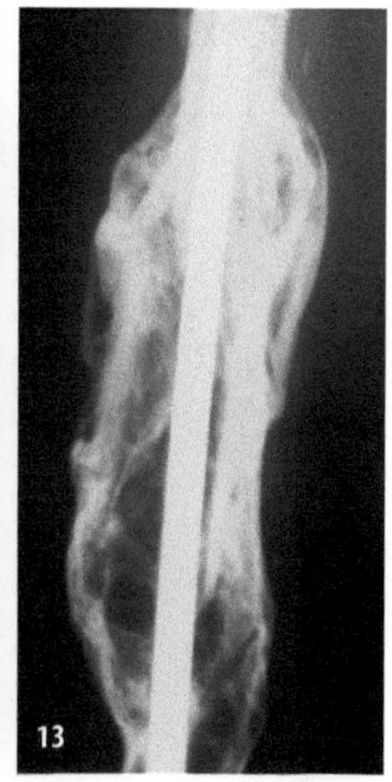

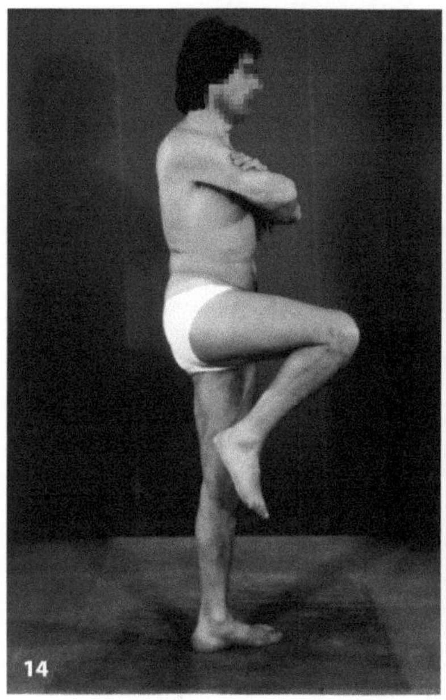

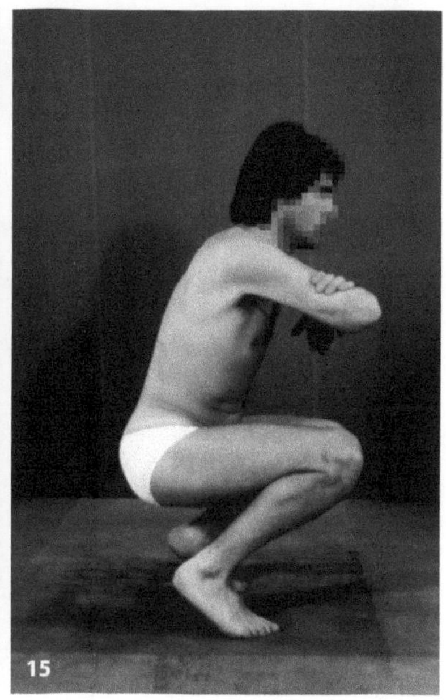

**Fig. 12.14.** Clinical results after 12 months

**Fig. 12.15.** Clinical results after 12 months

## Case 4: 22-Year-Old Female Patient with Bilateral Femur Fractures, Car Accident

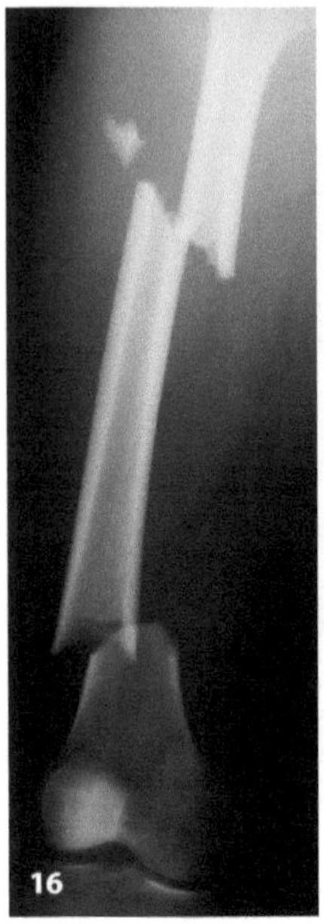


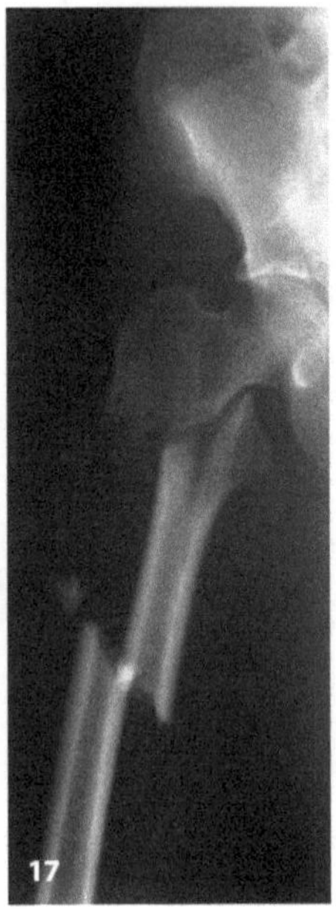


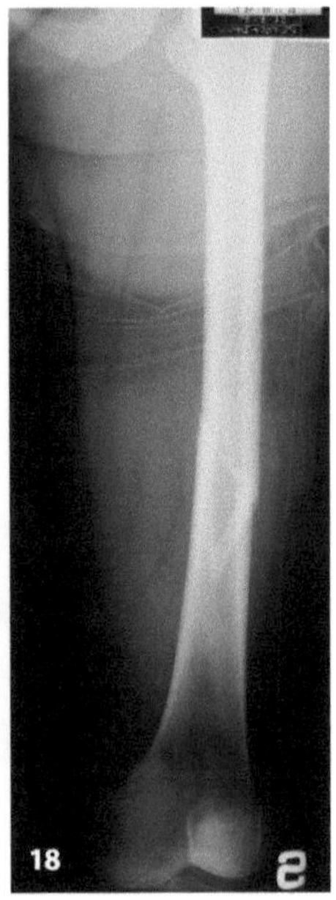


**Fig. 12.16.** Right AO classification 32C2

**Fig. 12.17.** Right AO classification 32C2

**Fig. 12.18.** Left AO classification 32A1

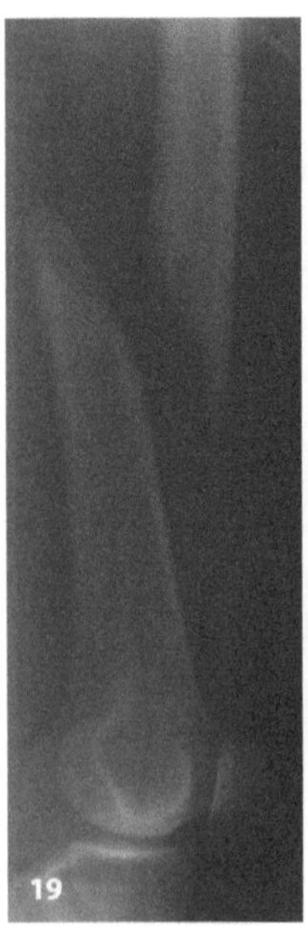


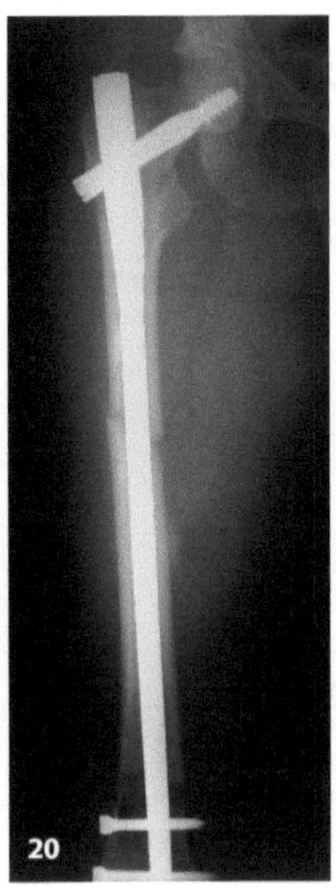


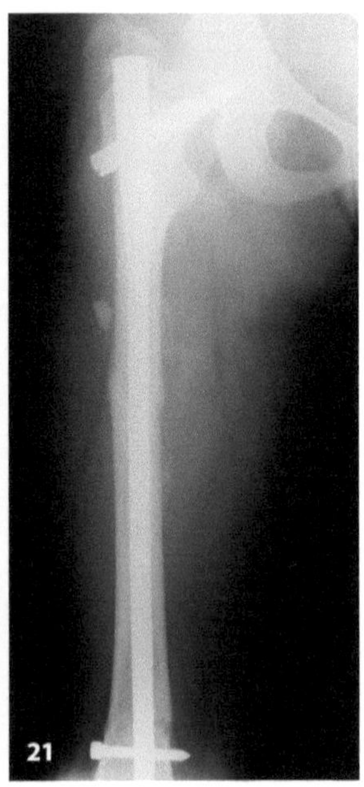


**Fig. 12.19.** Left AO classification 32A1

**Fig. 12.20.** Right postoperative view after static LGN

**Fig. 12.21.** Right, 3-month follow-up

**Fig. 12.22.** Right, 3-month follow-up

**Fig. 12.23.** Right, 3-month follow-up

**Fig. 12.24.** Left, postoperative view

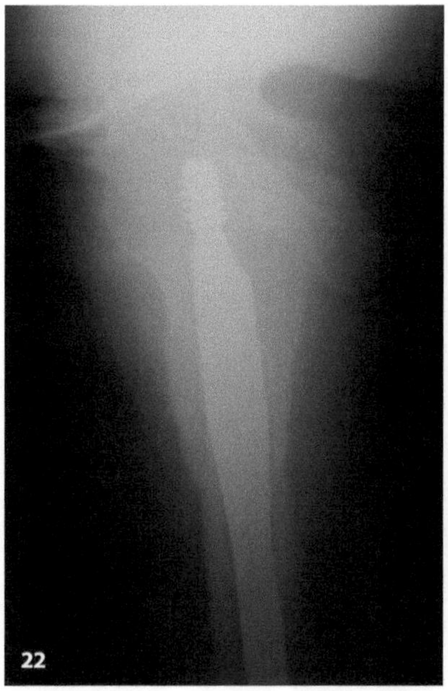


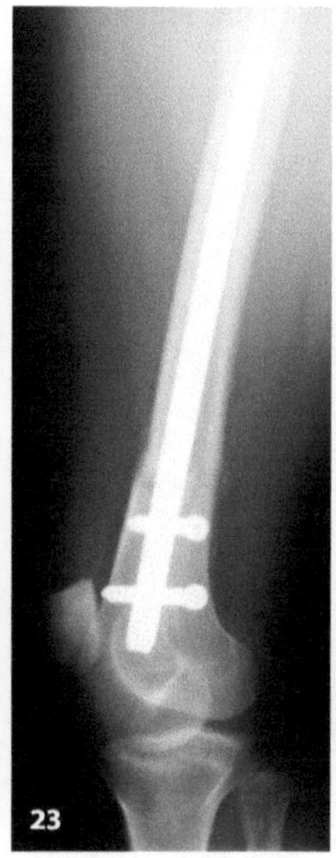


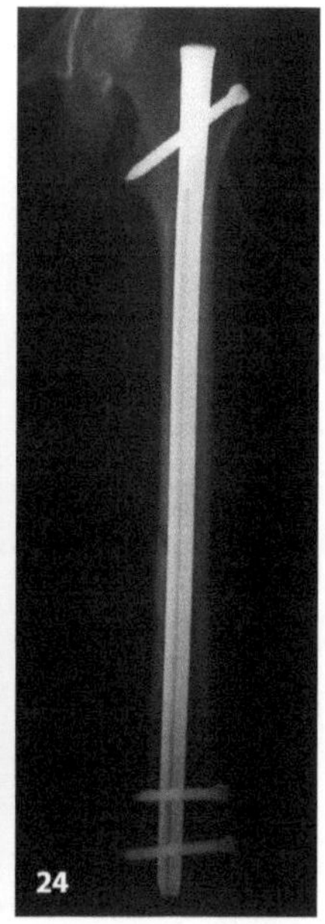


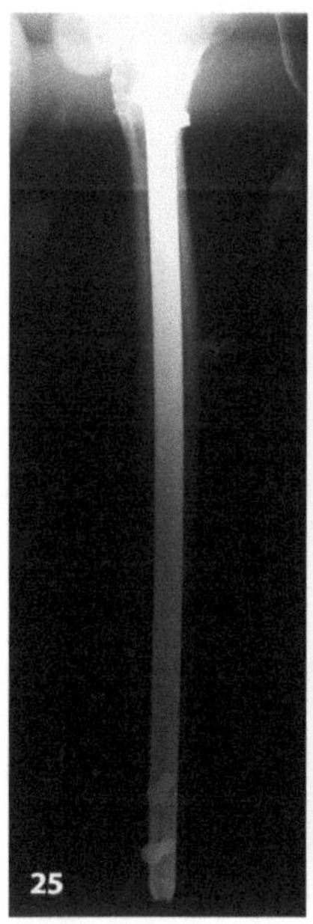


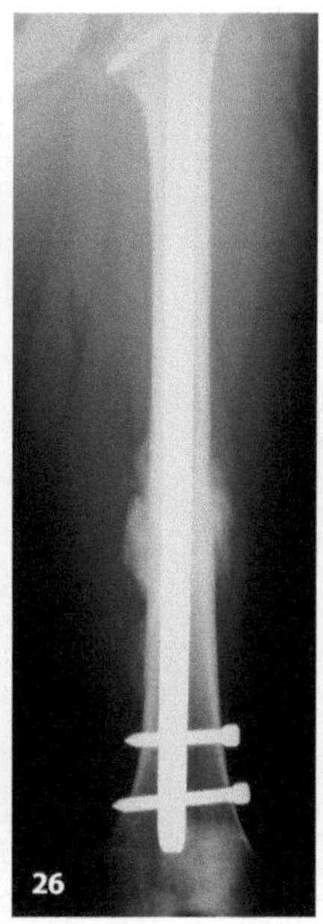


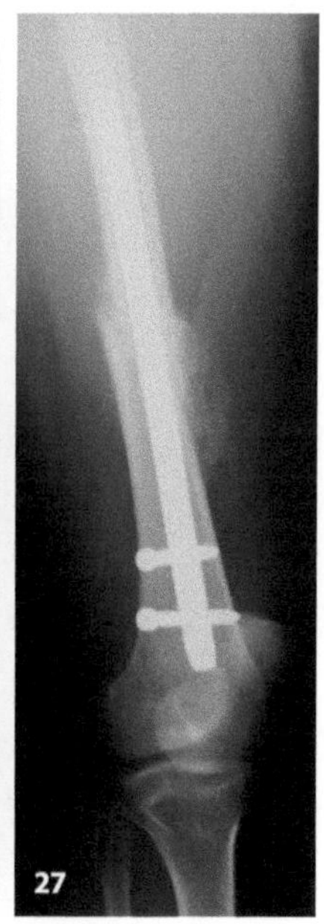


**Fig. 12.25.** Left, postoperative view

**Fig. 12.26.** Left, 3-month follow-up

**Fig. 12.27.** Left, 3-month follow-up

## Case 5: 20-Year-Old Male Patient, Motorcycle Accident

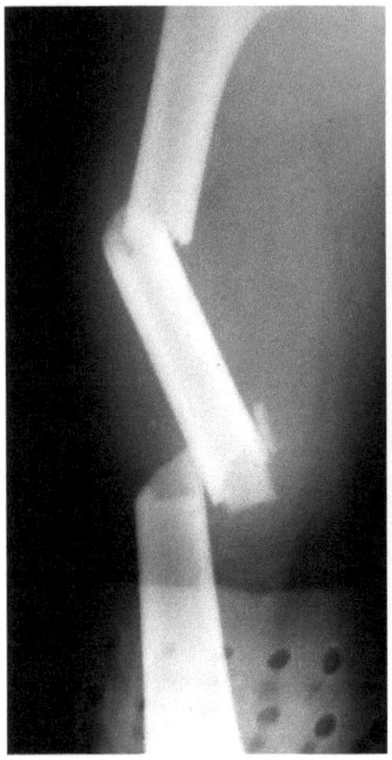

**Fig. 12.28.** AO classification 32C2

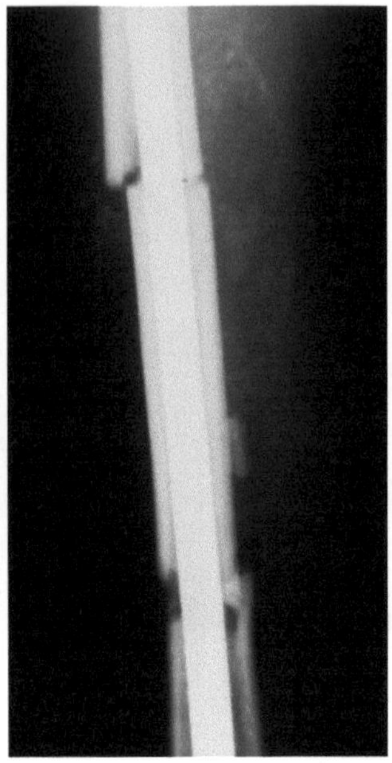

**Fig. 12.29.** One-month follow-up after static GK

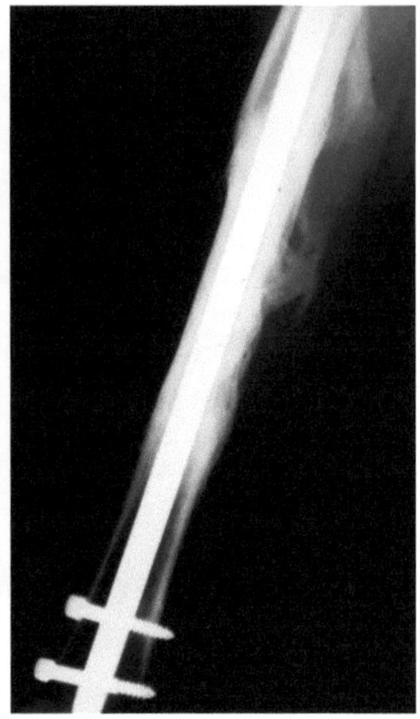

**Fig. 12.30.** Five-month follow-up

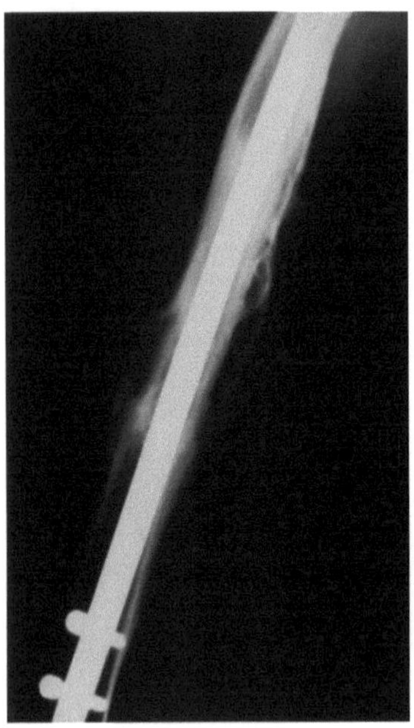

**Fig. 12.31.** Five-month follow-up

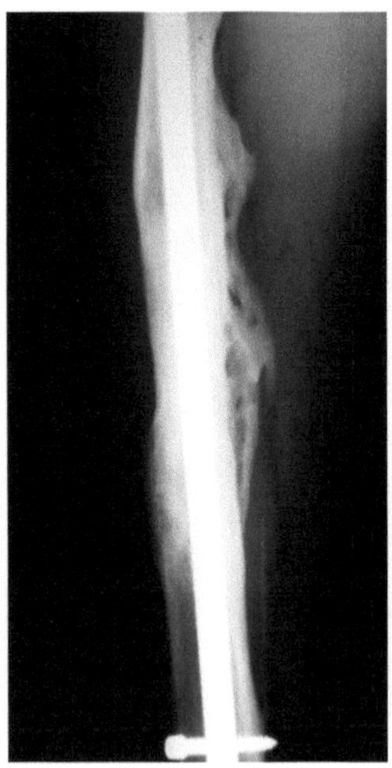

**Fig. 12.32.** Eighteen-month follow-up

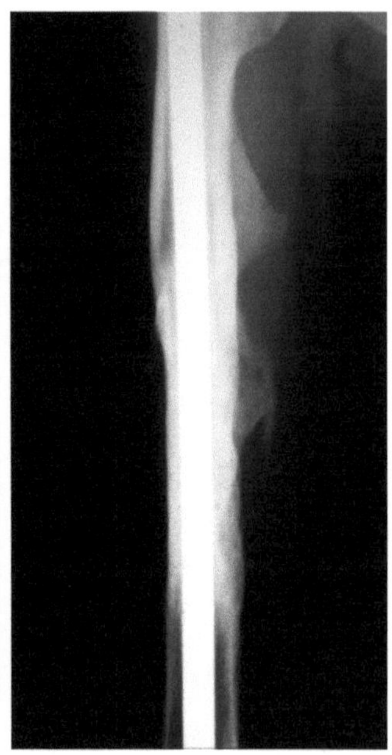

**Fig. 12.33.** Eighteen-month follow-up

## Case 6: 35-Year-Old Female Patient, Car Accident

**Fig. 12.34.** AO classification 32B1

**Fig. 12.35.** One-year follow-up after dynamic GK

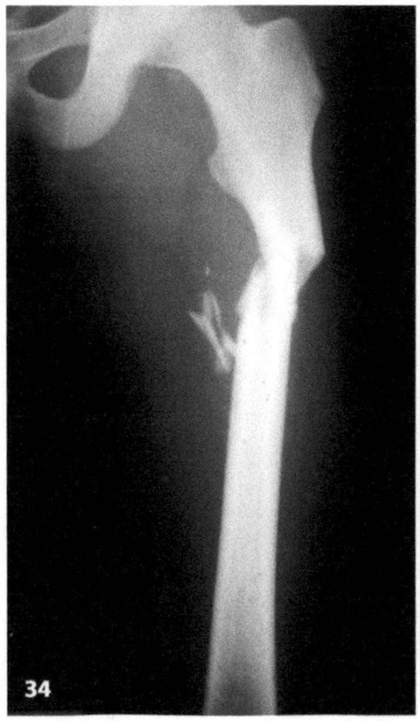

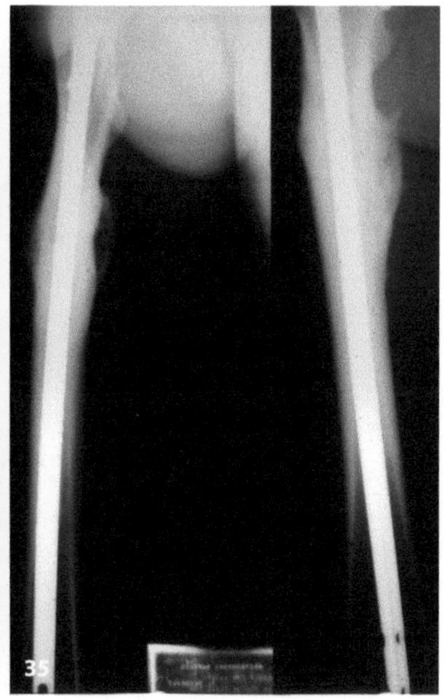

## Case 7: 45-Year-Old Female Patient, Car Accident

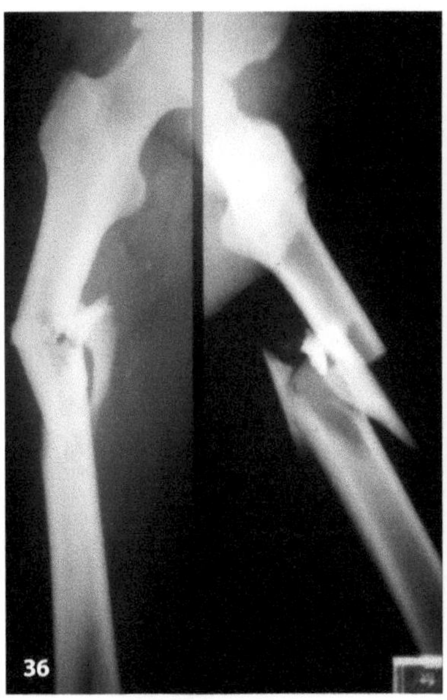

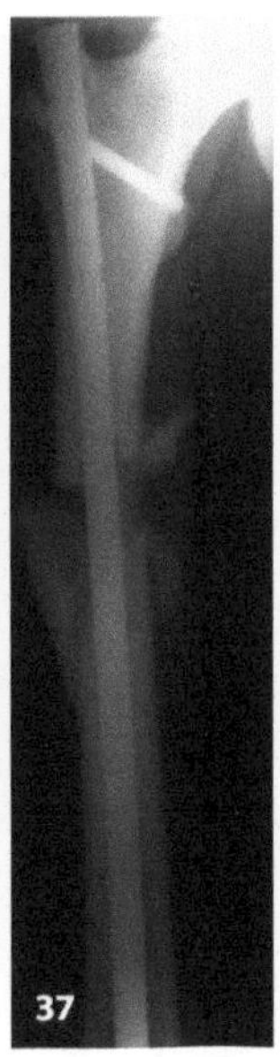

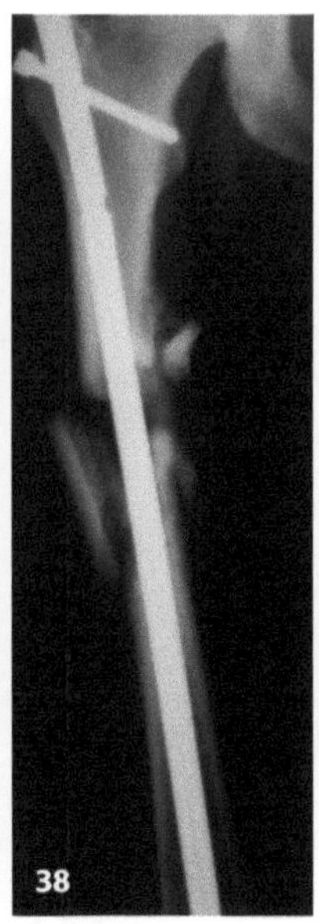

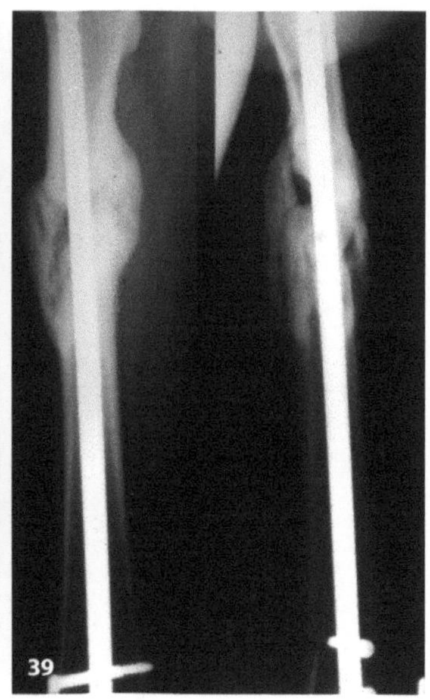

**Fig. 12.36.** AO classification 32C1

**Fig. 12.37.** One-month follow-up after static GK

**Fig. 12.38.** Three-month follow-up

**Fig. 12.39.** Six-month follow-up

## Case 8: 32-Year-Old Male Patient, Motorcycle Accident

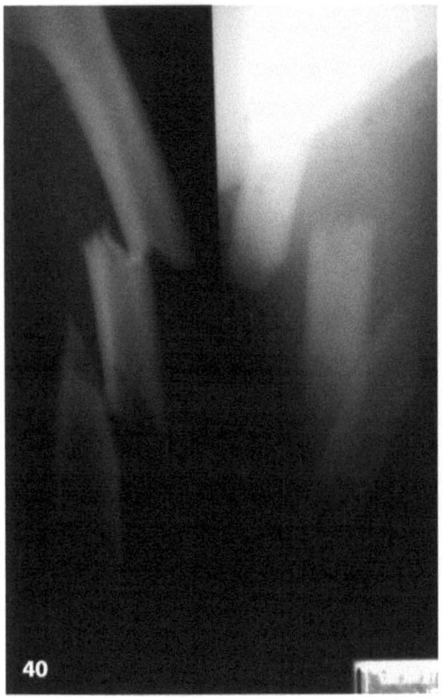

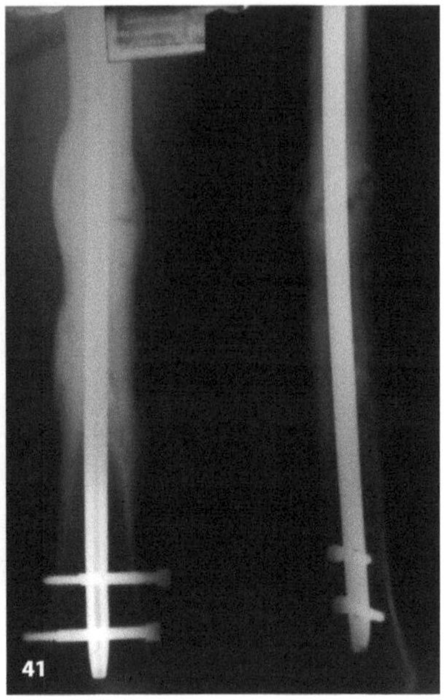

**Fig. 12.40.** AO classification 32C2

**Fig. 12.41.** Eight-month follow-up after static GK

## Case 9: 28-Year-Old Male Patient, Car Accident

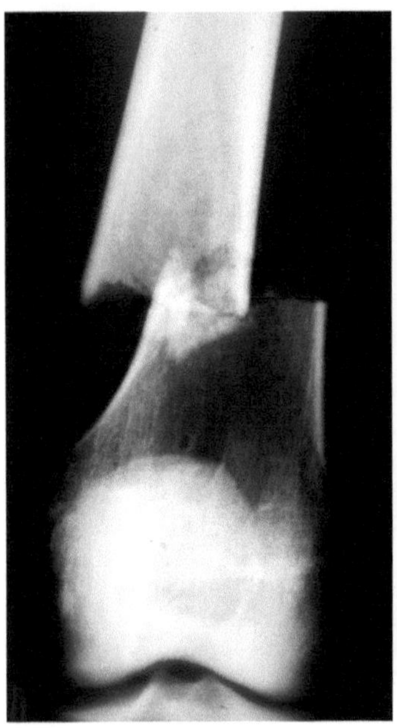

**Fig. 12.42.** AO classification 33A3

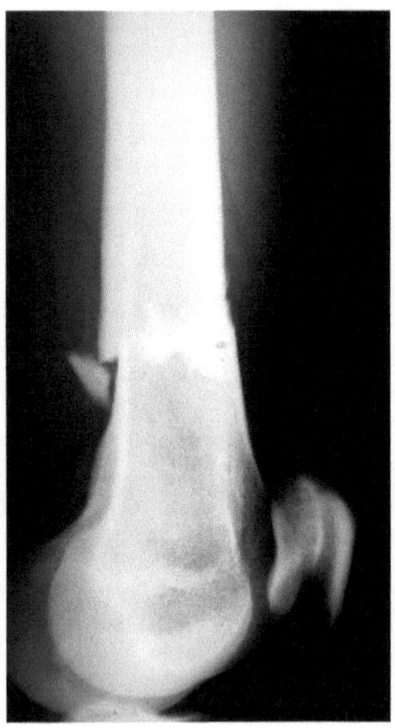

**Fig. 12.43.** AO classification 33A3

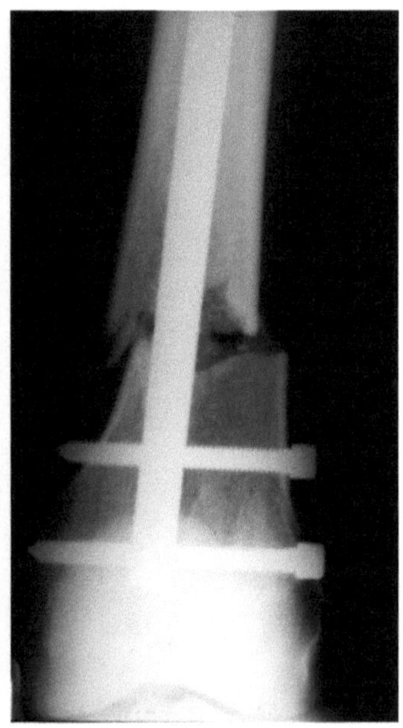

**Fig. 12.44.** Postoperative view after dynamic GK

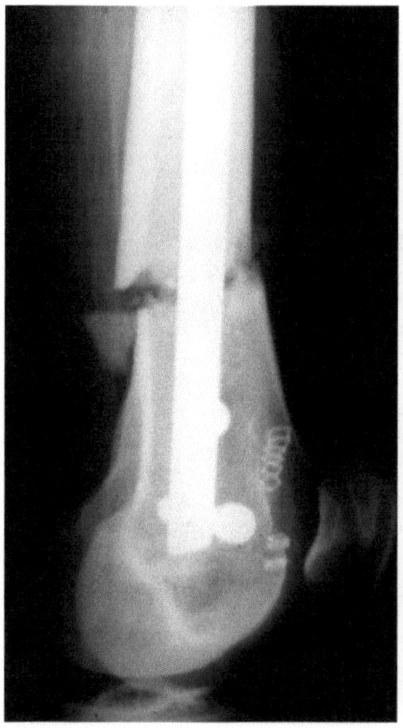

**Fig. 12.45.** Postoperative view after dynamic GK

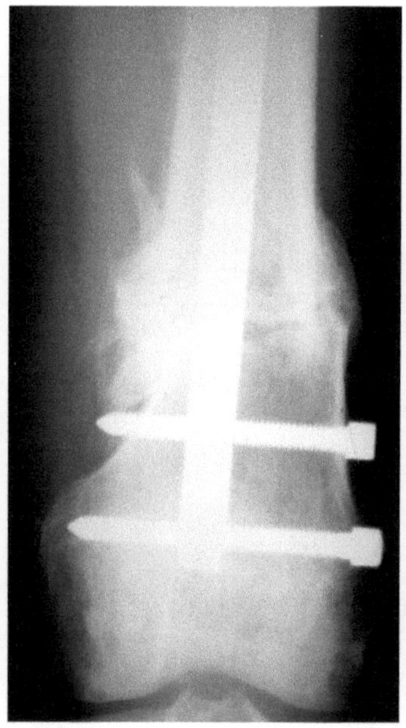

**Fig. 12.46.** Four-month follow-up

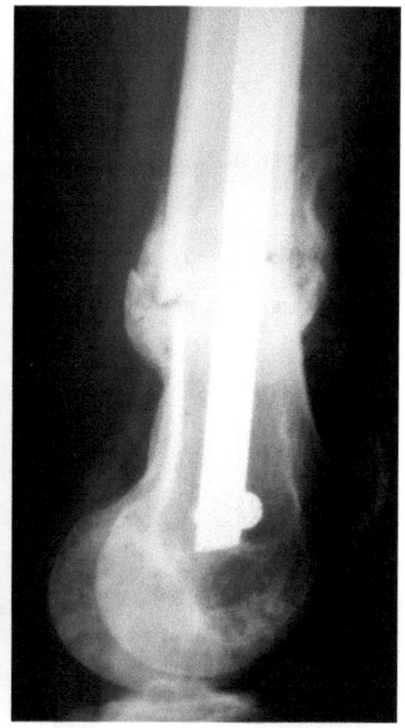

**Fig. 12.47.** Four-month follow-up

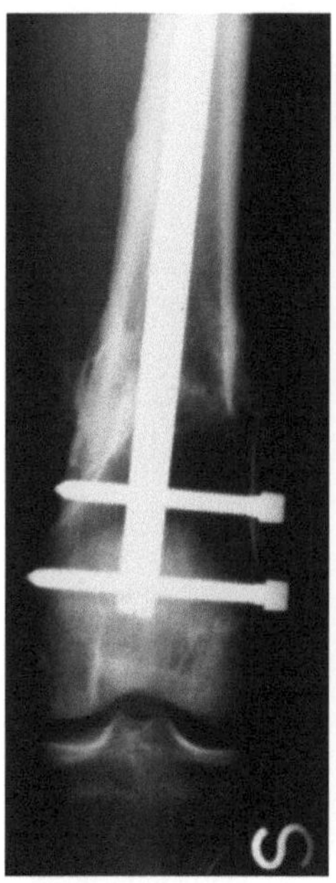

**Fig. 12.48.** Fourteen-month follow-up

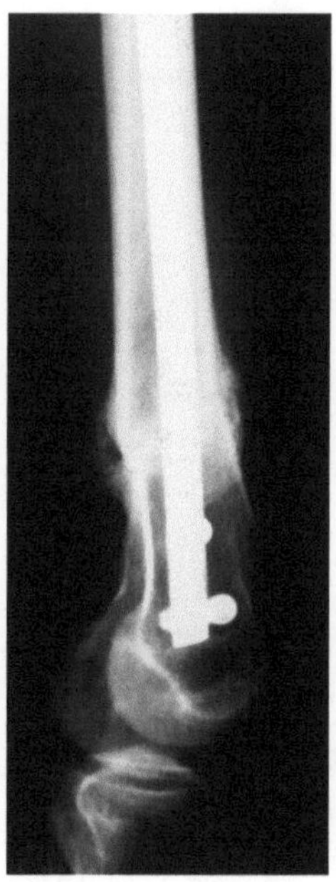

**Fig. 12.49.** Fourteen-month follow-up

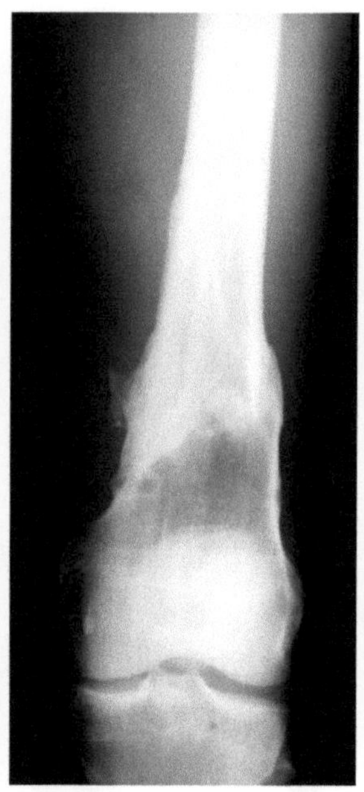

**Fig. 12.50.** Final view after nail removal

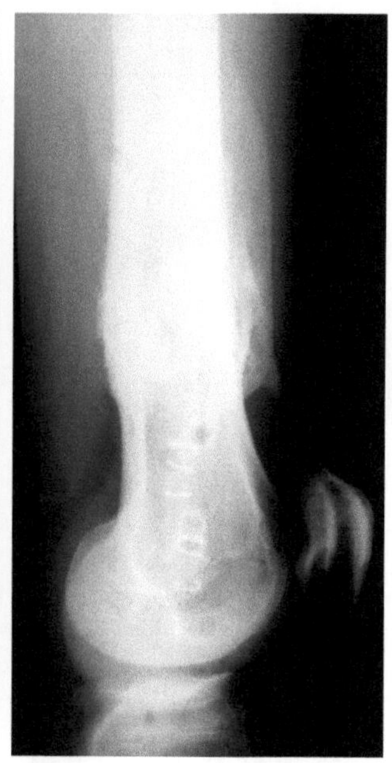

**Fig. 12.51.** Final view after nail removal

# Tibia

G. Taglang

## Case 1: 34-Year-Old Male Patient

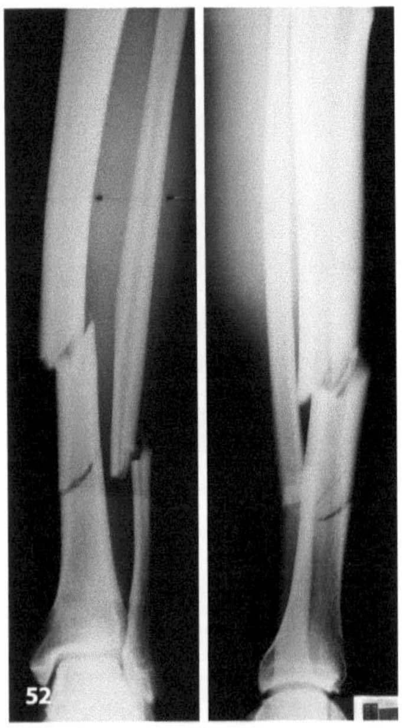

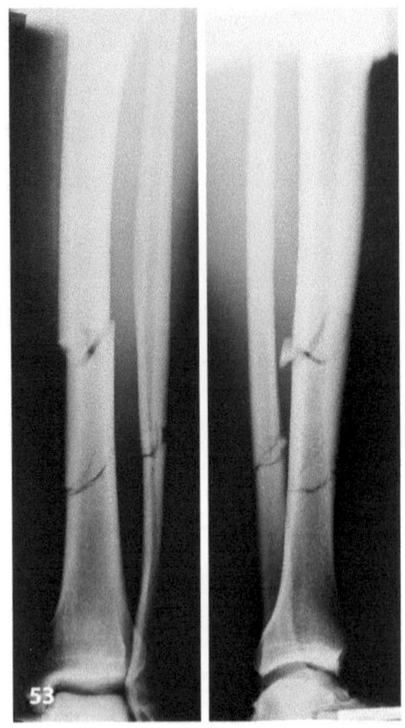

**Fig. 12.52.** Segmental fracture

**Fig. 12.53.** Reduction on the fracture table with the help of transcalcaneus traction

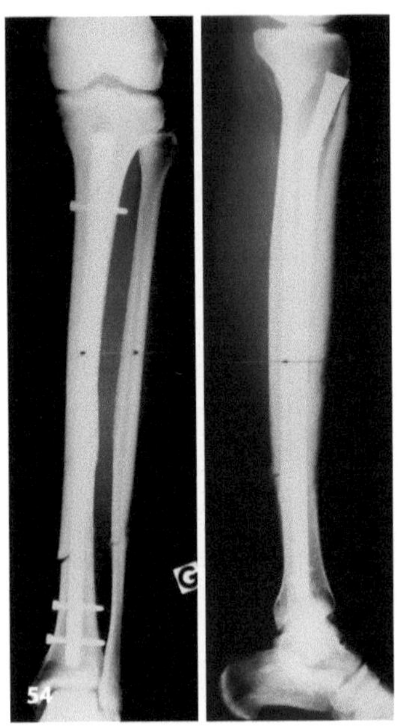

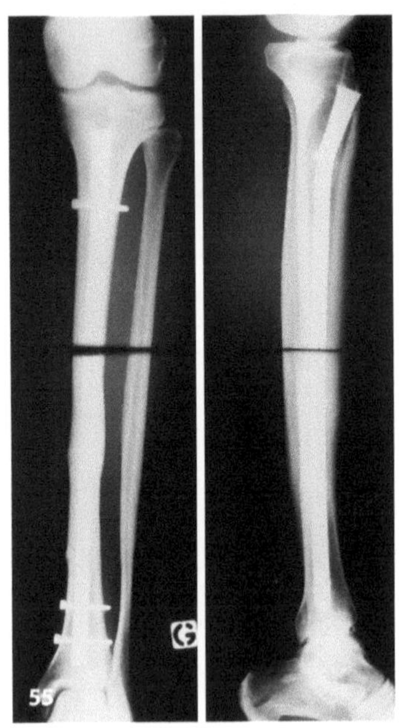

**Fig. 12.54.** Locking nail, static with three screws: one proximal transverse and two distal screws

**Fig. 12.55.** Immediate full weight-bearing was allowed. Follow-up after 7 months

## Case 2: 55-Year-Old Male Patient

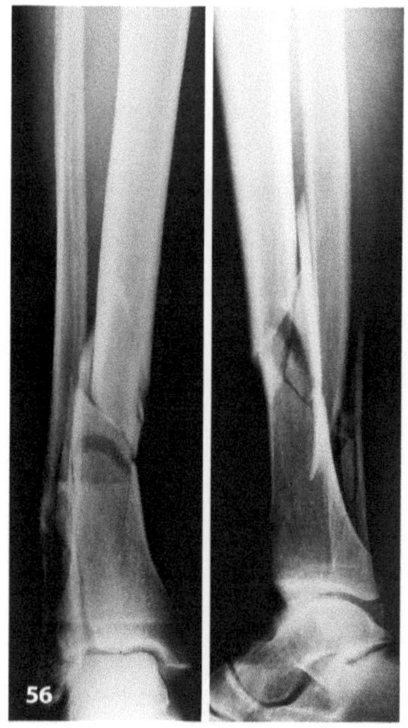

**Fig. 12.56.** Distal open Gustilo 2 fracture of tibia and fibula

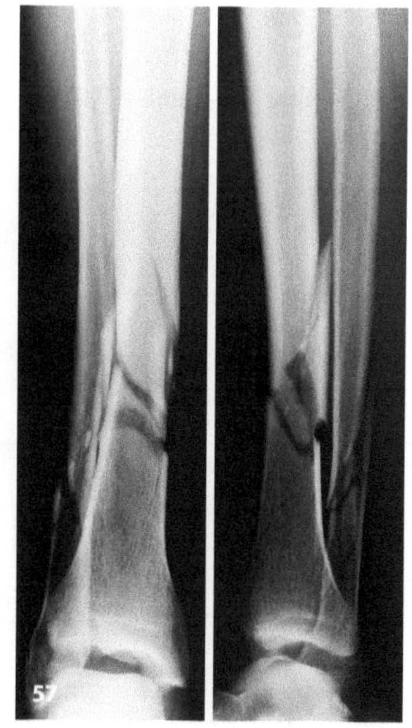

**Fig. 12.57.** Reduction on the fracture table, debridement of the wounds

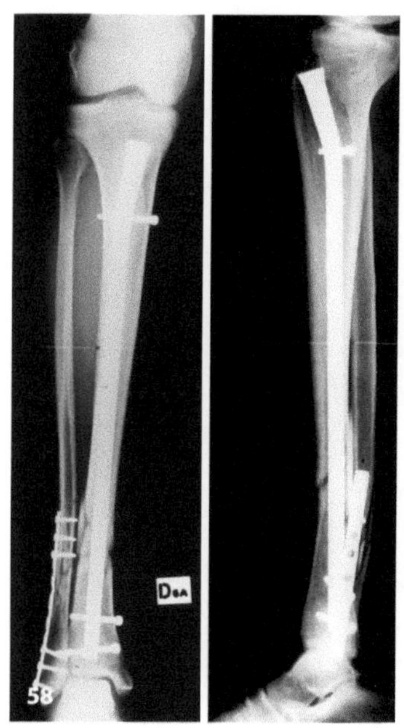

**Fig. 12.58.** Plating of the fibula and statically locked nail on the tibia. Distal end of the nail was cut

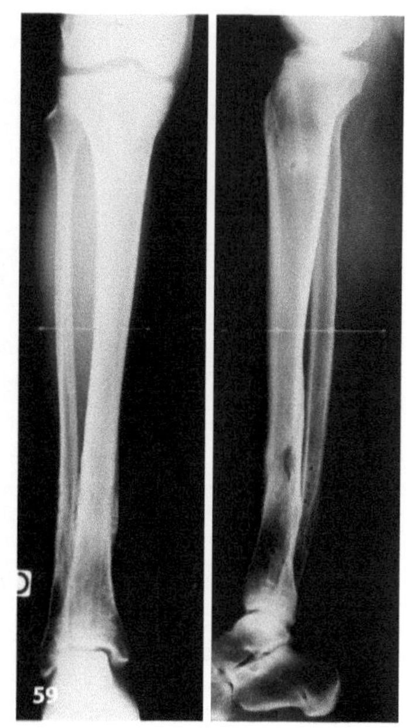

**Fig.12. 59.** Partial weight-bearing during the first 6 weeks and then full weight-bearing. End result 1.5 years later after hardware removal

# Gamma

G. TAGLANG

## Case 1: 74-Year-Old Female Patient

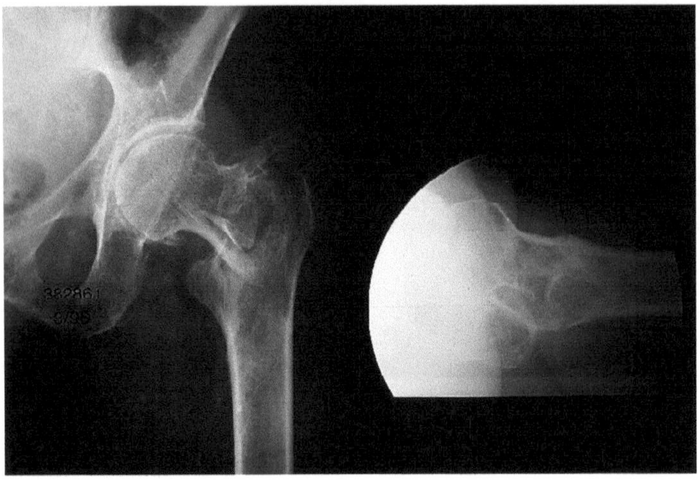

**Fig. 12.60.** Pertrochanteric fracture (basicervical)

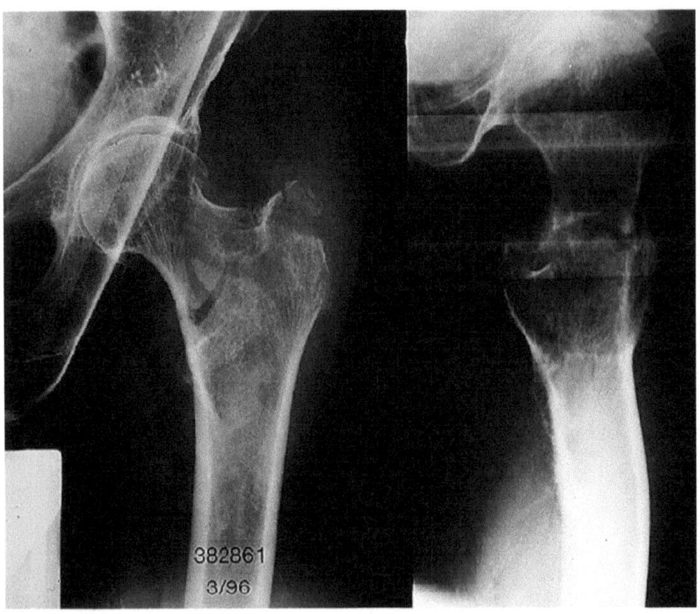


**Fig. 12.61.** Reduction on the fracture table (traction and internal rotation)

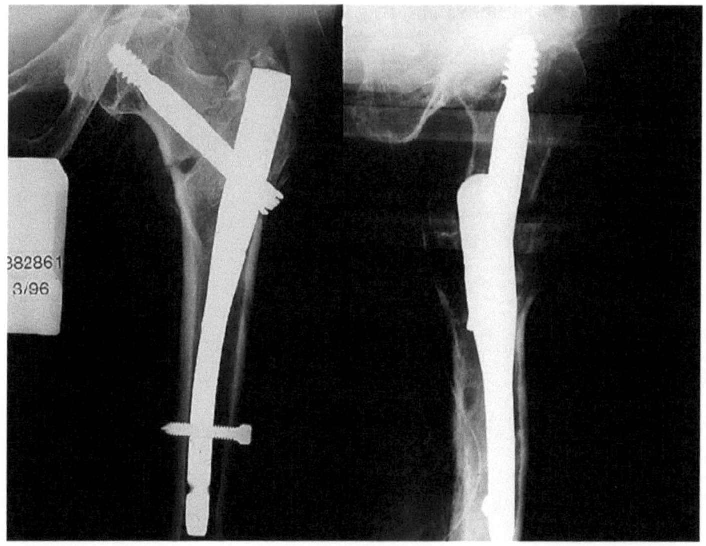

**Fig. 12.62.** Treatment with a standard gamma nail: 11 mm in diameter, 100-mm lag screw length, one single 30-mm distal screw. Immediate weight-bearing is allowed

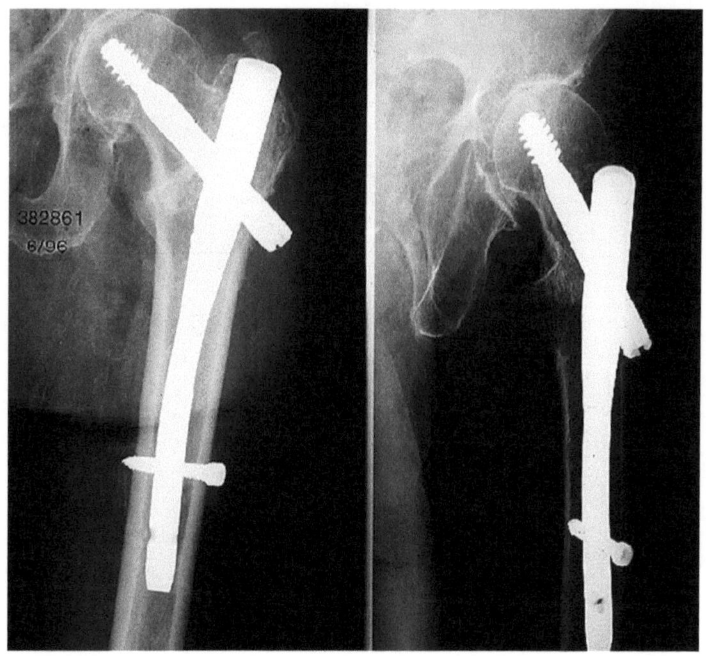

**Fig. 12.63.** Bony healing 3 months after surgery. Sliding of the lag screw

## Case 2: 88-Year-Old Female Patient

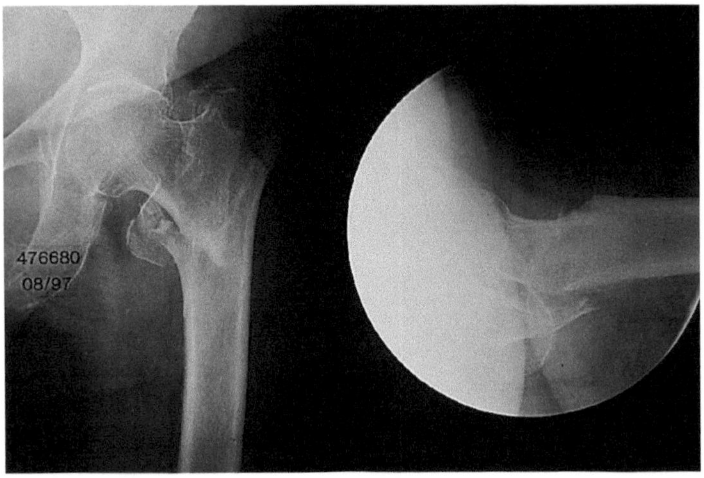


**Fig. 12.64.** Unstable intertrochanteric fracture

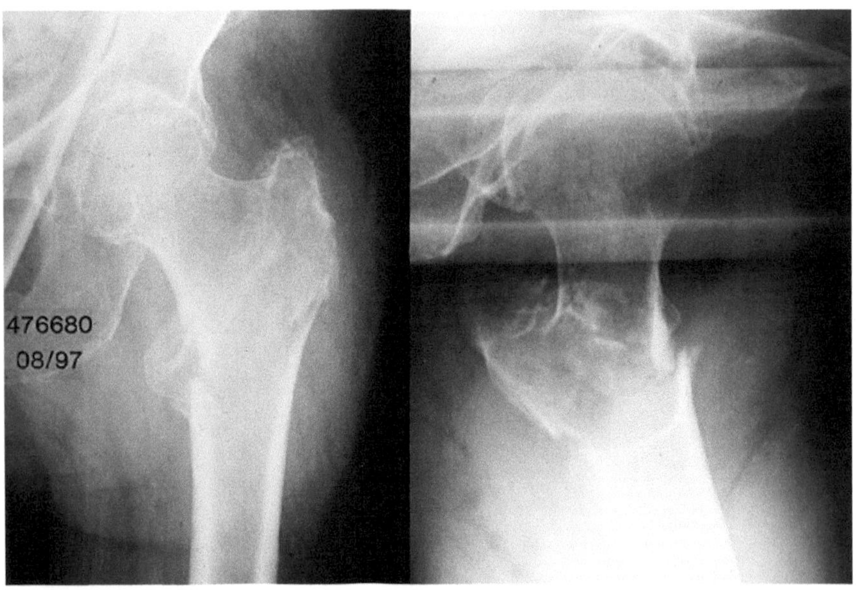


**Fig. 12.65.** Reduction on the fracture table

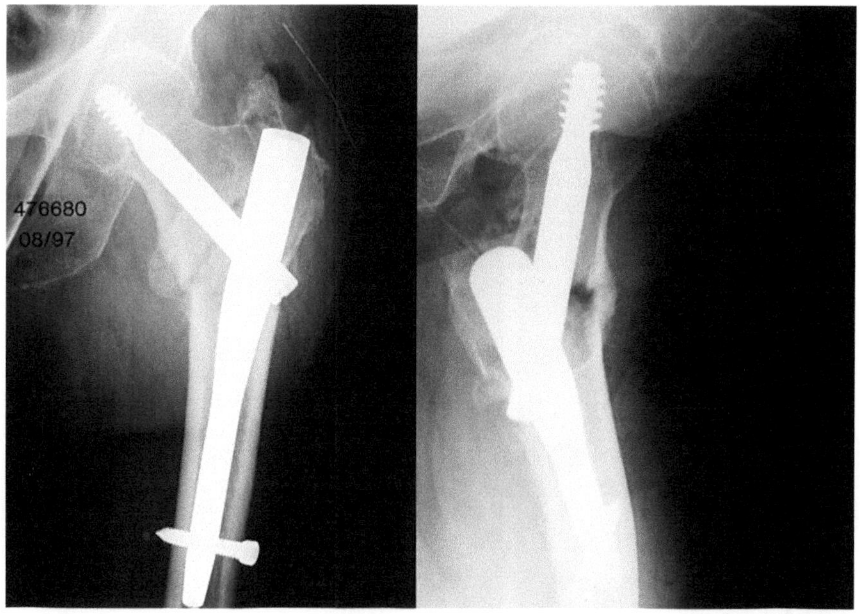


**Fig. 12.66.** Treatment with a trochanteric gamma nail (TGN): 130° angulation, 100-mm lag screw, distal locking screw 30 mm in length, TGN 11 mm in diameter

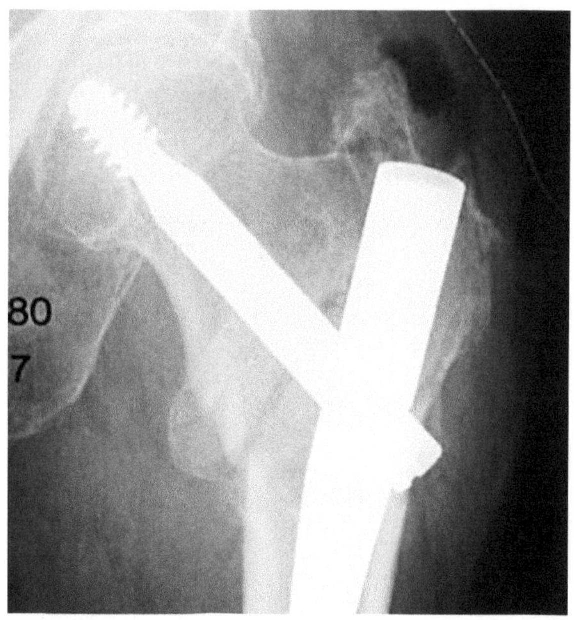

**Fig. 12.67.** Perfect positioning of the lag screw despite the point of entry being too lateral

## Case 3: 74-Year-Old Female Patient

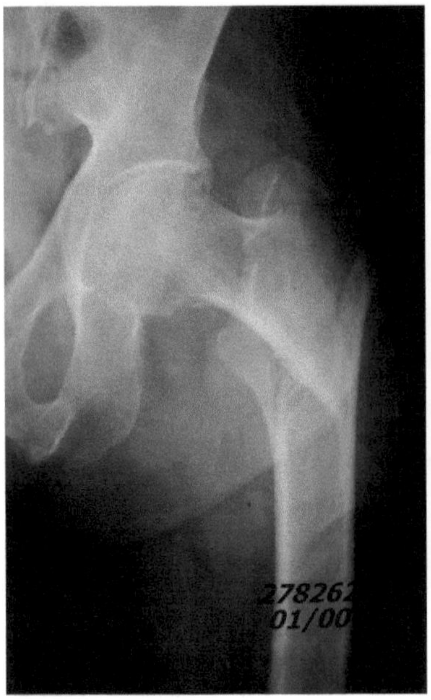

**Fig. 12.68.** Pertrochanteric fracture

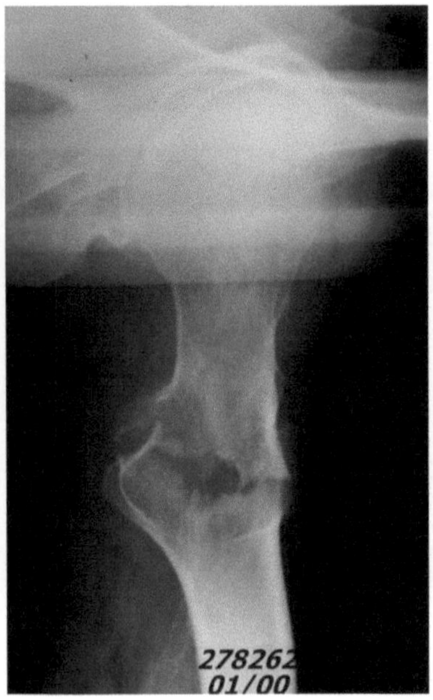

**Fig. 12.69.** The reduction on the lateral view is always important to avoid retroversion in the fracture line

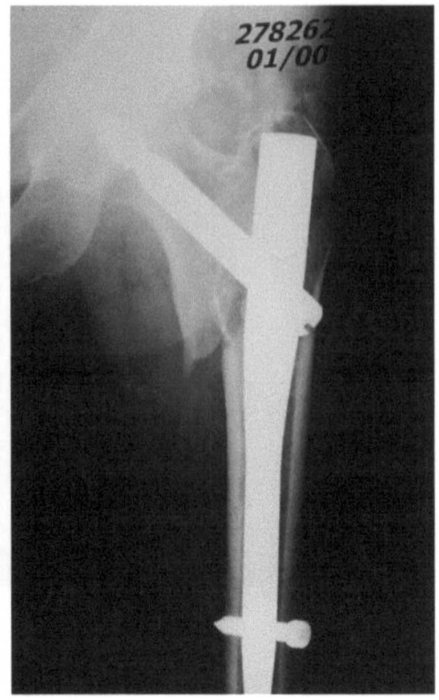

**Fig. 12.70.** Treatment with a trochanteric gamma nail: 130°, 100-mm lag screw, 30-mm distal screw. Immediate weight-bearing is allowed

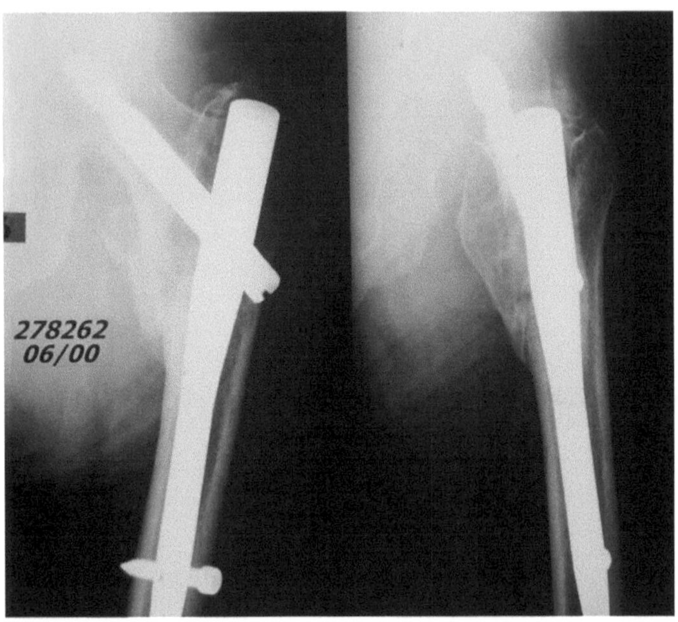


**Fig. 12.71.** Result 6 months after surgery. Complete range of motion of the hip joint

## Long Gamma

G. Taglang

### Case 1: 41-Year-Old Patient

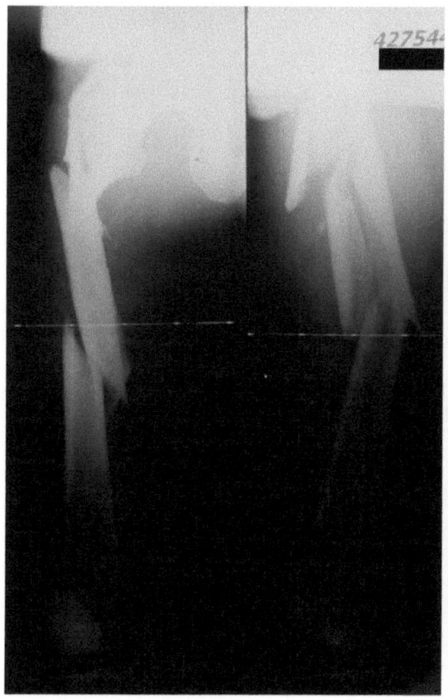

**Fig. 12.72.** Complex subtrochanteric fracture, RTA (Road Traffic Accident)

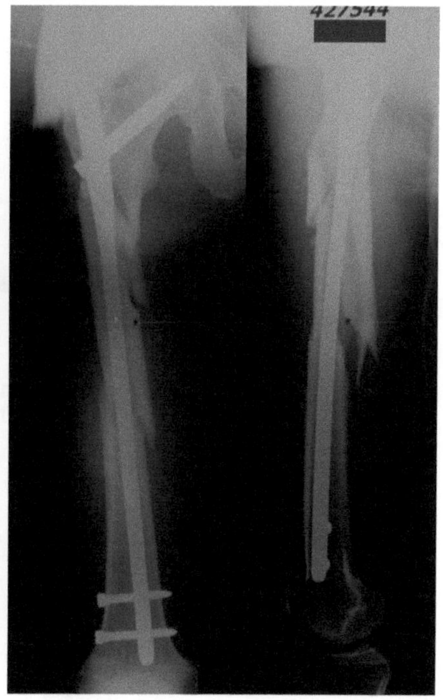

**Fig. 12.73.** Treatment with a long gamma nail 40 cm in length, immediate weight-bearing

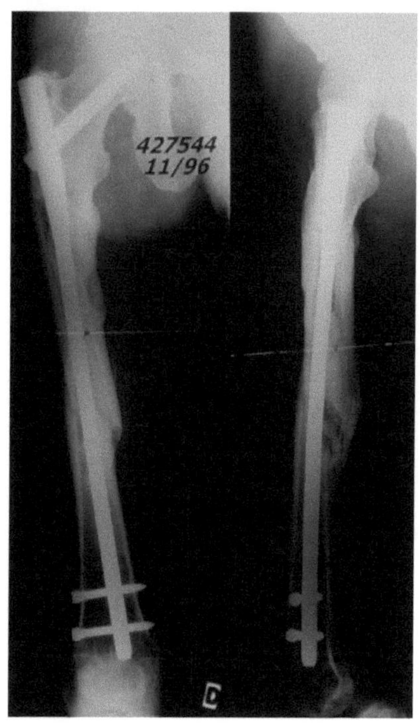

**Fig. 12.74.** Follow-up 8 months after surgery. Bony healing obtained

## Case 2: 42-Year-Old Patient, Car Accident

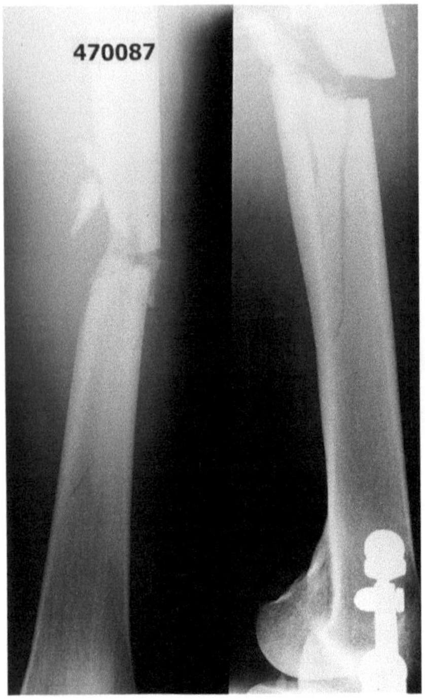


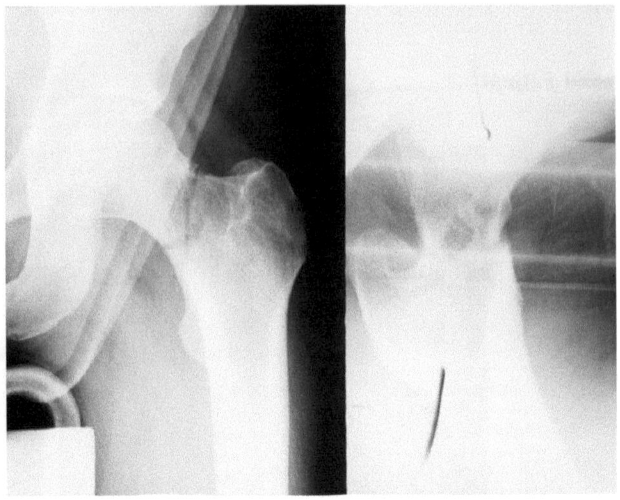

**Fig. 12.75.** Combined proximal and distal fractures left femur (on the fracture table)

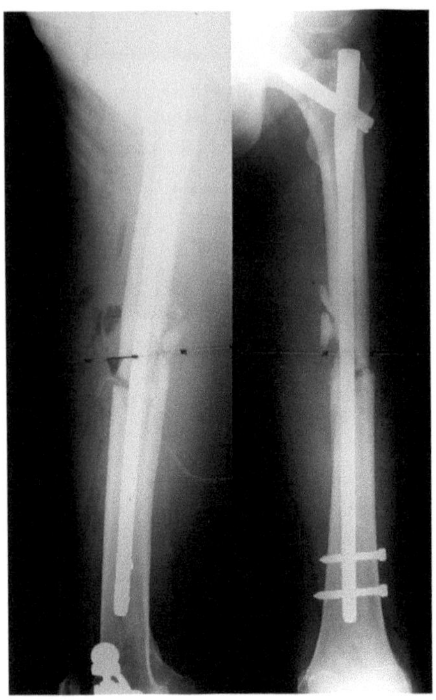

**Fig. 12.76.** Treatment with a long gamma nail (38 cm, 11 mm in diameter, 100-mm lag screw)

**Fig. 12.77.** Six months after surgery. Immediate weight-bearing was allowed after surgery

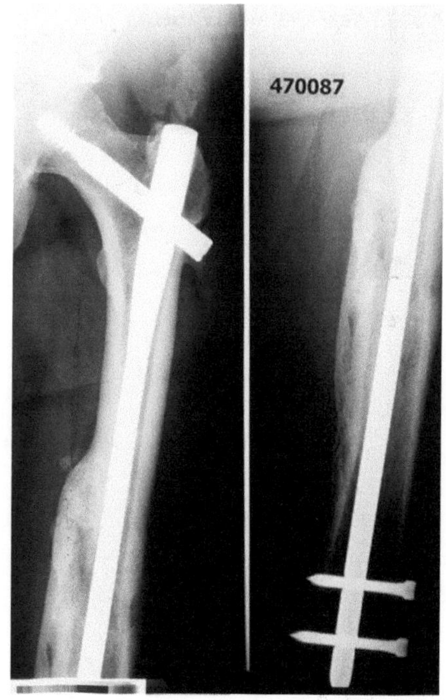


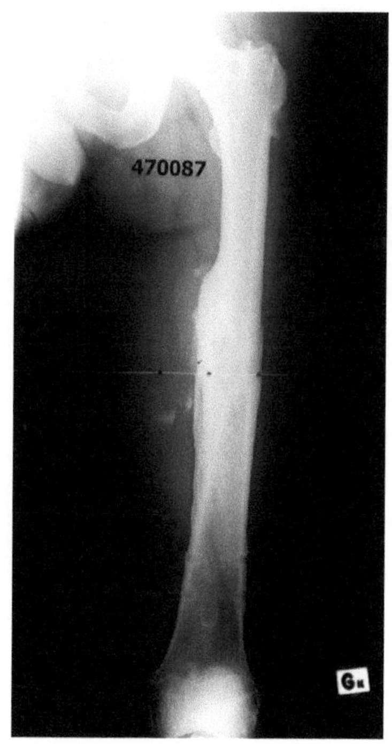


**Fig. 12.78.** End result 18 months after surgery (after hardware removal)

## Case 3: 71-Year-Old Male Patient

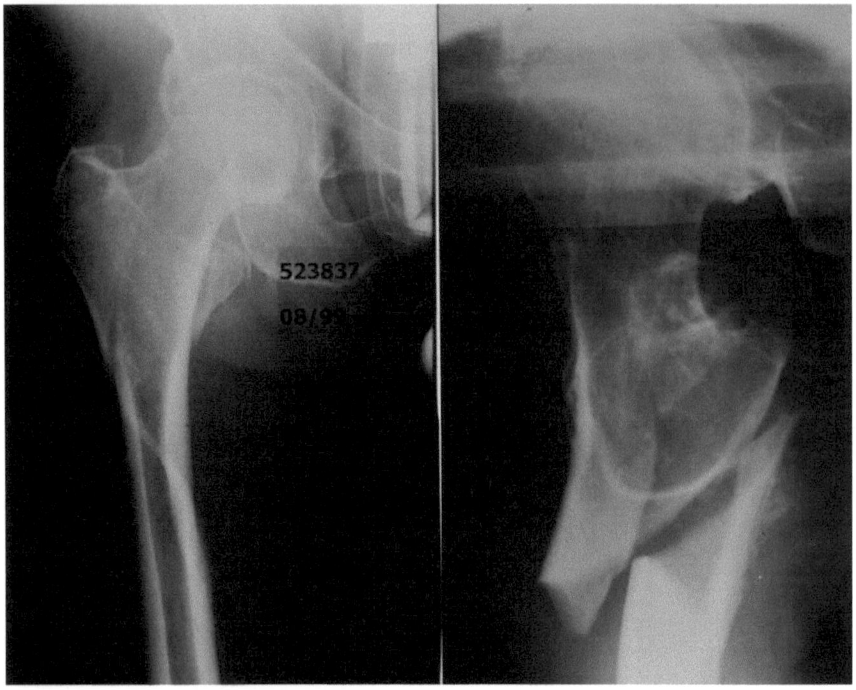


**Fig. 12.79.** Trochanteric fracture with extension to the diaphyseal area

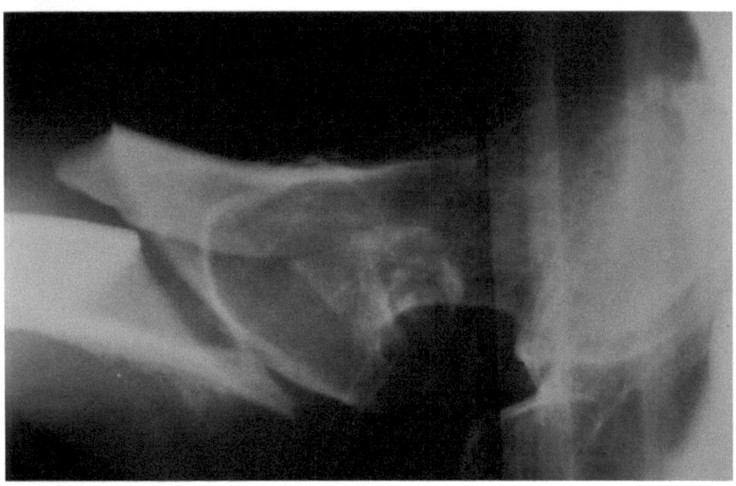

**Fig. 12.80.** Anterior displacement of the proximal fragment

**Fig. 12.81.** Reduction on the lateral view with a spatula

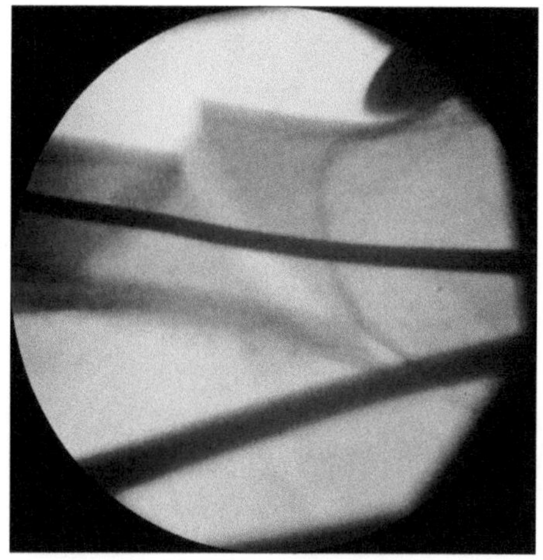

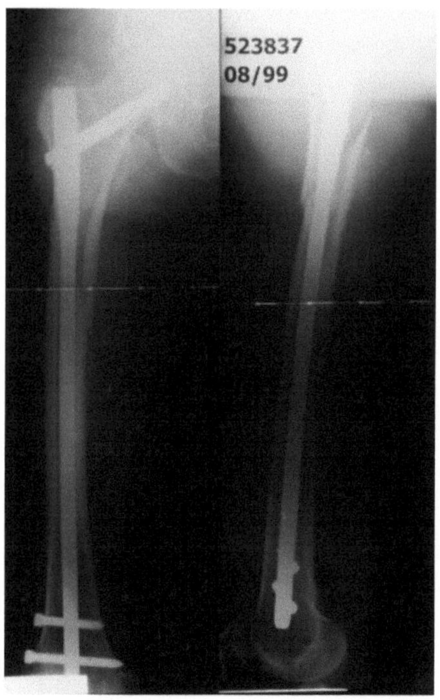


**Fig. 12.82.** Treatment with a 400-mm-long gamma nail. Immediate weight-bearing

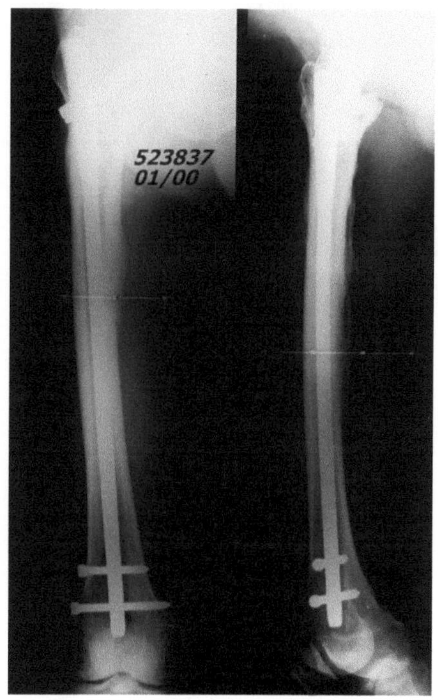


**Fig. 12.83.** Bony healing after 5 months

# Ulna

C. Lefèvre and D. Le Nen

## Case 1: 48-Year-Old Male Patient, Double Ulna Shaft Fracture

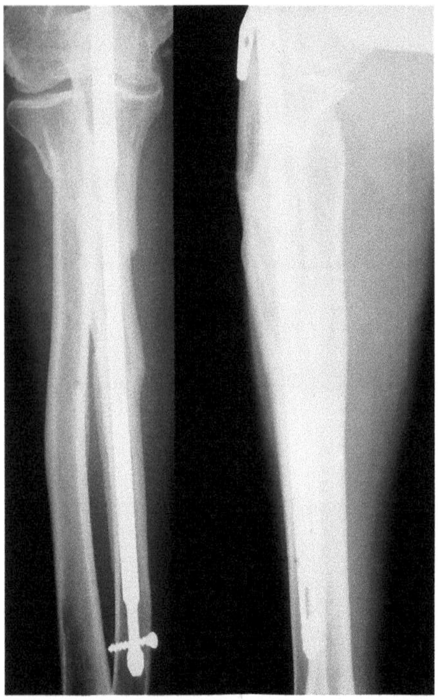

**Fig. 12.84.** Locking nailing in compression

## Case 2: 35-Year-Old Male Patient, Monteggia Fracture

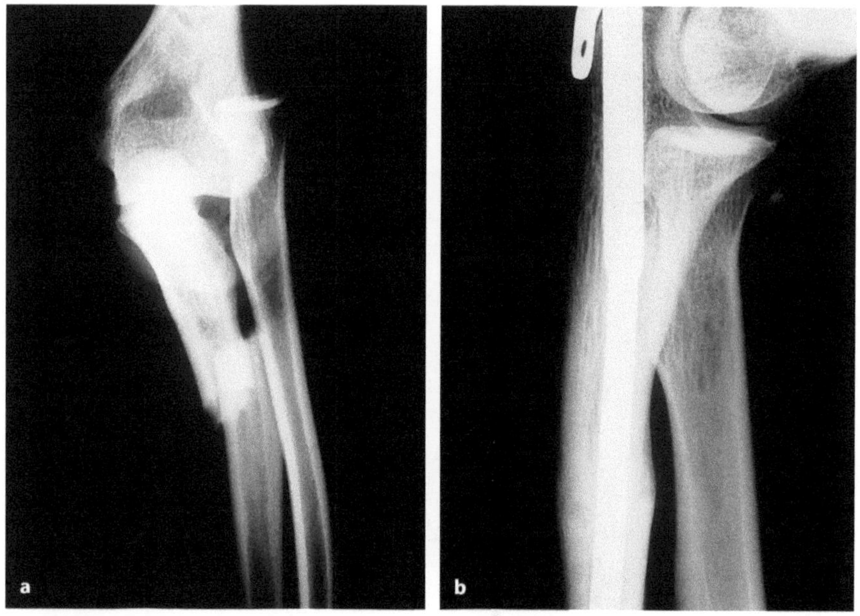

**Fig. 12.85. a, b** Monteggia fracture. Locking nailing in compression

## Case 3: 25-Year-Old Male Patient, Malunion of the Right Distal Radius

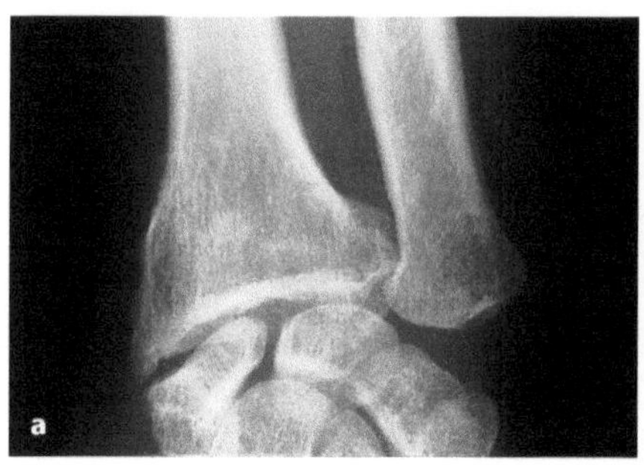

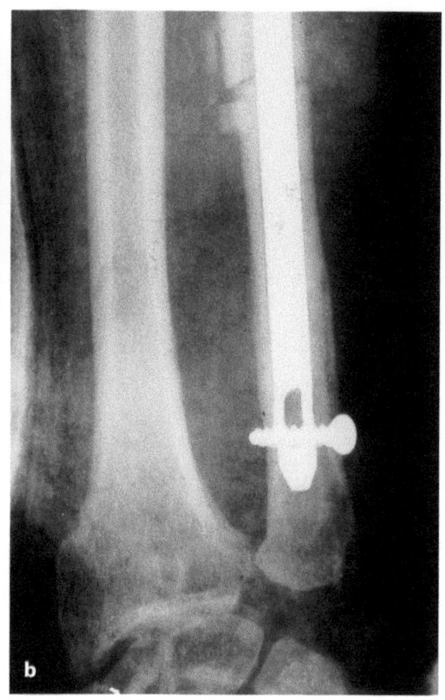

**Fig. 12.86. a** Internal overpression syndrome of the wrist in relation with a malunion of the distal radius. **b** Shortening osteotomy with locking nailing in compression of the ulna. Restoration of a correct ulna/radial index

## Case 4: 28-Year-Old Female Patient, Right Kienböck Disease

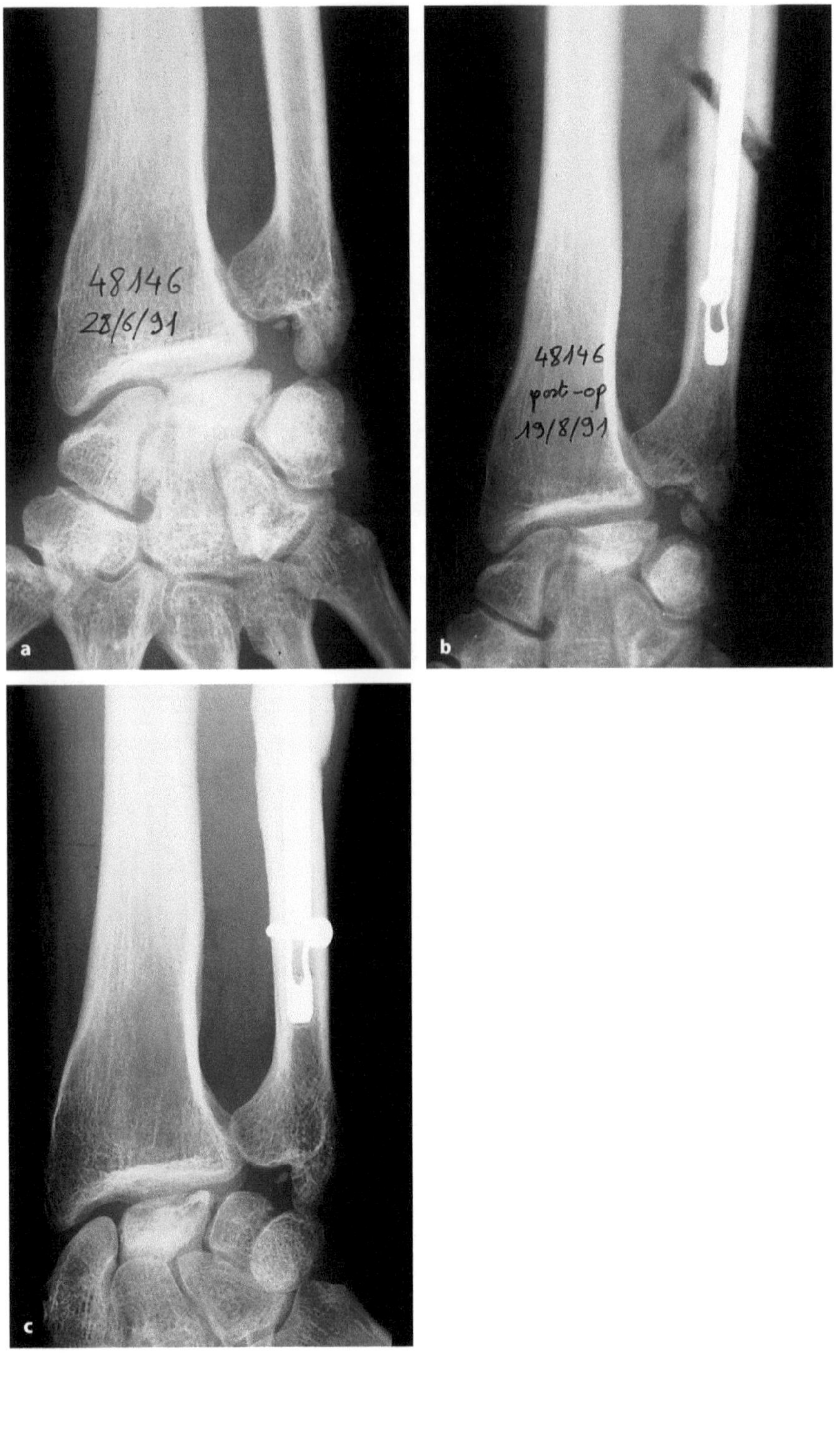


**Fig. 12.87.** **a** Kienböck disease. **b** Lengthening osteotomy of ulna locking nailing in distraction. **c** Restoration of a correct ulna/radial index

## Case 5: 38-Year-Old Male Patient: Open Comminutive Fracture of Both Bones of the Forearm

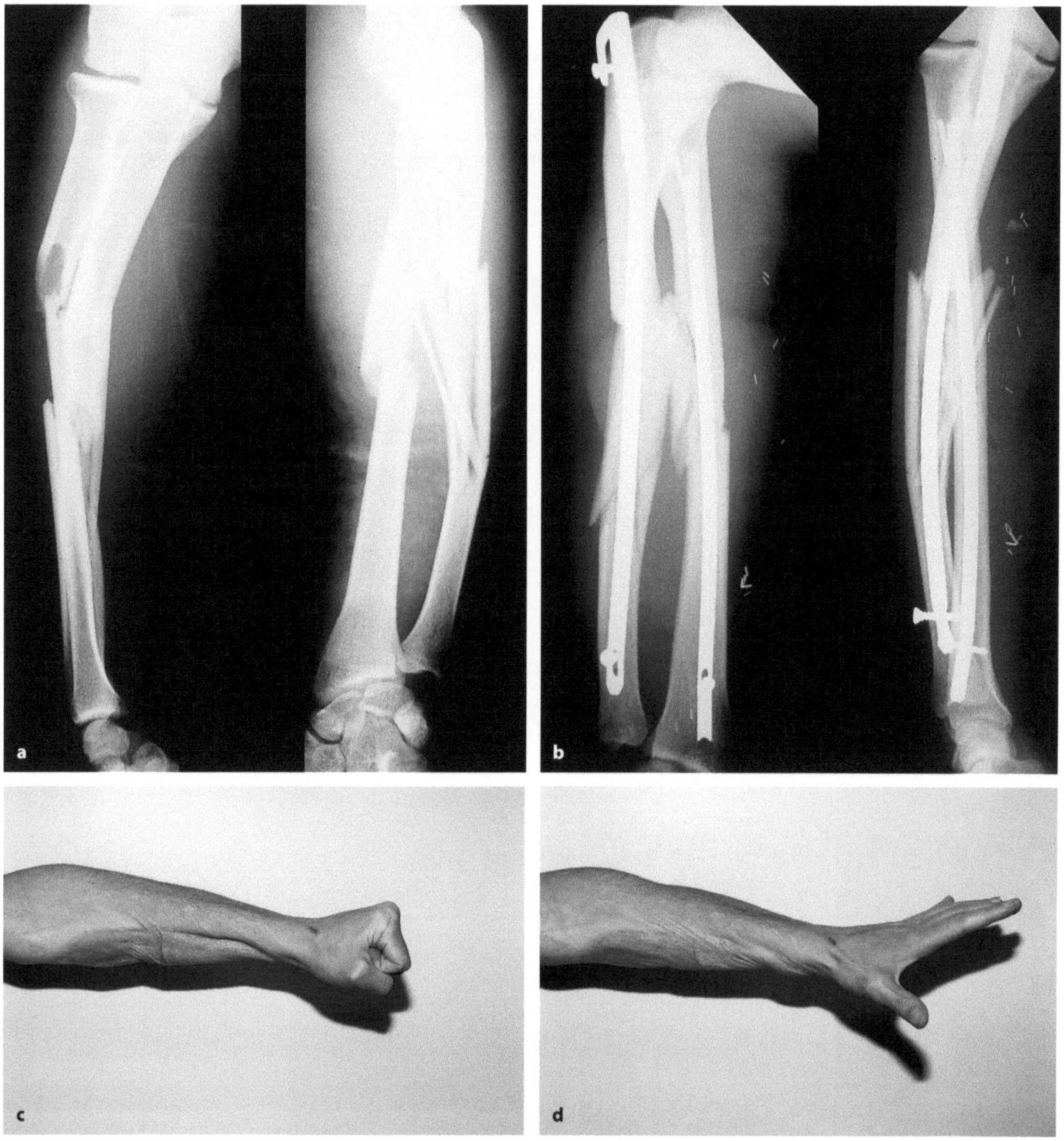

**Fig. 12.88. a** Crush syndrome of the forearm with massive flexor muscle necrosis. **b** Double locking nailing ulna and radius. Free gracilis muscle flap. **c, d** Final functional results

## Humerus

H. Seidel

### Case 1: 72-Year-Old Female Patient

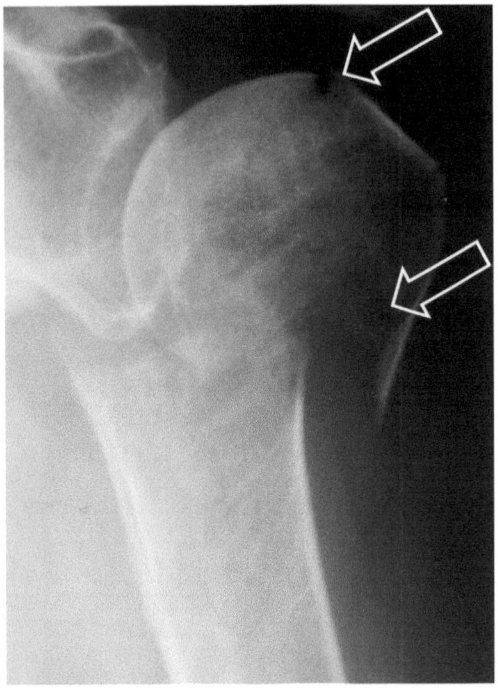

**Fig. 12.89.** Proximal humeral fracture. Subcapital fracture, section S1 and fracture of major tubercle, section A1 (*arrows*)

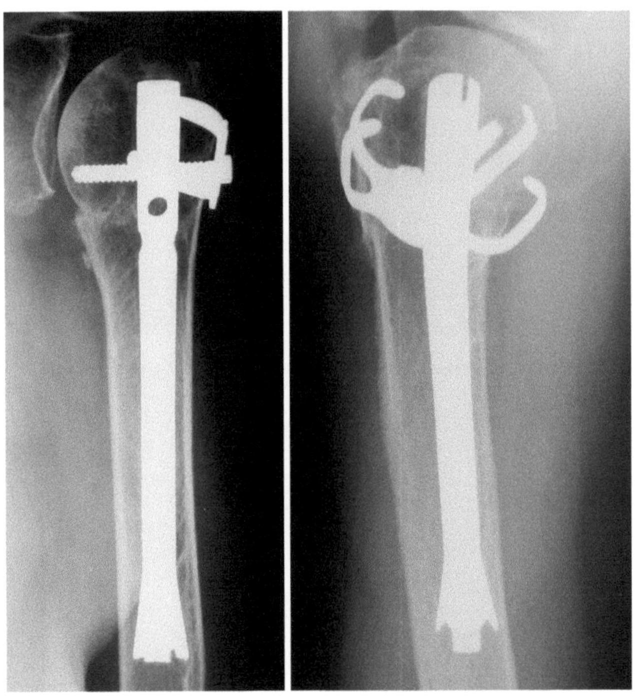

**Fig. 12.90.** Stable reconstruction with humeral locking nail and lateral washer

## Case 2: 74-Year-Old Female Patient

**Fig. 12.91.** Proximal comminuted humeral fracture, sections S1–S3

**Fig. 12.92.** Stabilization with humeral locking nail. Proximal locking with two screws. Distal locking with expansion screw (DS)

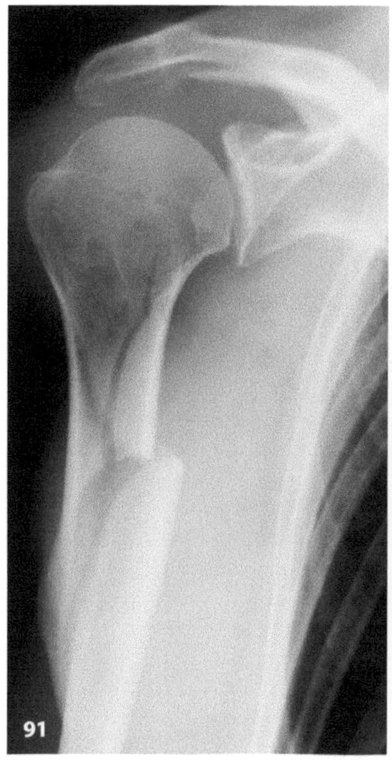


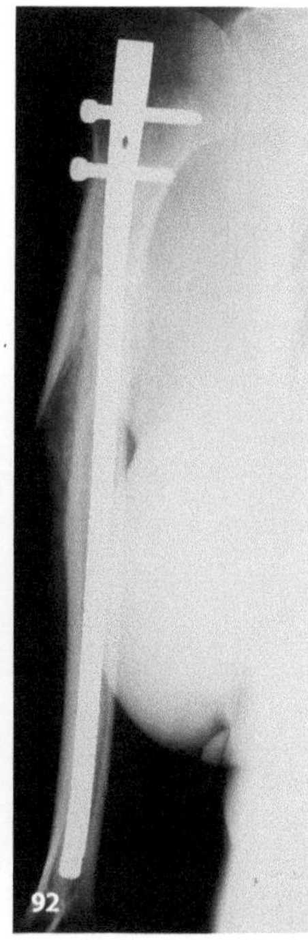


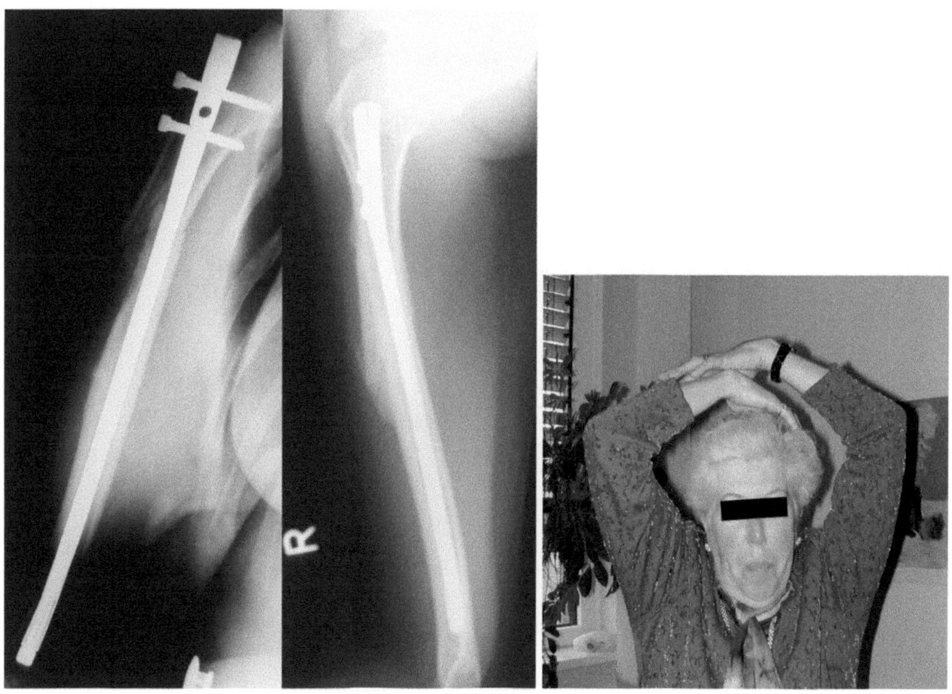


**Fig. 12.93.** Fracture consolidation after 6 months. Excellent function of shoulder and elbow with nail

## Case 3: 30-Year-Old Male Patient

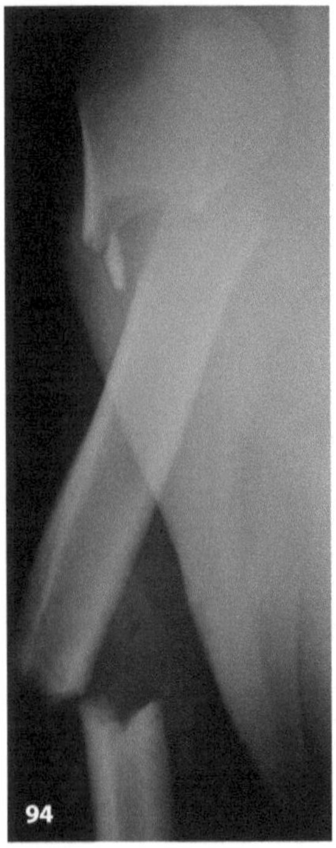


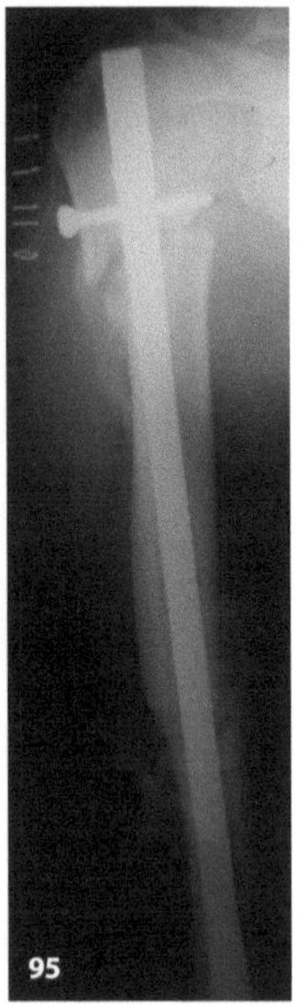


**Fig. 12.94.** Two-segment fracture, section S1 and section S3, 6 months of orthopedic treatment

**Fig. 12.95.** Open stabilization with humeral locking nail

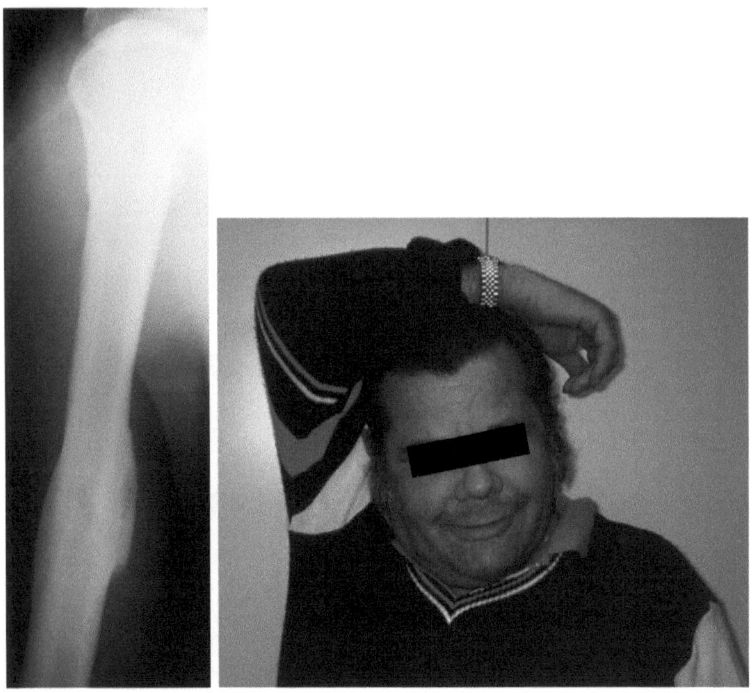

**Fig. 12.96.** Consolidation of both fractures 8 months after nailing. Full function of shoulder and elbow after removal of the nail

## Case 4: 32-Year-Old Male Patient

**Fig. 12.97.** Distal comminuted humeral fracture, section S4

**Fig. 12.98.** Distal comminuted humeral fracture, section S4. Open stabilization with HLN

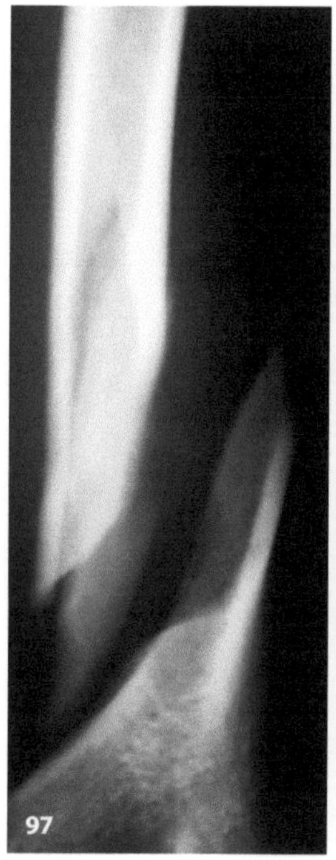

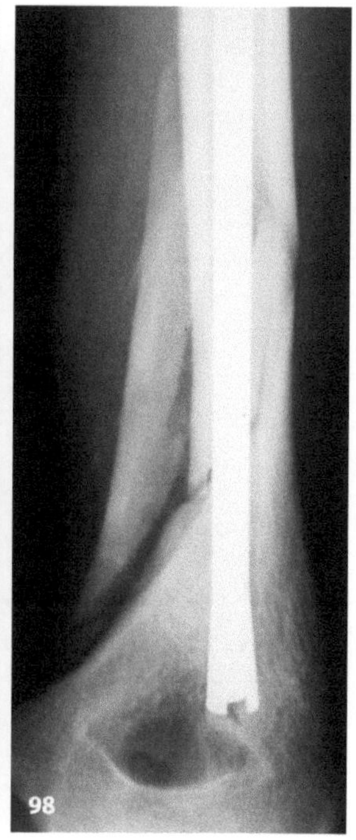

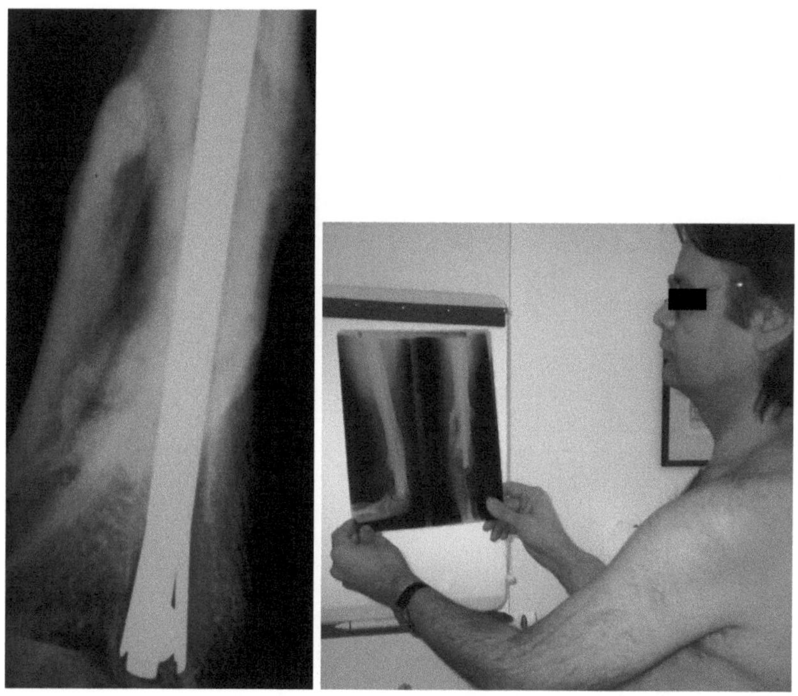

**Fig. 12.99.** Consolidation 3 months after nailing

## Case 5: 28-Year-Old Male Patient

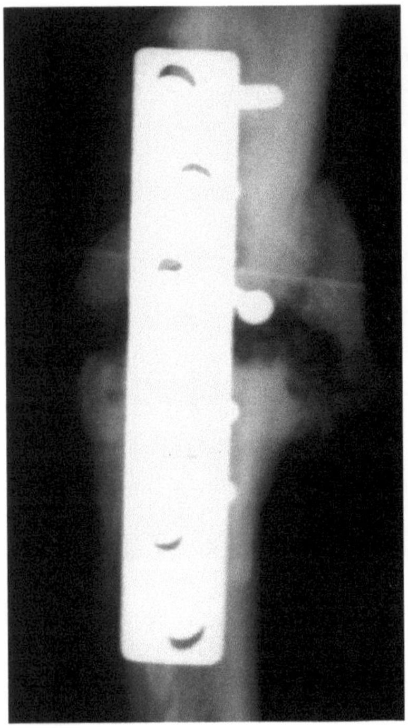

**Fig. 12.100.** Humeral pseudarthrosis with plate, section S4, 8 months following plate

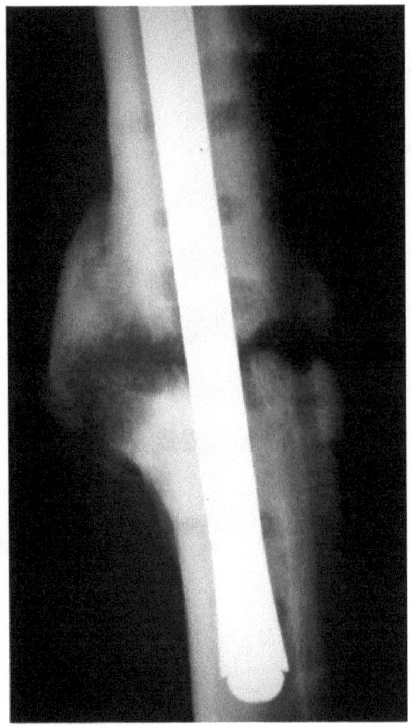

**Fig. 12.101.** Reoperation with humeral locking nail and reaming

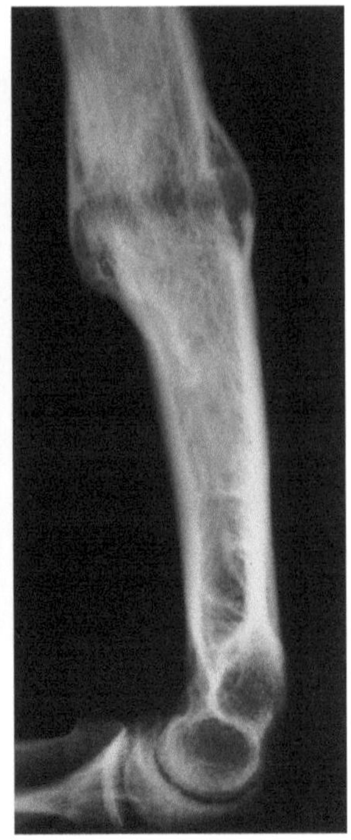

**Fig. 12.102.** Consolidation 2 years later

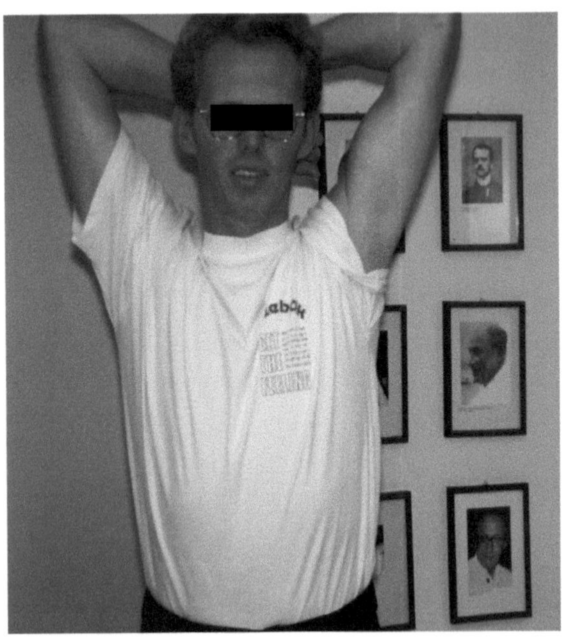

**Fig. 12.103.** Good function of shoulder and elbow after nail removal

# Subject Index

Druck- und Bindearbeiten: Stürtz AG, Würzburg

MIX
Papier aus verantwortungsvollen Quellen
Paper from responsible sources
FSC® C105338

If you have any concerns about our products,
you can contact us on
**ProductSafety@springernature.com**

In case Publisher is established outside the EU,
the EU authorized representative is:
**Springer Nature Customer Service Center GmbH**
**Europaplatz 3, 69115 Heidelberg, Germany**

Printed by Libri Plureos GmbH
in Hamburg, Germany